Handbook
of
LIPIDOLOGY

Handbook
of
LIPIDOLOGY

Tapan Ghose

MD DNB (Med) DNB (Cardio) FNB MNAMS FCSI FIMSA FACC FSCAI

Director and Head
Department of Cardiology
Paras Hospitals, Gurgaon, Haryana, India

Foreword
Upendra Kaul

JAYPEE *The Health Sciences Publisher*
New Delhi | London | Philadelphia | Panama

Jaypee Brothers Medical Publishers (P) Ltd.

Headquarters
Jaypee Brothers Medical Publishers (P) Ltd.
4838/24, Ansari Road, Daryaganj
New Delhi 110 002, India
Phone: +91-11-43574357
Fax: +91-11-43574314
E-mail: jaypee@jaypeebrothers.com

Overseas Offices

J.P. Medical Ltd.
83, Victoria Street, London
SW1H 0HW (UK)
Phone: +44-20 3170 8910
Fax: +44(0) 20 3008 6180
E-mail: info@jpmedpub.com

JP Medical Inc.
325, Chestnut Street
Suite 412
Philadelphia, PA 19106, USA
Phone: +1 267-519-9789
E-mail: support@jpmedus.com

Jaypee Brothers Medical Publishers (P) Ltd.
Bhotahity, Kathmandu, Nepal
Phone: +977-9741283608
E-mail: kathmandu@jaypeebrothers.com

Jaypee-Highlights Medical Publishers Inc.
City of Knowledge, Bld. 237, Clayton
Panama City, Panama
Phone: +1 507-301-0496
Fax: +1 507-301-0499
E-mail: cservice@jphmedical.com

Jaypee Brothers Medical Publishers (P) Ltd.
17/1-B, Babar Road, Block-B, Shaymali
Mohammadpur, Dhaka-1207
Bangladesh
Mobile: +08801912003485
E-mail: jaypeedhaka@gmail.com

Website: www.jaypeebrothers.com
Website: www.jaypeedigital.com

© 2016, Jaypee Brothers Medical Publishers

Inquiries for bulk sales may be solicited at: jaypee@jaypeebrothers.com

Handbook of Lipidology

First Edition: **2016**

ISBN: 978-93-5250-195-3

Printed at Replika Press Pvt. Ltd.

Dedicated to

The memory of
Mrs Purna Laxmi Ghose (Mother)
Mrs Rekha Chaudhuri (Mother in Law)
Mr GC Ghose (Father)
Dr Amitav Ganguly (Friend)
Dr Dinesh Chakraborty (Childhood Mentor)
and
All those patients who have left us

Contributors

Aijaz H Mansoor MD DNB
Senior Consultant, Department of Cardiology
Modern Hospital
Srinagar, Jammu and Kashmir, India

A Misra MD
Director
Fortis C-DOC Centre of Excellence for Diabetes
Metabolic Diseases and Endocrinology
Fortis Flt Lt Rajan Dhall Hospital
New Delhi, India

Anjali Arora MD
Incharge, Lipid Clinic
Sir Ganga Ram Hospital
New Delhi, India

Ashok Kumar Parida MD DNB MNAMS FACC
Senior Consultant and Head
Department of Cardiology
The Mission Hospital
Durgapur, West Bengal, India

Baridalyne Nongkynrih MD
Additional Professor
Centre for Community Medicine
All India Institute of Medical Sciences (AIIMS)
New Delhi, India

Bharat Bhusan Kukreti MD DM
Senior Consultant
Department of Cardiology
Paras Hospitals
Gurgaon, Haryana, India

Dheeraj Deo Bhatt MD DM
Consultant, Department of Cardiology
Fortis Flt Lt Rajan Dhall Hospital
New Delhi, India

DJ Dutta MD DM FESC
Professor of Cardiology
Assam Medical College
Dibrugarh, Assam, India

D Dev MD
Associate Professor
Department of Medicine
Silchar Medical College
Silchar, Assam, India

Dipti Sharma MD PGT (Endocrinology)
Professor and Head
Department of Endocrinology
Gauhati Medical College
Guwahati, Assam, India

Harsh Wardhan MD DM
Former Professor and Head
Department of Cardiology
Ram Monohar Lohia Hospital
Head, Department of Cardiology
Primus Super Speciality Hospital
New Delhi, India

Jeet Ram MD
Senior Resident
Department of Cardiology
All India Institute of Medical Sciences (AIIMS)
New Delhi, India

Kuntal Bhattacharyya MD DM
Consultant
Rabindranath Tagore International Institute
of Cardiac Sciences
Kolkata, West Bengal, India

Kushal Madan PhD
Consultant
Department of Cardiology
Sir Ganga Ram Hospital
New Delhi, India

Moushumi Lodh MD
Senior Consultant, Laboratory Services
The Mission Hospital
Durgapur, West Bengal, India

Rahul Nagpal MD
Director and Head
Department of Pediatrics
Fortis Flt Lt Rajan Dhall Hospital
New Delhi, India

Ritu Rani MSc (Clinical Research)
Research Associate
Department of Cardiology
Paras Hospitals
Gurgaon, Haryana, India

Roohi Khan MD
Associate Consultant
Department of Pediatrics
Fortis Flt Lt Rajan Dhall Hospital
New Delhi, India

Sandeep Singh MD DM
Professor of Cardiology
All India Institute of Medical Sciences (AIIMS)
New Delhi, India

Sanjeev Gulati MD DNB DM DNB FISN FIAP FRCP
Director
Department of Nephrology
Fortis Escorts Heart Institute and Fortis Flt Lt
Rajan Dhall Hospital
New Delhi, India

Sanjeev Kumar Gupta MD
Professor
Centre for Community Medicine
All India Institute of Medical Sciences (AIIMS)
New Delhi, India

Satya Nand Pathak MD DM
Consultant
Department of Cardiology
Paras Hospitals
Gurgaon, Haryana, India

SC Manchanda MD DM
Former Professor and Head
Department of Cardiology
All India Institute of Medical Sciences (AIIMS)
Senior Consultant
Department of Cardiology
Sir Ganga Ram Hospital, New Delhi, India

Sekhar Chakravarty MD
Professor
Department of Pathology
Vice Principal
Silchar Medical College
Silchar, Assam, India

Suchitra Behl MD ABIM
Consultant
Fortis C-DOC Centre of Excellence for Diabetes
Metabolic Diseases and Endocrinology
Fortis Flt Lt Rajan Dhall Hospital
New Delhi, India

Sudhir S Shetkar MD DM
Senior Resident
Department of Cardiology
All India Institute of Medical Sciences (AIIMS)
New Delhi, India

Sundeep Mishra MD DM
Professor
Department of Cardiology
All India Institute of Medical Sciences (AIIMS)
New Delhi, India

Sunil Kumar Verma MD DM
Assistant Professor
Department of Cardiology
All India Institute of Medical Sciences (AIIMS)
New Delhi, India

Supertiksh Yadav MD DM
Consultant
Department of Cardiology
Paras Hospitals
Gurgaon, Haryana, India

Tapan Ghose MD DNB DNB FNB MNAMS FCSI
FIMSA FACC FSCAI
Director and Head
Department of Cardiology
Paras Hospitals
Gurgaon, Haryana, India

Upendra Singh MD DM
Consultant
Department of Nephrology
Fortis Escorts Heart Institute
New Delhi, India

Foreword

My association with Dr Tapan Ghose, the worthy Editor of this handbook, has been of more than 18 years. He joined my team in Batra Hospital and Medical Research Centre, New Delhi, India, as a senior resident in the year 1997. Since then, he never looked behind and groomed into a mature cardiologist, adept in coronary and noncoronary interventions of international standards with numerous publications to this credit. He accompanied me to Fortis Network of Hospitals and helped me in setting up the Department at the Vasant Kunj facility and, finally, moved to his present place of work as Director Cardiology, Paras Hospital with my blessings.

His academic interests have been various including lipidology and management of lipid disorders. The first study on the efficacy of atorvastatin in this region was conducted and published by him under my guidance in 2000. It is, therefore, very logical that he has come out with a comprehensive *Handbook of Lipidology*. The book covers various aspects of the subject starting from history, molecular biology to various drugs and management of individual disorders precisely. It would become a very good and useful reference book on the subject for postgraduate students and clinicians, in general. I am sure Dr Ghose will come out with the updates of this handbook in the times to come.

Upendra Kaul
MD DM FCSI FSCAI FACC FAMS
Awardee of Padma Shri and Dr BC Roy Award
Executive Director and Dean, Cardiology
Fortis Escorts Heart Institute
and Fortis, Vasant Kunj
New Delhi, India

Preface

Coronary heart disease is the leading cause of death in the world. Each day, 30,000 people leave this planet because of coronary heart disease. Amongst the well-studied nine risk factors, dyslipidemia has the highest population-atributable risk factor and is modifiable. Since the initial description of thrombus as the cause of acute myocardial infarction by James B Herrick, many advances have taken place in the field of lipidology. One landmark achievement in the human history is the discovery of statin group of drugs. After penicillin and aspirin, these drugs are the third group of agents, which have an impact on the event-free survival of mankind.

There is an immense need of a comprehensive handbook on lipidology for the busy clinicians, which can serve as a desktop reference. Initially, I approached many people who are the known contributors from various countries, for this handbook. All of them had a long waiting time. Then, I approached leading physicians, who are involved in the day-to-day management of lipid disorders. All the contributors have tried to simplify the complex subject of lipidology into easily understandable language for the practitioners.

If a single life is saved and if a single episode of myocardial infarction or stroke is averted with the help of this handbook, then it would be presumed to be successful in serving its purpose.

Tapan Ghose

Acknowledgments

This work is the result of contribution made by many individuals.

I sincerely thank all the contributors of the various chapters of this handbook. In spite of being successful clinicians, all of them have taken out precious time from their busy work schedule for writing the chapters.

I would like to thank Prof Upendra Kaul, my mentor, for his constant guidance, help and for writing the Foreword for this handbook. This would not have been possible without his help.

I also thank Mr Manoj Sharma, Mr Priyawart Kumar, Ms Monika and Mr Praveen for helping me in the preparation of the manuscript. I sincerely thank all the team members of M/s Jaypee Brothers Medical Publishers (P) Ltd., New Delhi, India, for their direct and indirect contribution to this handbook.

I also thank Mr SL Choudhury for his literary help and guidance. I would like to thank my brothers Mr Manik, Mr Ratan, Mr Swapan and Mr Tarun for their constant encouragement.

Finally, I would like to acknowledge the constant help of my wife, Dr Sutapa, and son, Tuhin, for their help, tolerating my irregular work schedule and helping me in spite of disturbing their many weekends.

Contents

CHAPTER 1

History of the Dyslipidemia Research

Tapan Ghose and Ritu Rani

- The beginning
- Lipid and atherosclerosis
- Lipid-modifying therapeutic agents
- Statins—a landmark molecule in athero-sclerosis management
- The future

THE BEGINNING

Ancient Indian literature (*Bhagavad Gita*, 3500 BC) mentioned the role of dietary fat and its implication on the human body and mind. This is possibly the oldest document available on diet and phenotype.[1] The concept of dietary fat and changes in the composition of the human body existed even in the biblical times.[2]

Thirteen Nobel Prizes have been awarded to the scientists who were involved in cholesterol research. Pure cholesterol was first obtained from gallstone by a French physician and chemist Francois Pelletier in 1784.[3] The name "cholesterin" was given to it by a French chemist Michel E. Chevreul.[4] The molecular formula of cholesterol was established by Friedrich Reinitzer, an Austrian botanist, in 1888.[5] The cholesterol molecule has four rings and a tetracyclic skeleton. Heinrich O. Wieland and Adolf Windaus received the Noble Prize in chemistry in 1927 and 1928, respectively, for describing the structure of cholesterol.[6] In 1939, Carl Muller, a Norwegian clinician, first made a genetic connection between cholesterol and heart attacks.[7]

The citric acid cycle, which is also known as tricarboxylic acid cycle (TCA cycle) or the Krebs cycle,[8] was identified in 1937 by Hans Adolf Krebs while he was working at the University of Sheffield. This is a series of biochemical reactions used by all aerobic organisms to generate energy. The acetate derived from carbohydrates, fats and proteins is oxidized into carbon dioxide and chemical energy in the form of adenosine triphosphate. He was awarded the Nobel Prize for this important discovery in 1953.[9] Michael S. Brown and Joseph L. Goldstein jointly received the Nobel Prize in physiology or medicine in 1985 for their discoveries on the cholesterol metabolism and the treatment of diseases caused by abnormally elevated cholesterol.[10] Dr. D.S. Fredrickson, who is known as the founding father of lipidology, discovered Tangier disease and cholesteryl ester storage diseases; these are genetic conditions caused by aberrant lipid metabolism. His identification of various apolipoprotein components led to our current understanding of lipid transport and physiology.[11]

LIPID AND ATHEROSCLEROSIS

The first hint that cholesterol is related to atherosclerosis was given by Windaus in 1910.[12] He reported that atherosclerosis plaque from aortas of human subjects possess 20-fold higher concentration of cholesterol than the normal aortas.

The cholesterol–coronary connection was unfolded in the early 1950s by John Gofman at the University of California. He found that not only the high cholesterol level in blood but also the elevated low-density lipoprotein (LDL) is the reason of heart attack. In the case of elevated level of high-density lipoprotein (HDL), the chance of heart attack is very less.[13]

National Heart Institute in Framingham carried out the Framingham Heart Study, which provides evidence that people with high blood cholesterol level at the time of baseline measurement were more prone to experience a myocardial infarction (MI), and it also revealed that the risk of MI was increased by a number of factors such as smoking and high blood pressure. The Framingham Heart Study established the risk factor concept in medicine. This study is also considered the mother of evidence-based medicine.[14]

The cholesterol biosynthesis pathway was described by four biochemists—Konrad E. Bloch, Feodor Lynen, John Cornforth and George Popják in 1950. James B. Herrick described for the first time in 1912 that coronary thrombosis was the cause of acute MI.[15]

LIPID-MODIFYING THERAPEUTIC AGENTS

Triparanol was the first cholesterol-lowering agent that inhibits cholesterol synthesis, which was introduced in the United States in 1959. It was withdrawn from the market in early 1960s because of serious side effects, such as cataracts. In cholesterol synthesis, triparanol inhibits the final stage, which results in the accumulation of sterols.[16]

In 1955, a Canadian pathologist Rudolf Altschul discovered the cholesterol-lowering properties of nicotinic acid.[17] Clofibrate was synthesized at Imperial Chemical Industries in England in 1958 and in 1960 fibrates—derivatives of clofibrate—were synthesized; they were safer than clofibrate.[18] After that, cholestyramine is highly effective in the treatment of many patients with hypercholesterolemia, but it is not tolerated by all patients.[19]

STATINS: A LANDMARK MOLECULE IN ATHEROSCLEROSIS MANAGEMENT

In April 1971, citrinin was isolated from a broth culture of mold that had strong inhibitory activity. Citrinin strongly inhibited 3-hydroxy-3-methylglutaryl-coenzyme A (HMGCoA) reductase and lowered serum cholesterol levels in rat, but the research was suspended because of its toxicity to the kidneys.

Dr. Endo Akiro and colleague work at Daichi Sankeyo, Japan, led to the discovery of a new drug called statin. After penicillin and aspirin, statins are the highest selling molecule in the world and possibly the most important life-saving discovery in human history.[20]

In 1973, three active metabolites were isolated from a broth culture of blue–green mold, *Penicillium citrinum*. These metabolites show potent activity to inhibit cholesterol synthesis both in vivo and in vitro. The most active product of these three was ML-236B and later it was given the name compactin.

3-Hydroxy-3-methylglutaryl-coenzyme A reductase is the rate-limiting enzyme in cholesterol biosynthesis. Compactin and HMG-CoA are structurally similar. Compactin is an extremely potent inhibitor of HMG-CoA reductase. In 1976, two studies were published reporting the discovery and characterization of compactin, as the first statin.

Sankyo, Japan, started a phase 1 clinical trial for compactin in November 1978. In phase 2 of the trial, compactin was administered to subjects with serious cases of hypercholesterolemia at 12 hospitals. All the participating hospitals reported positively on the remarkable efficacy and excellent safety profile of compactin (1979).

However, in August 1980 the clinical development of compactin was called off, as the drug caused lymphoma in dogs at dosage.

In July 1976, Merck Research Laboratories signed a confidentiality agreement with Sankyo and obtained samples of compactin and experimental data. Under the direction of Alfred Albert, Merck set out to find its own statins. In February 1979, Merck reported the isolation of a statin very similar to compactin in chemical structure. This was named mevinolin, which was derived from the fungus *Aspergillus terreus*.

Merck began preliminary clinical studies of lovastatin in April 1980, but after 5 months, in September 1980, they discontinued the clinical trials because of the possibility that compactin-induced cancers in dogs.

Scandinavian Simvastatin Survival Study is the most important study that established the role of statins in the secondary prevention of coronary artery disease (CAD) mortality. Subsequent studies have shown that statins are beneficial in primary prevention of CAD and also in acute coronary syndrome. Nonlipid modifying beneficial properties of statins are termed pleiotropic effect. Statins have been shown to regress atherosclerotic plaque.[21]

Statin has been tested in large phase 3 trials, and this class of drug has been shown to be beneficial in primary and secondary prevention, in acute coronary syndrome and in acute MI. Strong data derived from these trials have prompted the revision of guidelines from time to time.

The Jupiter trial, which began in 2003, was directed by Paul Ridker of Brigham and Women's Hospital. Inflammatory biomarkers C-reactive protein (CRP) levels are strong, independent predictors of cardiovascular risk and can enhance risk stratification. Role of statn in population with mildly elevated LDL-C or elevated high sensitivity C reactive protein (hs CRP) was evaluated in this trial.

The Jupiter trial enrolled 17,802 apparently healthy middle-aged men and women with CRP levels over 2.0 mg/L, and LDL <130 mg/dL. They were randomly assigned to receive rosuvastatin 20 mg daily or placebo. The primary end point of the trial was combination of nonfatal MI, stroke, arterial revascularization, hospitalization for unstable angina or cardiovascular death. Rosuvastatin lowered CRP (37%), LDL (50%), nonfatal MI (55%), nonfatal stroke (48%), hospitalization and revascularization (47%), all-cause mortality (20%) and benefited women and minority subgroups at 1.9 years. Rosuvastatin was tolerated relatively well, with a small rise in incidence of diabetes mellitus. The Jupiter data suggest that patients with high levels of CRP should receive statins. Approximately 4.3% of the population satisfies Jupiter inclusion criteria.[22]

The risk–benefit ratio clearly favors the use of statin for the primary and secondary prevention of CAD. Apolipoprotein A-1 (Apo A-1) Milano, a genetic variant of Apo A-1, has been showed to be beneficial in regression of atherosclerosis.[23] Nicotinic acid derivatives have been shown not to be beneficial in the treatment of atherosclerotic disorder as a sole agent.[24] Nicotinic acid has been shown to be inferior to high-dose statin alone. Merck has withdrawn the molecule from the market recently. Fibric acid in addition to high dose statin. The HDL targeting by a class of drugs called cholesteryl ester transport protein (CETP) inhibitors raised the LDL-Cholesterol substantially, yet there was no clinical benefit.[25]

THE FUTURE

PCSK-9 is the enzyme that is responsible for LDL receptor degradation. Humanized propro-tein convertase sub-tilisin–kexin type 9 (PCSK9) antibodies prevents the degradation of the LDL-C receptors. The receptors are available for recycling and transporting more LDL-C to liver for metabolic degradation. Injection of PCSK-9 monoclonal antibodies have shown to reduce LDL-C when added to maximally tolerated dose of statin. Trials have shown 39 to 62% reduction of LDL-C with alirocumab and 47 to 56% of LDL-C with evolocumab. 37% of patients receiving evlocumab and 24% of patients receiving alirocumab reached LDL below 25 mg per deciliter. Based on the results of phase 3 clinical trials the US FDA has approved the use of these two agents, recently. Injectable formulation and lack of evidence of mortality reduction are the current limitation of these agents. The potential targets include adults with primary hypercholesterolemia (nonfamilial or heterozygous familial), mixed dyslipidemia (including those with type 2 diabetes mellitus), statins intolerance.[26,27,28] Phase 3 trial has been completed with one agent evolocumab.

REFERENCES

1. Bhagavad Gita (3500 BC), The three division of material existence, chapter 17 verses 5, 6, 7, Available from: www.bhagavad-gita.org
2. Davidson H. The Bible Diet (Maker's Diet). In: Longe JL (Ed). The Gale Encyclopedia of Diets: A Guide to Health and Nutrition. Farmington Hills, MI: Thomson Gale; 2008. pp. 643-6.
3. Annales de Chimie et de Physique. 1816;2:339-72. From page 346: Je nommerai cholesterine, de χολη, bile, et στερεος, solide, la substance cristallisée des calculs biliares humains (I will name cholesterine—from χολη (bile) and στερεος (solid)—the crystalized substance from human gallstones ...).
4. Chevreul ME. 1816. Recherches chimiques sur les corps gras, et particulièrement sur leurs combi-naisons avec les alcalis. Sixième mémoire. Examen des graisses d'homme, de mouton, de boeuf, de jaguar et d'oie (Chemical researches on fatty substances, and particularly on their combinations o filippos ine kapios with alkalis. Sixth memoir. Study of human, sheep, beef, jaguar and goose fat).
5. Reinitzer F. Contributions to the knowledge of cholesterol. Mon Chem. 1888;9:421-41.
6. Bernhard W. Remembering Heinrich Wieland (1877–1957) portrait of an organic chemist and founder of modern biochemistry. Med Res Rev. 1993;12(3):195-274.
7. Müller C. Angina pectoris in hereditary xanthomatosis. Arch. Intern. Med. 1939;64:675-700.
8. Krebs HA, Weitzman PDJ. Krebs' Citric Acid Cycle: Half a Century and Still Turning. London: Biochemical Society; 1987.
9. The Nobel Prize in Physiology or Medicine 1953. The Nobel Foundation. Available from http://www.nobelprize.org/nobel_prizes/medicine/laureates/1953/ [Accessed October 2011]
10. Brown MS, Goldstein JL. A receptor-mediated pathway for cholesterol homeostatis. Science. 1985;232:34-47.
11. Fredrickson DS, Altrocchi PH, Avioli LV, et al. Tangier disease. Ann Intern Med. 1961;55:1016-31.
12. Windaus A. Ueber der Gehalt normaler und atheromatoser Aorten an Cholesterol und Cholesterin-ester. Z Physiol Chemie. 1910;67:174.

13. Gofman JW, Lindgren FT, Elliott H, et al. The role of lipids and lipoproteins in atherosclerosis. Science. 1950;111:166-71.
14. Mahmood L, Wang V. The Framingham heart study and the epidemiology of cardiovascular disease: a historical perspective (fee required). Lancet. 2013;27:61752-3.
15. Bloch K. Speech at the Nobel Banquet Stockholm, December 10, 1964.
16. Blohm TR, MacKenzie RD. Specific inhibition of cholesterol biosynthesis by a synthetic compound (MER-29). Arch Biochem Biophys. 1959;85(1):245-9.
17. Altschulr H, Stephen JD. Influence of nicotinic acid on serum cholesterol in man. Arch Biochem Biophys. 1955; 54(2):558-9.
18. Thorp JM, Warig WS. Modification of metabolism and distribution of lipids by ethyl chlorophenoxy-isobutyrate. Nature. 1962;194:948-9.
19. Bergen SS, Jr, Van Itallie TB, Tennent DM, et al. Effect of an anion exchange resin on serum cholesterol in man. Proc Soc Exp Biol Med. 1959;102:676-9.
20. Endo A. A gift from nature: the birth of the statins. Nat Med. 2008;14:1050-52.
21. Scandinavian Simvastatin Survival Study Group. Randomised trial of cholesterol lowering in 4444 patients with coronary heart disease: the Scandinavian Simvastatin Survival Study (4S). Lancet. 1994;344:1383-9.
22. Ridker PM, Danielson E, Fonseca FAH, et al. Glynn RJ for the JUPITER Study Group. Rosuvastatin to prevent vascular events in men and women with elevated C-reactive protein. N Engl J Med. 2008;359:2195-2207.
23. Nissen SE, Tsunoda T, Tuzcu EM, et al. Effect of recombinant ApoA-I Milano on coronary atherosclerosis in patients with acute coronary syndromes. JAMA. 2003;290(17):2292-300. doi:10.1001/jama.290.17.2292
24. Carlson LA. Nicotinic acid: the broad-spectrum lipid drug. A 50th anniversary review. Intern Med. 2005;258:94-114.
25. Nicholls SJ, Brewer HB, Kastelein JJ, et al. Effects of the CETP inhibitor evacetrapib administered as monotherapy or in combination with statins on HDL and LDL cholesterol: a randomized controlled trial. JAMA. 2011;306(19):2099-2109. doi:10.1001/jama.2011.1649
26. Horton JD, Cohen JC, Hobbs HH. Molecular biology of PCSK9: its role in LDL metabolism. Trends Biochem Sci. 2007;32(2):71-7.
27. Cho L, Rocco M, Colquhoun D, et al. Design and rational of the GAUSS-2 study trial: a double-blind, ezetimibe-controlled phase 3 study of the efficacy and tolerability of evolocumab (AMF145) in subjects with hypercholesterolemia who are intolerant of statin therapy. Clin Cardiol. 2014;37:131-9.
28. Reducing LDL with PCSK9 Inhibitors—The Clinical Benefit of Lipid Drugs Brendan M. Everett, M.D., M.P.H., Robert J. Smith, M.D., and William R. Hiatt, M.D. DOI: 10.1056/NEJMp1508120

Epidemiology of Lipid Disorders

Baridalyne Nongkynrih and Sanjeev Kumar Gupta

- Introduction: Definition and risk factors
- Global burden of dyslipidemia
- Epidemiology of dyslipidemia in South-East Asian region
- Epidemiology of dyslipidemia in India
- Prevention and control measures
- Conclusion

INTRODUCTION

Dyslipidemia is a disorder of lipoprotein metabolism, which may be manifested by the elevation of total cholesterol, low-density lipoprotein (LDL) cholesterol and triglyceride and a decrease in high-density lipoprotein (HDL) cholesterol levels. Low-density lipoprotein (LDL) cholesterol makes up 60–70% of the total serum cholesterol; HDL cholesterol contributes to 20–30% and very low-density lipoproteins (VLDLs), which are triglyceride-rich lipoproteins, make up 10–15 % of the total serum cholesterol.

According to National Cholesterol Education Program (NCEP) Adult Treatment Panel III (ATP III) guidelines, dyslipidemia is defined by the presence of high total cholesterol (≥200 mg/dL), high LDL cholesterol (≥130 mg/dL), low HDL cholesterol (<40 mg/dL), high non-HDL cholesterol (≥160 mg/dL), high cholesterol remnants [VLDL cholesterol = total – (HDL+LDL) cholesterol ≥ 25 mg/dL] or high triglycerides (≥150 mg/dL) (Table 2.1).[1]

There are well-known causes of elevated serum triglycerides (Box 2.1). Multiple factors usually coexist in the same individual; hence, it is difficult to attribute the contribution of any single factor to the development of lipid disorders. Most of the factors are modifiable; therefore, primary prevention of emergence of these risk factors is crucial in order to reduce the long-term morbidity and mortality associated with cardiovascular diseases (CVDs).

The description of dyslipidemia would be incomplete without a brief mention of metabolic syndrome.

Metabolic syndrome is defined by a cluster of interrelated risk factors that increase the risk of coronary heart disease (CHD), other forms of CVDs and diabetes mellitus type 2. Its main components are dyslipidemia (elevated triglycerides, low HDLs), elevation of arterial blood pressure and high blood glucose, abdominal obesity and/or insulin resistance (Table 2.2).

Box 2.1: Causes of elevated serum triglycerides

Overweight and obesity

Physical inactivity

Cigarette smoking

Excess alcohol intake

Very high-carbohydrate diets (>60% of total energy)

Other diseases (type 2 diabetes, chronic renal failure, nephrotic syndrome)

Certain drugs (corticosteroids, protease inhibitors for HIV, beta-adrenergic blocking agents, estrogens)

Genetic factors

Source: National Cholesterol Education Program. Third Report of the National Cholesterol Education Program (NCEP) Expert Panel on Detection, Evaluation, and Treatment of High Blood Cholesterol in Adults (Adult Treatment Panel III). National Heart, Lung, and Blood Institute, National Institutes of Health NIH Publication No. 02-5215, September 2002ATP-III)

Table 2.1: ATP-III classification of total cholesterol, LDL cholesterol and HDL cholesterol

Total cholesterol (mg/dL)		LDL cholesterol (mg/dL)		HDL cholesterol (mg/dL)	
<200	Desirable	<100	Optimal	<40	Low
200–239	Borderline high	100–129	Near optimal/above optimal	≥60	High
≥240	High	130–159	Borderline high		
		160–189	High		
		≥190	Very high		

ATP III, Adult Treatment Panel III; LDL, low-density lipoprotein; HDL, high-density lipoprotein.

Table 2.2: Clinical identification of the metabolic syndrome[1] (ATP III)

Risk factor	Defining level
Abdominal obesity	Waist circumference
Men	>102 cm
Women	>88 cm
Triglycerides	≥150 mg/dL
HDL cholesterol	
Men	<40 mg/dL
Women	<50 mg/dL
Blood pressure	≥130/85 mmHg
Fasting glucose	≥6.1 mmol/L (110 mg/dL)

ATP III, Adult Treatment Panel III; HDL, high-density lipoprotein.

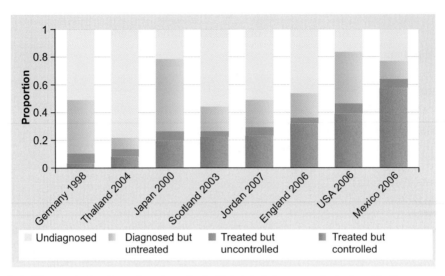

Figure 2.1: Diagnosis, treatment and control of high total serum cholesterol in the population aged 40–79 in eight countries with different income levels, 1998–2007

GLOBAL BURDEN OF DYSLIPIDEMIA

Cholesterol levels usually increase steadily with age, more so in women and stabilize after middle age. A high cholesterol level increases the risks of heart disease and stroke. High cholesterol is estimated to cause 18% of global cerebrovascular disease (mostly nonfatal events), and 56% of global ischemic heart disease.[2] Overall, raised cholesterol is estimated to cause 2.6 million deaths (4.5% of total) and 29.7 million disability-adjusted life years (DALYS), or 2.0% of total DALYS. A 10% reduction in serum cholesterol in men aged 40 has been reported to result in a 50% reduction in heart disease within 5 years; the same serum cholesterol reduction for men aged 70 can result in an average 20% reduction in heart disease occurrence in the next 5 years.[3]

Dyslipidemia as such is not usually reported in isolation, but often as a component of metabolic risk factors for noncommunicable diseases (NCDs). A recent study conducted by the World Health Organization (WHO) in 2011 (Fig. 2.1) among the largest ever number of subjects, representing 147 million people in eight countries (England, Germany, Japan, Jordan, Mexico, Scotland, Thailand and USA), showed that the proportion of people with undiagnosed high serum cholesterol was highest in Thailand [78%; 95% confidence interval (CI): 74–82] as compared to other countries, and the proportion of diagnosed but untreated was also highest in 9% in Thailand (95% CI: 8–11).[4] Therefore, the burden of dyslipidemia, as reflected by high serum cholesterol levels, needs to be seen as a health problem not only in the high-income countries, but also emerging in low- and middle-income countries.

EPIDEMIOLOGY OF DYSLIPIDEMIA IN SOUTH-EAST ASIA REGION

According to WHO reports, in 2008 the prevalence of raised cholesterol (≥190 mg/dL) in the South-East Asia region (SEAR) was 29% (Fig. 2.2). Although the proportion in SEAR maybe less as compared to other regions, the burden is substantial because SEAR includes Indian

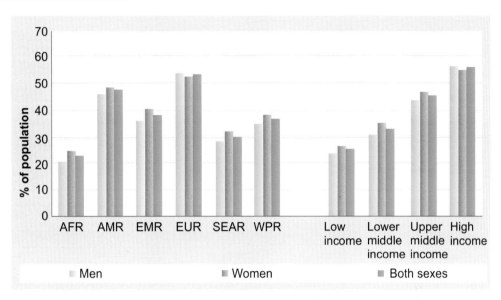

Figure 2.2: Proportion of population above 25 years (age adjusted) with raised cholesterol (≥190 mg/dL) in different WHO regions, 2008

subcontinent, which is the second largest populated country in the world, therefore translating to large number of affected individuals.[3]

The most recent NCD global report by the WHO released in September 2011 provides country profiles on various risk factors of NCDs, including mean cholesterol levels for almost three decades (Fig. 2.3).[5]

The mean total serum cholesterol in all the countries of SEAR is above 4 mmol/L (154 mg/dL)* in both males and females. It is to be noted that there is an increasing trend in all the countries of SEAR during 1998-2000, with the exception of Bangladesh and Nepal, which shows a slight decrease in the prevalence. In DPR Korea, India, Maldives, Myanmar and Sri Lanka, the prevalence is seen more in women as compared to men. If the present trend continues, the burden of dyslipidemia is expected to increase in the SEAR with serious consequences in terms of morbidity, mortality and healthcare cost. Data also shows that 56% of the adult population in Thailand had raised serum cholesterol levels.

EPIDEMIOLOGY OF DYSLIPIDEMIA IN INDIA

Dyslipidemia in Adults

India is undergoing a demographic transition. The increase in life expectancy, improving lifestyle and growing economy are all welcoming changes for a developing nation; however, the flip side of development is the emergence of "lifestyle" diseases. Obesity, diabetes and lipid disorders are now more frequently seen as compared to three decades ago. There are various studies in India since the early 1990s to show that the problem is on the rise. Data on the prevalence of dyslipidemias is available from various parts of the country. Most of the information is

---

* Total cholesterol & HDL cholesterol mmol/L = mg/dL × 0.026.

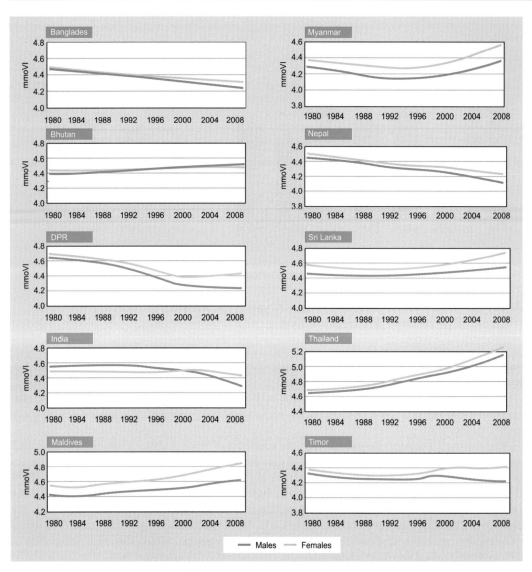

Figure 2.3: Mean total cholesterol levels in the countries of WHO—South-East Asia Region[5]

available from urban population, but there are some studies from rural India which show that the problem exists in rural India as well.

Dyslipidemia among Adults in Urban India

In North India, the Jaipur Heart Watch, which is a series of cross-sectional epidemiological studies (JHW1, JHW2, JHW3, JHW4) was carried out in Rajasthan from 1992 to 2005 to determine cardiovascular risk factors in urban population. In this study, dyslipidemia was defined according to NCEP ATP III guidelines. It was reported that in all cohorts, the prevalence of various forms of lipid abnormalities increased with age. There was a sharp increase in dyslipidemias from JHW1 to JHW2. However, about 25% of study subjects had total serum cholesterol level above 200 mg/dL in all the four cohorts. The prevalence was seen to be similar in both sexes.[6] Besides, there are studies from other parts of the country, such as Haryana,[7] Mumbai[8] and Calcutta,[9] which have reported high serum cholesterol levels and variants of lipid disorders in urban areas.

One of the landmark studies in India on risk factors of NCDs was a multicentric study carried out by the Indian Council of Medical Research (ICMR) in 2005–2006 in a representative population of 7500 adults above 15 years in six centers (Chennai, Delhi, Dibrugarh, Ballabgarh, Nagpur and Trivandrum). In this study, the WHO STEPS surveillance method was used to estimate the risk factors for NCDs of which estimation of lipids was included. The mean total serum cholesterol level was seen to be 4.7 mmol/L (180.9 mg/dL) in urban men and women. Twenty-three percent men and 27% women had total serum cholesterol levels above the cutoff limit of ≥5.2 mmol/L (200 mg/dL). In all these centers, the proportion of subjects with total serum cholesterol levels ≥5.2 mmol/L (200 mg/dL) increased with increasing age. The proportion of men with HDL cholesterol ≤0.9 mmol/L (35 mg/dL) was 37.5% and 26% women in all populations. The prevalence of dyslipidemia (Fig. 2.4), which included individuals with elevated total serum cholesterol and triglyceride levels, also reported low HDL levels. Overall, there were 4.1% men and 2.7% women with dyslipidemia in all populations. The highest proportions among men were seen in Trivandrum (6.2%) and women in Delhi (4.2%).[10]

Dyslipidemia in Rural India

Information about lipid disorders in rural India is scarce since few studies have been carried out in rural areas. It is often thought that the rural population is relatively "healthier" as compared to their urban counterparts because of increased physical activity and healthy diet. However, the ICMR study showed that the mean total cholesterol level was seen to be similar in both urban and rural areas. The prevalence of dyslipidemia was 3% in rural men, which was highest in Trivandrum (Fig. 2.4).[10]

The Indian Migration Study carried out in 2005–2007 also provides some information about the proportion of rural persons with lipid disorders. In this study of 1983 rural participants, risk factors for NCDs were estimated. It was reported that the mean total serum cholesterol was 4.5 mmol/L (173.2 mg/dL) in men and 4.7 mmol/L (180.9 mg/dL) in women. The proportion

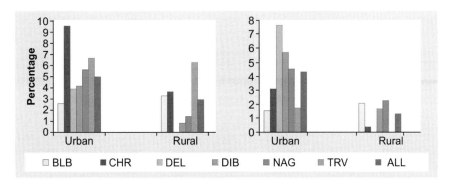

Figure 2.4: Proportion (%) of men and women with dyslipidemia according to Center and Population[9]

of men with high ratio of total serum cholesterol to HDL cholesterol (≥4.5 or 173.2 mg/dL)[‡] was 33.0% and 34.6% in women. High triglyceride concentration (≥1.69 mmol/L or 147 mg/dL) was seen in 27% in both men and women.[11]

Therefore, there is evidence to show that dyslipidemia is not restricted to urban areas alone, but it is also a reality in rural India.

Dyslipidemia in Children

One of the disturbing trends currently is the increase in the presence of risk factors for NCDs in children and young adults reflected in obesity, deranged lipid profiles and blood sugar levels. In India there are enough studies to show that lipid disorders are not restricted to adults only, but are also seen in children.

A study conducted among 2640 school children aged 12–19 years, from 16 schools in Chennai, from different parts of the city, including government and private schools, showed that 65% of normal weight children and adolescents had at least one cardiometabolic risk factor.[12] The most common cardiometabolic abnormality was low HDL cholesterol, followed by elevated triglycerides. Obesity and dyslipidemia are also reported from various studies among urban school children in Delhi.[13,14] There is sufficient evidence to show that obesity and associated lipid abnormalities are becoming a universal phenomenon seen across children in urban Indian, and therefore cannot be ignored.

PREVENTION AND CONTROL MEASURES

Primary prevention: The aim of primary prevention is to prevent the development of risk factors for dyslipidemia, which could lead to serious/fatal cardiovascular consequences. As has been discussed earlier, many of the factors for lipid disorders are modifiable, such as dietary habits, overweight and obesity, tobacco and alcohol. These factors argue strongly for the role of primary prevention through lifestyle changes. The NCEP guidelines also affirm the validity of *lifestyle changes as first-line therapy for primary prevention*.

In addition, clinical trials of cholesterol-lowering drugs support the efficacy of clinical primary prevention in higher risk individuals (Table 2.3). It was seen that there is a reduction in major coronary events by about 31–37% with the use of statins.

Dyslipidemia is often undiagnosed, especially in young adults. Therefore, early detection by routine screening has to be performed. According to ACEP guidelines, routine serum cholesterol testing should begin in young adulthood (≥20 years of age).[1] In countries like India because of lack of awareness and limitation of resources, screening at such an early age may not be possible. The National Programme for Prevention and Control of Cancer, Diabetes, CVD and Stroke,[15] which was recently launched by the Ministry of Health & Family Welfare, Government of India in 2008 recommends "opportunistic screening" for all individuals above the age of 30 years who come in contact with any healthcare facility, both in the rural and urban areas.

Secondary prevention: Secondary prevention is applicable to those who have had CHD. Individuals with established CHD are highly susceptible to develop recurrent CHD. Trials demonstrate that reduction in LDL cholesterol levels significantly reduces risk for recurrent major coronary events in individuals with established CHD (Table 2.4).

[‡]Triglycerides mmol/L = mg/dL × 0.0115.

Table 2.3: Major primary prevention trials with statins

Study	WOSCOPS	AFCAPS/TexCAPS
Persons	6595	6605
Duration	4.9 years	5 years
Drug (dose/day)	Pravastatin 40 mg	Lovastatin 40 mg
Baseline LDL-C (mg/dL)	192	150
LDL-C change	−26%*	−25%*
Major coronary events	−31%*	−37%*
Revascularization	−37%*	−33%*
Coronary mortality	−33%*	NS
Total mortality	−22*	NS

Source: National Cholesterol Education Program. Third Report of the National Cholesterol Education Program (NCEP) Expert Panel on Detection, Evaluation, and Treatment of High Blood Cholesterol in Adults (Adult Treatment Panel III). National Heart, Lung, and Blood Institute, National Institutes of Health NIH Publication No. 02-5215, September 2002.
*Statistically significant.
LDL-C, low-density lipoprotein cholesterol.

Table 2.4: Major secondary prevention trials with statins: morbidity and mortality results

Study	4S	CARE	LIPID
Persons	4444	4159	9014
Duration	5.4 years	5 years	5 years
Drug (dose/day)	Simvastatin	Pravastatin 40 mg	Pravastatin 40 mg
Baseline LDL-C (mg/dL)	188	139	150
LDL-C change	−35%*	−27%*	−25%*
Major coronary events	−35%*	−25%*	−29%*
Revascularization	−37%*	−27%*	−24%*
Coronary mortality	−42%*	−24%*	−24%*
Total mortality	−30%*	−9%	−23%*
Stroke	−27%*	−31%*	−19%*

Source: National Cholesterol Education Program. Third Report of the National Cholesterol Education Program (NCEP) Expert Panel on Detection, Evaluation, and Treatment of High Blood Cholesterol in Adults (Adult Treatment Panel III). National Heart, Lung, and Blood Institute, National Institutes of Health NIH Publication No. 02-5215, September 2002.
*Statistically significant.
LDL-C, low-density lipoprotein cholesterol.

Recommendations: According to the ATP III guidelines,[1] in young adults aged 20 and above, optimal LDL cholesterol levels deserve attention. When LDL cholesterol concentrations range from 100 to 129 mg/dL, young adults should be encouraged to modify life habits to minimize long-term risk. In those with borderline high LDL cholesterol (130–159 mg/dL), clinical attention through therapeutic lifestyle changes is needed both to lower LDL cholesterol and to minimize other risk factors. If LDL cholesterol is high (160–189 mg/dL), more intensive clinical intervention should be initiated, with emphasis on therapeutic lifestyle changes. However, if LDL cholesterol remains elevated despite therapeutic lifestyle changes, particularly when LDL cholesterol is ≥190 mg/dL, consideration should be given to long-term management with LDL-lowering drugs.

CONCLUSION

Noncommunicable diseases are emerging as a major public health problem in South-East Asia, and dyslipidemia is one of the major contributing risk factors. Raised total serum cholesterol is a major cause of disease burden as a risk factor for ischemic heart disease and stroke. There is evidence to show that about one-fourth of the Indian population have serum cholesterol levels above the cutoff limits, with both urban and rural population in India manifesting equally high levels of dyslipidemia. An alarming trend is seen among children as well where obesity and lipid disorders are on the rise, especially in urban children. Therefore, there is an urgent need to take steps to prevent and control the increasing trend of dyslipidemia in India. It is essential to create awareness among the population about the importance of a healthy lifestyle, routine screening and timely management to prevent the onset of catastrophic and debilitating consequences.

REFERENCES

1. National Cholesterol Education Program. Third Report of the National Cholesterol Education Program (NCEP) Expert Panel on Detection, Evaluation, and Treatment of High Blood Cholesterol in Adults (Adult Treatment Panel III). National Heart, Lung, and Blood Institute, National Institutes of Health NIH Publication No. 02-5215, September 2002.
2. World Health Organization. Diet related risk factors;2002. Available from: http://who.int/whr/2002/chapter4/en/index4.html [Accessed May 2, 2012]
3. World Health Organization. Global Health Observatory. Raised Cholesterol: observations and trends 2011. Available from: http://www.who.int/gho/ncd/risk_factors/cholesterol_text/en/index.html [Accessed May 2, 2012].
4. Roth GA, Fihn SD, Mokdad AH, et al. High total serum cholesterol, medication coverage and therapeutic control: an analysis of national health examination survey data from eight countries. Bull World Health Organ. 2011;89(2):92-101.
5. World Health Organization. Noncommunicable diseases country profiles 2011. WHO Global Report. Available from: http://www.who.int/nmh/publications/ncd_profiles2011/en/index.html [Accessed May 2, 2012].
6. Gupta R, Guptha S, Agrawal A, et al. Secular trends in cholesterol lipoproteins and triglycerides and prevalence of dyslipidemias in an urban Indian population. Lipids Health Dis. 2008;7:40.
7. Nongkynrih B, Acharya A, Ramakrishnan L, et al. Profile of biochemical risk factors for non communicable diseases in urban, rural and periurban Haryana, India. J Assoc Physicians India. 2008;56:165-70.

8. Sawant AM, Shetty D, Mankeshwar R, et al. Prevalence of dyslipidemia in young adult Indian population. J Assoc Physicians India. 2008;56:99-102.
9. Ghosh A. Anthropometric, metabolic, and dietary fatty acids characteristics in lean and obese dyslipidemic Asian Indian women in Calcutta. Food Nutr Bull. 2007;28(4):399-405.
10. Indian Council Medical Research: Sentinel Health Monitoring Centers in India: Biochemical Risk Factor Survey for Non-communicable Diseases 2005–2006. Available from: http://whoindia.org/ LinkFiles/NMH_Resources_NCD_Risk_step_3_report.pdf [Accessed May 2, 2012].
11. Kinra S, Bowen LJ, Lyngdoh T, et al. Sociodemographic patterning of non-communicable disease risk factors in rural India: a cross sectional study. BMJ. 2010 Sep 27;341:c4974. doi: 10.1136/bmj.c4974.
12. Ramachandran A, Snehalatha C, Yamuna A, et al. Insulin resistance and clustering of cardiometabolic risk factors in urban teenagers in southern India. Diabetes Care. 2007;30(7):1828-33.
13. Kaur S, Kapil U. Dyslipidemia amongst obese children in National Capital Territory (NCT) of Delhi. Indian J Pediatr. 2011;78:55-7.
14. Gupta DK, Shah P, Misra A, et al. Secular trends in prevalence of overweight and obesity from 2006 to 2009 in urban Asian Indian adolescents aged 14–17 years. PLoS One. 2011;6(2):e17221.
15. National Programme for Prevention and Control of Cancer, Diabetes, CVD and Stroke Ministry of Health & Family Welfare, Government of India; Operational Guidelines 2010.. Available from: http://health.bih.nic.in/Docs/Guidelines-NPCDCS.pdf [Accessed May 2, 2012]

Biochemical Basis of Dyslipidemia

Moushumi Lodh and Ashok Kumar Parida

- Apolipoproteins
- Cholesterol metabolism
- Small and dense LDL
- Lipoprotein metabolism

- Lipoprotein oxidation
- Current guidelines and expert panel recommendations

Dyslipidemia is a common metabolic disorder that may result from abnormalities in the synthesis, processing and catabolism of lipoprotein particles. Elevated plasma total cholesterol,[1] triglyceride (TG),[2] low-density lipoprotein cholesterol (LDL-C)[3] and apolipoprotein B (ApoB),[4] together with decreased levels of ApoA1[4] and high-density lipoprotein cholesterol (HDL-C),[5] are associated with an increased risk of coronary artery disease (CAD). A number of epidemiological studies have shown that, in addition to environmental factors, genetic mechanisms may play a role in determining susceptibility to dyslipidemia.[6] The heritability estimates of the interindividual variation in plasma lipid phenotypes from both twin and family studies are in the range of 40–60%,[7] suggesting a considerable genetic contribution, and discovery of the genes that contribute to these changes may lead to a better understanding of these processes.

APOLIPOPROTEINS

Cholesterol, in both free and esterified forms, and TGs are the two main lipids in plasma. They are transported in lipoproteins, pseudomicellar lipid–protein complexes, differentiated on the basis of their constituent apolipoproteins.[8]

The apolipoproteins, ApoB-100/48, ApoA-I, ApoA-II, ApoE and the ApoCs, are integral components of lipoproteins. Apolipoprotein B is a component of all atherogenic lipoproteins (chylomicron remnants, very low-density lipoprotein [VLDL] and their remnants, intermediate-density lipoprotein (IDL), lipoprotein(a) [Lp(a)] and LDL), whereas ApoA-I and ApoA-II are components of HDL. Apolipoprotein A-I and ApoC-I are involved in the activation of lecithin:cholesterol acyltransferase (LCAT), which mediate the reverse cholesterol transport from peripheral tissues to the liver.[9-11] Apolipoprotein CII stimulates LPL-mediated hydrolysis of chylomicrons and VLDL.[12,13] Apolipoprotein E is the ligand for the cellular uptake of IDL and chylomicron remnants.[14-16] Apolipoprotein B-100, an approximately 550 kDa nonexchangeable protein, is the major apolipoprotein component of the atherogenic lipoproteins (VLDL, LDL, IDL) and contains the ligands for the cellular uptake of LDL via its receptor. Plasma ApoB concentration levels are more discriminating than other plasma lipids and lipoproteins in patients with coronary heart disease (CHD),[4,17] prospective studies of Plasma Apo B levels reported variable predictivity of CHD.[18] Apolipoprotein B-48, is a product of a novel mRNA editing mechanism, where an amino acid codon is converted to a stop codon, giving an expression product that lacks the LDL receptor-binding domain.[19,20] Apolipoprotein B-48 is a truncated form of ApoB, present in chylomicrons.

Apolipoprotein CIII is a major component of TG-rich lipoproteins (TRLs) (chylomicrons and VLDL) and a minor component of HDL. The mature 79-amino acid ApoCIII protein is synthesized predominantly in the liver, but also to a lesser extent in the intestine. Apolipoprotein CIII is a noncompetitive inhibitor of lipoprotein lipase, thus suggesting an important role in the catabolism of TRLs.[21] Apolipoprotein A-V is a secreted protein present in human serum and is associated with specific lipoprotein particles. It was detectable in VLDL, HDL and chylomicrons. Plasma ApoCIII correlates with plasma TG level,[22,23] while ApoA-V, which occurs at low levels,[24] appears to be antilipemic.[25] Human ApoA1/C3/A5 gene, candidate region for hyperlipidemia, in particular for hypertriglyceridemia and atherosclerosis, resides in the ApoA1/C3/A4/A5 gene cluster, a short region on chromosome 11q23–q24.[25-27]

Evidence from major epidemiologic studies (e.g., INTERHEART, ISIS, AMORIS, Apolipoprotein-related Mortality Risk) and clinical trials (e.g., AFCAPS/TexCAPS, CARDS, IDEAL) strongly supports the use of apolipoproteins, particularly ApoB, to inform both population- and patient-based assessments and decision making in cardiovascular prevention.[28] The World Health Organization (WHO)–International Federation of Clinical Chemistry (IFCC) has now developed standardized methods for the measurement of ApoB and ApoA-I,[29] and population results have subsequently been reported.[30] The prospective Québec Cardiovascular Study[31] and other investigations have demonstrated the importance of ApoB in estimating coronary risk. Recently, the large prospective AMORIS study[32] showed that the age-adjusted values of ApoB and the ApoB/ApoA-I ratio were strongly and positively related to increased risk of fatal myocardial infarction in men and women. In multivariate analyses, ApoB was a stronger predictor of risk than LDL cholesterol in both men and women. This study suggests that ApoB and the ApoB/ApoA-I ratio should be regarded as highly predictive in evaluating cardiac risk. ApoB might be of greatest value in the diagnosis and treatment of persons with normal or low concentrations of LDL cholesterol.[32] For example, patients with type 2 diabetes mellitus frequently have hypertriglyceridemia together with hyper-ApoB, an atherogenic lipid profile that is often unappreciated because of concomitant low or normal levels of LDL cholesterol.[33]

CHOLESTEROL METABOLISM

Adequate stores of cholesterol are vital and achieved through exogenous sources and endogenous pathways of cholesterol metabolism. Ingestion of cholesterol and its active absorption in the gut and enterohepatic recirculation of bile acids from the gut back to the liver are referred to as exogenous pathways of cholesterol metabolism. Synthesis of cholesterol within the liver and reverse transport of cholesterol from the blood back to the liver, either by the direct or indirect pathways, is considered the endogenous component of cholesterol metabolism.[34]

The direct pathway utilizes HDL receptors, such as scavenger receptor BI that mediates the selective uptake of cholesterol from HDL. The second mechanism is the indirect one, mediated by cholesterol ester transfer protein (CETP). This protein exchanges TGs of VLDL with cholesterol esters of HDL. The VLDL is then processed to LDL and removed from the circulation by the LDL receptor pathway. The TGs are not stable in HDL but degraded by hepatic lipase (HL), converting them to small HDL particles where they are capable of picking up cholesterol from cells by interaction with the ATP-binding cassette transporter A1 (ABCA1) and then unloading their cholesterol content back to the liver by the direct pathway. Because cholesterol is not water soluble, its transport through the blood requires it to be carried by water-soluble lipoproteins. Apolipoprotein B (ApoB) is the primary apolipoproteins of LDL. It is responsible for delivering cholesterol to tissues and acts as a ligand for LDL receptors in various cells throughout the body, thus allowing the influx of cholesterol into the cells. Apolipoprotein A-I, on the other hand, is the major protein component of HDL. This protein has the exact opposite effect of ApoB and promotes cholesterol efflux from tissues and reverse transport to the liver for excretion.[35]

When the cholesterol pool is depleted, the liver can replenish its supply of cholesterol in two ways. First, it can do so by increasing the activity of HMG-CoA reductase, the rate-controlling enzyme for the production of cholesterol, and secondly by absorbing more cholesterol from the blood by upregulation of LDL receptors. However, if cholesterol synthesis is blocked by statins, then the only way for the liver to obtain more cholesterol is by further upregulation of LDL receptors, causing even greater clearance of LDL from the blood.

Lipoprotein(a) is a plasma lipoprotein consisting of a cholesterol-rich LDL particle with one molecule of ApoB100 and an additional protein, apolipoprotein A, attached via a disulfide bond.[36] Elevated Lp(a) levels can potentially increase the risk of CVD via (i) prothrombotic/antifibrinolytic effects as ApoA possesses structural homology with plasminogen and plasmin, but has no fibrinolytic activity and (ii) accelerated atherogenesis as a result of intimal deposition of Lp(a) cholesterol, or both. The largest epidemiological study to date on Lp(a) assessed individual records of 126,634 participants in 36 prospective studies.[37] Lipoprotein(a) concentration was weakly correlated with several known risk factors: positively with total and non-HDL cholesterol, ApoB100 and inversely with $\log_e$ TGs. Lipoprotein(a) levels were 12% [95% confidence interval (CI): 8–16%] higher in women and 11% (4–17%) lower in people with diabetes.[37]

Plasma concentrations of Lp(a) are determined chiefly by rates of hepatic synthesis of ApoA: although the site of formation of Lp(a) has not been definitively identified, evidence suggests that ApoA adducts extracellularly and covalently to ApoB100-containing lipoproteins, predominantly LDL.[38,39] Apolipoprotein A genotype, which determines both the synthetic rate and size of the ApoA moiety of Lp(a), alone accounts for 90% of plasma concentrations of Lp(a).[38,40,41] As hepatic secretion rates are lower for large ApoA isoforms, and as most individuals are heterozygous for two different isoforms, the smallest isoform typically predominates in plasma. Lipoprotein(a) is thought to be catabolized primarily by hepatic and renal pathways, but these metabolic routes do not appear to govern plasma Lp(a) levels. After transfer from plasma into the arterial intima, Lp(a) may be more avidly retained than LDL as it binds to the extracellular matrix not only through ApoA, but also via its ApoB component,[42] thereby contributing cholesterol to the expanding atherosclerotic plaque. In vitro, Lp(a) binds to several extracellular matrix proteins, including fibrin[43] and defensins, a family of 29–35 amino acid peptides that are released by neutrophils during inflammation and severe infection.[44]

It is likely that defensins, such as lipoprotein lipase, provide a bridge between Lp(a) and the extracellular matrix.

Through its ApoA moiety, Lp(a) also interacts with the β2-integrin Mac-1, thereby promoting the adhesion of monocytes and their transendothelial migration.[45] In atherosclerotic coronary arteries, Lp(a) was found to localize in close proximity to Mac-1 on infiltrating mononuclear cells. Lipoprotein(a) has also been shown to bind pro-inflammatory-oxidized phospholipids[46] and is a preferential carrier of oxidized phospholipids in human plasma. Lipoprotein(a) also contains lipoprotein-associated phospholipase A2 (equally referred to as Paf-acetylhydrolase), which may cleave oxidized fatty acids at the sn-2 position in oxidized phospholipids to yield short-chain fatty acids and lysolecithin.[47]

Apolipoprotein A, a homologue of the fibrinolytic proenzyme plasminogen, impairs fibrinolysis.[48] Essential to fibrin clot, lysis is a number of plasmin-dependent, positive feedback reactions that enhance the efficiency of plasminogen activation, including the plasmin-mediated conversion of Glu-plasminogen to Lys-plasminogen. It has been observed that the ApoA component of Lp(a) inhibits the key positive feedback step involving conversion of plasmin-mediated Glu-plasminogen to Lys-plasminogen.[49] Lipoprotein(a) may also enhance coagulation by inhibiting the function of tissue factor pathway inhibitor.[50] Finally, small isoforms of ApoA have been observed to possess elevated potency in inhibiting fibrinolysis and thereby promoting thrombosis.[51] A recent meta-analysis demonstrated a twofold increase in the risk of CHD and ischemic stroke in subjects with small ApoA phenotypes.[52] Furthermore, prospective findings in the Bruneck study have revealed a significant association, specifically between small ApoA phenotypes and advanced atherosclerotic disease involving a component of plaque thrombosis.[53] In summary, elevated Lp(a) levels may promote atherosclerosis via Lp(a)-derived cholesterol entrapment in the intima, via inflammatory cell recruitment and/or via the binding of pro-inflammatory-oxidized phospholipids. The prothrombotic, antifibrinolytic actions of ApoA are expressed on the one hand as inhibition of fibrinolysis with enhancement of clot stabilization and on the other as enhanced coagulation via the inhibition of tissue factor pathway inhibitor.[54-56] It forms a link between genetics and two major explanations of the pathogenesis of atherosclerosis: the fibrin-deposition theory of Rokitansky and the lipid hypothesis of Virchow.[57]

SMALL AND DENSE LDL

Results from the Québec Cardiovascular Study have indicated that persons displaying elevated plasma concentrations of insulin and ApoB together with small and dense LDL particles showed a remarkable increase in CHD risk.[58] The small and dense LDL phenotype rarely occurs as an isolated disorder. It is most frequently accompanied by hypertriglyceridemia, reduced HDL-cholesterol levels, abdominal obesity and insulin resistance (all of which are components of the metabolic syndrome) and by a series of other metabolic alterations predictive of an impaired endothelial function and increased susceptibility to thrombosis. In a prospective, nested case-control study of subjects with childhood-onset type 1 diabetes (Pittsburgh Epidemiology of Diabetes Complications Study),[59] univariate analyses showed that both lipid mass and particle concentrations (NMR spectroscopy) of all VLDL subclasses, small LDL, medium LDL and medium HDL were increased in CAD cases compared with controls, whereas large HDL was decreased. Mean LDL and HDL particle sizes were less in CAD cases.[59] These changes in the nuclear magnetic resonance spectroscopy (NMR) lipoprotein subclass profile predictably increased the risk of cardiovascular disease, but were not fully apparent in the conventional lipid panel.[60]

LIPOPROTEIN METABOLISM

Triglycerides are predominantly carried in fasting conditions in VLDLs and their remnants, and postprandially in chylomicrons and their remnants. The generic term "triglyceride-rich lipoprotein remnants," therefore relates to chylomicron and VLDL particles that have undergone dynamic remodeling in the plasma after secretion from the intestine (chylomicrons) or liver (VLDL) (Fig. 3.1).[61]

This remodeling results in a spectrum of particles that are heterogeneous in size, hydrated density and have lipid and protein composition.[62] Remodeled chylomicrons and VLDL are atherogenic, primarily as a result of their progressive enrichment with cholesterol and depletion of TGs in the plasma compartment. This process also results in progressive reduction in their size. Upon entry into the circulation, chylomicrons (containing ApoB-48) produced by the small intestine, and VLDL (containing ApoB-100) produced by the liver undergo LPL-mediated lipolysis mainly in peripheral tissues, notably adipose tissue and muscle. Intravascular remodeling of TRL equally involves the actions of lipid transfer proteins [CETP, phospholipid transfer protein (PLTP)], HL and endothelial lipase, with the formation of remnant particles. Triglyceride-rich

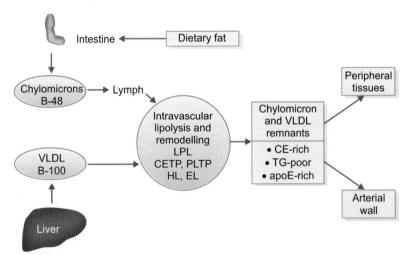

Figure 3.1: CETP facilitates transfer of cholesteryl ester from HDL to VLDL, IDL and LDL and allows triacylglycerol to transfer in the opposite direction. Much of the cholesteryl ester formed by LCAT in HDL finds its way to the liver via VLDL remnants. Simultaneously, the HDL2 that has been enriched with triacylglycerol unloads this cargo in the liver after reaction with hepatic lipase and is recycled as HDL3

Abbreviations: apo, apolipoprotein; CETP, cholesteryl ester transfer protein; EL, endothelial lipase; FFA, free fatty acids; HL, hepatic lipase; LDL, low-density lipoprotein; LPL, lipoprotein lipase; LRP, lipoprotein receptor-related protein; PLTP, phospholipid transfer protein; TRL, triglyceride-rich lipoprotein; VLDL, very-low density lipoprotein; IDL, intermediate-density lipoprotein.

Source: Adapted from Chapman MJ, Ginsberg HN, Amarenco P, et al. (for the European Atherosclerosis Society Consensus Panel). Triglyceride-rich lipoproteins and high-density lipoprotein cholesterol in patients at high risk of cardiovascular disease: evidence and guidance for management. Euro Heart J;doi:10.1093/eurheartj/ehr112 [European Heart Journal Advance Access published April 29, 2011].

lipoprotein remnants are typically enriched in cholesterol and ApoE, but depleted in TG; they are principally catabolized in the liver upon uptake through the lipoprotein receptor-related protein and LDL receptor pathways. Triglyceride-rich lipoprotein remnants can contribute either directly to plaque formation following penetration of the arterial wall at sites of enhanced endothelial permeability[63] or potentially indirectly following liberation of lipolytic products (such as free fatty acid and lysolecithin), which may activate proinflammatory signaling pathways in endothelial cells.[62,63]

The ApoB-containing lipoproteins and the ApoA-I/A-II lipoprotein classes are closely interrelated via several metabolic pathways (Fig. 3.2).[61]

De novo production of nascent HDL (discs) occurs in the liver and small intestine through the production of ApoA-I (the major HDL protein) and lipidation (with cholesterol and phospholipids) of this protein by the ABCA1 in these organs. Upon secretion, LCAT esterifies cholesterol on these discs, which matures into spherical particles (due to the formation of a hydrophobic core resulting from generation of cholesteryl esters by LCAT). High-density lipoprotein, a highly dynamic pool of heterogeneous particles,[64] undergoes extensive interconversion through TG lipolysis (HL), phospholipid hydrolysis (endothelial lipase, EL), fusion (PLTP) and lipid exchange among the HDL subpopulations (CETP). Cholesterol ester transfer protein also mediates major lipid transfer and exchange between HDL and TRLs (VLDL, chylomicrons) and their remnants

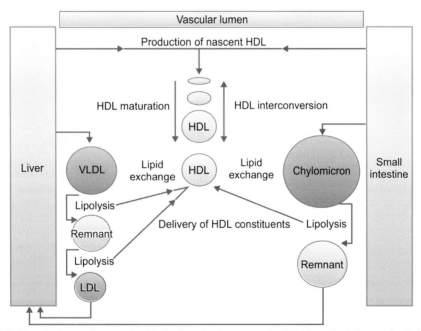

Figure 3.2: Metabolic pathways for high-density lipoprotein (HDL) and triglyceride-rich lipoprotein (TRL) remnants highlight their close interrelationship
Source: Adapted from Adapted from Chapman MJ, Ginsberg HN, Amarenco P, et al. (for the European Atherosclerosis Society Consensus Panel). Triglyceride-rich lipoproteins and high-density lipoprotein cholesterol in patients at high risk of cardiovascular disease: evidence and guidance for management. Euro Heart J;doi:10.1093/eurheartj/ehr112 [European Heart Journal Advance Access published April 29, 2011].

[VLDL remnants one-fourth IDLs, chylomicron remnants]. During this process, cholesteryl esters are transferred from HDL to VLDL and TGs move from VLDL to HDL.[65] Cholesterol efflux from macrophages represents only a small fraction of overall flux through the reverse cholesterol transport pathway, it is probably the component that is most relevant to atheroprotection.[66] The pathways known to mediate cholesterol efflux from macrophages are ABCA1, ABCG1, scavenger receptor B1 and aqueous diffusion.[67]

Chylomicrons also act as cholesteryl ester acceptors from LDL and HDL during the postprandial phase.[68] A second route that contributes to the plasma HDL pool involves hydrolysis of TGs in VLDL, IDL and chylomicrons. In this process, which is catalyzed by LPL, phospholipids and several apolipoproteins (such as ApoCI, CII, CIII, AV) are transferred to HDL. Phospholipid transfer protein contributes significantly to this remodeling process.[61]

Hepatic lipase is hypothesized to directly couple HDL lipid metabolism to tissue/cellular lipid metabolism (Fig. 3.3).[69]

The potential significance of the HL pathway is that it provides the hepatocytes with a mechanism for the uptake of a subset of phospholipids enriched with unsaturated fatty acids and may allow the uptake of cholesteryl ester, free cholesterol and phospholipid without catabolism of HDL apolipoproteins. Hepatic lipase can hydrolyze TG and phospholipid in all lipopro-

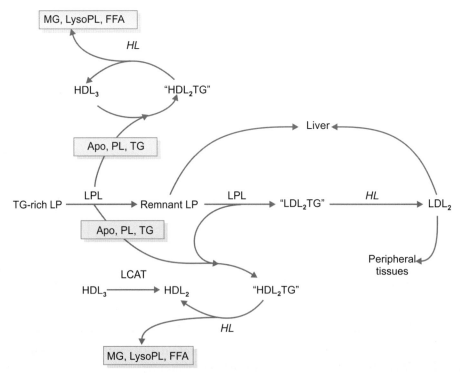

Figure 3.3: Metabolic scheme showing the multiple steps in lipoprotein metabolism catalyzed by hepatic lipase

Abbreviations: MG, monoglycerides; lysoPL, lysophospholipid; FFA, free fatty acid; PL, phospholipid; TG, triglyceride; apo, apolipoproteins; LP, lipoprotein, LPL, lipoprotein lipase; LCAT, lecithin cholesterol acyltransferase; HL, hepatic lipase.[69]

teins, but is predominant in the conversion of intermediate density lipoproteins to LDL and the conversion of postprandial TG-rich HDL into the postabsorptive TG-poor HDL. It has been suggested that enzymatically inactive HL can play a role in hepatic lipoprotein uptake forming a "bridge" by binding to the lipoprotein and to the cell surface. This raises the interesting possibility that production and secretion of mutant-inactive HL could promote clearance of VLDL remnants. Human HL deficiency in the context of a second factor causing hyperlipidemia is strongly associated with premature CAD.[69]

The lipid triad (increased levels of TGs, low levels of HDL cholesterol and increased small and dense LDL particles) results from hepatic uptake of free fatty acids from adipose tissues, with hepatic overproduction of VLDL ApoB. Triglycerides in VLDL are then exchanged for cholesteryl esters in LDL and HDL by CETP, and TGs in the core of these lipoproteins are hydrolyzed by lipoprotein lipase. These processes result in smaller, denser LDL particles, which have greater propensity to elicit oxidative arterial wall injury.[70,71] In patients with increased numbers of small, dense LDL particles, the total number of LDL particles may be higher than the LDL cholesterol level, because LDL particles differ in their cholesterol contents. Conversely, there is a 1:1 relationship between ApoB levels and the total number of atherogenic particles.[72]

LIPOPROTEIN OXIDATION

Atherosclerosis results from a combination of abnormalities in lipoprotein metabolism, oxidative stress, chronic inflammation and susceptibility to thrombosis. All of these processes contribute individually, or more commonly in aggregate, in the clinical expression of cardiovascular disease.[73,74] The term oxidized low-density lipoprotein (OxLDL) was traditionally used to describe LDL modified by exposure to copper ions, which catalyzed lipid peroxidation. The term OxLDL in a generic sense, however, additionally describes a broad array of chemical, biological and immunological entities, ranging from measurement of conjugated dienes, susceptibility of LDL to oxidation, ApoB–immune complexes and autoantibodies to various epitopes of OxLDL.[75] Oxidized low-density lipoprotein is proinflammatory and proatherogenic and is intimately involved in the initiation, progression and, potentially, in the destabilization of atherosclerotic lesions.[76] Therefore, it may be a unifying factor that can influence underlying risk in lipid disorders, inflammation and thrombosis. Use of OxLDL biomarkers, however, shows promise in diagnosing preclinical atherosclerosis in asymptomatic individuals, monitoring active disease and predicting cardiovascular outcomes.

Most cardiovascular risk factors generate oxidative stress in the vessel wall. As LDL traverses the subendothelial space it becomes oxidized, prior to advanced lesion formation, and may induce endothelial dysfunction, one of the earliest manifestations of atherosclerosis.[77] Most of OxLDL is present in the vessel wall rather than plasma (100-fold greater levels compared to plasma);[78] plasma levels may not necessarily reflect an association with all risk factors. Nonetheless, OxLDL levels have been associated with small and dense LDL [79,80] and the metabolic syndrome.[81] Studies have established that the OxPL/ApoB ratio is an independent predictor of the presence and extent of angiographically determined CAD in patients under 60 years old.[46] The influence of OxPL and lipoprotein(a) on CAD risk was diminished in patients over 60 years old, perhaps through the accumulation of additional risk factors that may have superseded the risk of OxPL/ApoB and lipoprotein(a), which can be elevated at birth in many subjects.[82] The utility of OxLDL-E06 in predicting progression of atherosclerosis was recently evaluated in the Bruneck study, a large prospective population-based survey of 40–79-year-old men and women initiated in 1990.[83]

CURRENT GUIDELINES AND EXPERT PANEL RECOMMENDATIONS

Mounting evidence has led expert panels to recommend consideration of Apo levels, particularly in patients with increased cardiometabolic risk, diabetic dyslipidemia or CHD. A consensus panel of the American Diabetes Association/American College of Cardiology Foundation recommended a goal ApoB level of <80 mg/dL for patients at highest risk and <90 mg/dL for patients at high risk.[84] The 2009 Canadian Cardiovascular Society/Canadian guidelines recommended an ApoB goal of <80 mg/dL, an LDL cholesterol level of <77 mg/dL or a 50% decline in LDL cholesterol levels from baseline in patients at high and moderate risk.[85] On the basis of recent (2000–2006) Third National Health and Nutrition Examination Survey population data, the ApoB treatment target should be <70 mg/dL for patients at high risk (i.e., those with CHD) and <90 mg/dL for those at moderately high risk.[86] National guidelines, recently published in Canada and the United States, address risk stratification and intervention based on individual lipid profiles and risk factors.[87-89] According to the SAFEHEART study, the risk of CVD is higher in those patients with an Lp(a) level >50 mg/dL and carrying a receptor-negative mutation in the LDLR gene compared with other less severe mutations.[90]

REFERENCES

1. Shekelle RB, Shryock AM, Paul O, et al. Diet, serum cholesterol, and death from coronary heart disease: The Western Electric study. N Engl J Med. 1981;304:65-70.
2. Austin MA. Plasma triglyceride as a risk factor for coronary heart disease: The epidemiologic evidence and beyond. Am J Epidemiol. 1989;129:24959.
3. März W, Scharnagl H, Winkler K, et al. Low-density lipoprotein triglycerides associated with low-grade systemic inflammation, adhesion molecules, and angiographic coronary artery disease: the Ludwigshafen Risk and Cardiovascular Health study. Circulation. 2004;110:3068-74.
4. Kwiterovich PO Jr, Coresh J, Smith HH, et al. Comparison of the plasma levels of apolipoproteins B and A-1 and other risk factors in men and women with premature coronary artery disease. Am J Cardiol. 1992;69:1015-21.
5. Hokanson JE, Austin MA. Plasma triglyceride level is a risk factor for cardiovascular disease independent of high-density lipoprotein cholesterol level: a meta-analysis of population-based prospective studies. J Cardiovasc Risk. 1996;3:213-319.
6. Yin RX, Li YY, Liu WY, et al. Interactions of the apolipoprotein A5 gene polymorphisms and alcohol consumption on serum lipid levels. PLoS ONE. 2011;6:e17954.
7. Heller DA, de Faire U, Pedersen NL, et al. Genetic and environmental influences on serum lipid levels in twins. N Engl J Med. 1993;328:1150-6.
8. Lee DM, Alaupovic P. Composition and concentration of apolipoproteins in very-low- and low-density lipoproteins of normal human plasma. Atherosclerosis. 1974;19:501-20.
9. Li Y, Yin R, Zhou Y, et al. Associations of the apolipoprotein A-I gene polymorphism and serum lipid levels in the Guangxi Hei Yi Zhuang and Han populations. Int J Mol Med. 2008;21:753-64.
10. Fielding CJ, Shore VG, Fielding PE. Lecithin cholesterol acyltransferase: effects of substrate composition upon enzyme activity. Biochim Biophys Acta. 1972;270:513.
11. Soutar AK, Garner CW, Baker HN, et al. Effect of the human apolipoproteins and phosphatidylcholine acyl donor on the activity of 1ecithin: cholesterol acyltransferase. Biochemistry. 1975;14:3057-64.
12. Havel RJ, Shore VG, Shore B, et al. Role of specific glycopeptides of human serum lipoproteins in the activation of lipoprotein lipase. Circ Res. 1970;27:595-600.
13. LaRosa JC, Levy RI, Herbert P, et al. A specific apoprotein activator for lipoprotein lipase. Biochem. Biophys Res Commun. 1970;41:57-62.
14. Utermann G, Jjaeschke M, Menzel J. Familial hyperlipoproteinemia type III: deficiency of a specific apolipoprotein (Apo E-III) in the very low density lipoproteins. FEBS Lett. 1975;56:352-5.
15. Rall SC Jr, Weisgraber KH, Innerarity TL, et al. Structural basis for receptor binding heterogeneity of apolipoprotein E from type III hyperlipoproteinemic subjects .Proc Natl Acad Sci USA. 1982;79:4696-4700.
16. Sherrill BC, Innerarity TL, Mahley RW. Steps of lipid metabolism. J Biol Chem. 1980;255:1804-07.

17. Pischon T, Cynthia J. Girman CJ, et al. Non high-density lipoprotein cholesterol and apolipoprotein B in the prediction of coronary heart disease in men. Circulation. 2005;112:3375-83.
18. Sigurdsson G, Baldursdottir A, Sigvaldason H, et al. Predictive value of apolipoproteins in a prospective survey of coronary artery disease in men. Am J Cardiol. 1992;69:1251-4.
19. Powell LM, Wallis SC, Pease RJ, et al. A novel form of tissue-specific RNA processing produces apolipoprotein-B48 in intestine. Cell. 1987;50(6):831-40.
20. Chen S-H, Habib G, Yang C-Y, et al. Apolipoprotein B-48 is the product of a messenger RNA with an organ-specific in-frame stop codon. Science. 1987;238:363-6.
21. Wang C, McConathy WJ, Kloer HU, et al. Modulation of lipoprotein lipase activity by apolipoproteins. J Clin Invest. 1985;75:384-90.
22. Ito Y, Azrolan N, O'Connell A, Walsh A, Breslow JL. Hypertriglyceridemia as a result of human apo CIII gene expression in transgenic mice. Science. 1990;249:790-93.
23. Aalto-Setälä K, Fisher EA, Chen X, et al. Mechanism of hypertriglyceridemia in human apolipoprotein (apo) CIII transgenic mice: diminished very low density lipoprotein fractional catabolic rate associated with increased apo CIII and reduced apo E on the particles. J Clin Invest. 1992;90:1889-1900.
24. O'Brien PJ, Alborn WE, Sloan HJ, et al. The novel apolipoprotein A5 is present in human serum, is associated with VLDL, HDL, and chylomicrons, and circulates at very low concentrations compared with other apolipoproteins. Clin Chem. 2005;51:351-9.
25. Pennacchio LA, Olivier M, Hubacek JA, et al. An apolipoprotein influencing triglycerides in humans and mice revealed by comparative sequencing. Science. 2001;294:169-73.
26. Bruns GA, Karanthasis SK, Breslow JL. Human apolipoprotein AI-CIII gene complex is located on chromosome 11. Arteriosclerosis. 1984;4:97-102.
27. Ordovas JM, Civeira F, Genest J Jr, et al. Restriction fragment length polymorphisms of the apolipoprotein A-I, CIII,A-IV gene locus. Relationships with lipids, apolipoproteins, and premature coronary artery disease. Atherosclerosis. 1991;87:75-86.
28. Jacobson TA. Opening a new lipid "Apo-thecary": incorporating apolipoproteins as potential risk factors and treatment targets to reduce cardiovascular risk. Mayo Clin Proc. 2011;86(8):762-80.
29. Marcovina SM, Albers JJ, Kennedy H, et al. International Federation of Clinical Chemistry standardization project for measurements of apolipoproteins A-I and B, IV: comparability of apolipoprotein B values by use of International Reference Material. Clin Chem. 1994;40:586-92.
30. Jungner I, Marcovina SM, Walldius G, et al. Apolipoprotein B and A-I values in 147576 Swedish males and females, standardized according to the World Health Organization-International Federation of Clinical Chemistry First International Reference Materials. Clin Chem. 1998;44(8, pt 1):1641-9.
31. Lamarche B, Moorjani S, Lupien PJ, et al. Apolipoprotein A-I and B levels and the risk of ischemic heart disease during a five-year follow-up of men in the Quebec Cardiovascular Study. Circulation. 1996;94:273-8.
32. Walldius G, Jungner I, Holme I, et al. High apolipoprotein B, low apolipoprotein A-I, and improvement in the prediction of fatal myocardial infarction (AMORIS study): a prospective study. Lancet. 2001;358:2026-33.
33. Sniderman AD, Scantlebury T, Cianflone K. Hypertriglyceridemic hyperapoB: the unappreciated atherogenic dyslipoproteinemia in type 2 diabetes mellitus. Ann Intern Med. 2001;135:447-59.
34. Russell DW. Cholesterol biosynthesis and metabolism. Cardiovasc Drugs Ther. 1992;6:103-10.
35. Hill SA, McQueen MJ. Reverse cholesterol transport—a review of the process and its clinical implications. Clin Biochem. 1997;30:517-25.
36. Scriver CR, Beaudet AL, Sly WS, et al. Lipoprotein(a). In: Scriver CR, Beaudet AL, Sly WS, Valle D (Eds). The Metabolic and Molecular Bases of Inherited Disease, 8th edition. New York: McGraw-Hill; 2001. pp. 2753-87.
37. Erqou S, Kaptoge S, Perry PL, et al. Lipoprotein(a) concentration and the risk of coronary heart disease, stroke, and nonvascular mortality. JAMA. 2009;302:412-23.
38. Rader DJ, Cain W, Ikewaki K, et al. The inverse association of plasma lipoprotein(a) concentrations with apolipoprotein(a) isoform size is not due to differences in Lp(a) catabolism but to differences in production rate. J Clin Invest. 1994;93:2758-63.
39. Koschinsky ML, Marcovina SM. Structure-function relationships in apolipoprotein(a): insights into lipoprotein(a) assembly and pathogenicity. Curr Opin Lipidol. 2004;15:167-74.
40. Marcovina SM, Koschinsky ML, Albers JJ, et al. Report of the National Heart, Lung, and Blood Institute Workshop on Lipoprotein(a) and Cardiovascular Disease: recent advances and future directions. Clin Chem. 2003;49:1785-96.
41. Ballantyne C, Koschinsky M, Marcovina SM. Lipoprotein(a). In: Ballantyne C (Ed). Clinical Lipidology: A Companion to Braunwauld's Heart Disease. Philadelphia: Saunders Elsevier; 2009. pp. 130-43.
42. Nielsen LB. Atherogenecity of lipoprotein(a) and oxidized low density lipoprotein: insight from in vivo studies of arterial wall influx, degradation and efflux. Atherosclerosis. 1999;143:229-43.

43. Lundstam U, Hurt-Camejo E, Olsson G, et al. Proteoglycans contribution to association of Lp(a) and LDL with smooth muscle cell extracellular matrix. Arterioscler Thromb Vasc Biol. 1999;19:1162-7.
44. Bdeir K, Cane W, Canziani G, et al. Defensin promotes the binding of lipoprotein(a) to vascular matrix. Blood. 1999;94:2007-19.
45. Sotiriou SN, Orlova VV, Al-Fakhri N, et al. Lipoprotein(a) in atherosclerotic plaques recruits inflammatory cells through interaction with Mac-1 integrin. FASEB J. 2006;20:559-61.
46. Tsimikas S, Brilakis ES, Miller ER, et al. Oxidized phospholipids, Lp(a) lipoprotein, and coronary artery disease. N Engl J Med. 2005;353:46-57.
47. Tsimikas S, Tsironis LD, Tselepis AD. New insights into the role of lipoprotein(a)-associated lipoprotein-associated phospholipase A2 in atherosclerosis and cardiovascular disease. Arterioscler Thromb Vasc Biol. 2007;27:2094-9.
48. Rouy D, Grailhe P, Nigon F, et al. Lipoprotein(a) impairs generation of plasmin by fibrin-bound tissue-type plasminogen activator. In vitro studies in a plasma milieu. Arterioscler Thromb. 1991;11:629-38.
49. Feric NT, Boffa MB, Johnston SM, et al. Apolipoprotein(a) inhibits the conversion of Glu-plasminogen to Lys-plasminogen: a novel mechanism for lipoprotein(a)-mediated inhibition of plasminogen activation. J Thromb Haemost. 2008;6:2113-20.
50. Pan S, Kleppe LS, Witt TA, et al. The effect of vascular smooth muscle cell-targeted expression of tissue factor pathway inhibitor in a murine model of arterial thrombosis. Thromb Haemost. 2004;92:495-502.
51. Hervio L, Chapman MJ, Thillet J, et al. Does apolipoprotein(a) heterogeneity influence lipoprotein(a) effects on fibrinolysis? Blood. 1993;82:392-7.
52. Erqou S, Thompson A, Di AE, et al. Apolipoprotein(a) isoforms and the risk of vascular disease: systematic review of 40 studies involving 58,000 participants. J Am Coll Cardiol. 2010;55:2160-67.
53. Kronenberg F, Kronenberg MF, Kiechl S, et al. Role of lipoprotein(a) and apolipoprotein(a) phenotype in atherogenesis: prospective results from the Bruneck study. Circulation. 1999;100:1154-60.
54. Nordestgaard BG, Chapman MJ, Ray K, et al. Lipoprotein(a) as a cardiovascular risk factor: current status. Euro Heart J. 2010; 31:2844-53.
55. Luthra K, Misra A, Srivastava LM. Lipoprotein(a): biology and role in atherosclerotic vascular disease. Curr Sci. 1999;76:1553-60.
56. Rhoads GG, Dahlen G, Berg K, et al. Lipoprotein(a) as a risk factor for myocardial infarction. J Am Med Assoc. 1986;256:2540-44.
57. Dahlen G. Lipoprotein(a) in cardiovascular disease: review article and viewpoint. Atherosclerosis. 1994;108:111-26.
58. Lamarche B, Lemieux I, Despres JP. The small, dense LDL phenotype and the risk of coronary heart disease: epidemiology, pathophysiology and therapeutic aspects. Diabetes Metab. 1999;25:199-211.
59. Soedamah-Muthu SS, Chang YF, Otvos J, et al. Lipoprotein subclass measurements by nuclear magnetic resonance spectroscopy improve the prediction of coronary artery disease in type 1 diabetes: a prospective report from the Pittsburgh Epidemiology of Diabetes Complications Study. Diabetologia. 2003;46:674-82.
60. Garvey WT, Kwon S, Zheng D, et al. Effects of insulin resistance and type 2 diabetes on lipoprotein subclass particle size and concentration determined by nuclear magnetic resonance. Diabetes. 2003;52:453-62.
61. ChapmanMJ, Ginsberg HN, Amarenco P, et al. (for the European Atherosclerosis Society Consensus Panel). Triglyceride-rich lipoproteins and high-density lipoprotein cholesterol in patients at high risk of cardiovascular disease: evidence and guidance for management. Euro Heart J; doi:10.1093/eurheartj/ehr112 [European Heart Journal Advance Access published April 29, 2011]
62. Ginsberg HN. New perspectives on atherogenesis: role of abnormal triglyceride-rich lipoprotein metabolism. Circulation. 2002;106:2137-42.
63. Twickler TB, Dallinga-Thie GM, Cohn JS, Chapman MJ. Elevated remnant-like particle cholesterol concentration: a characteristic feature of the atherogenic lipoprotein phenotype. Circulation. 2004;109:1918-25.
64. Rye KA, Bursill CA, Lambert G, et al. The metabolism and antiatherogenic properties of HDL. J Lipid Res. 2009;50(suppl):S195-S200.
65. Havel RJ. Triglyceride-rich lipoproteins and plasma lipid transport. Arterioscler Thromb Vasc Biol. 2010;30:9-19.
66. Cuchel M, Rader DJ. Macrophage reverse cholesterol transport: key to the regression of atherosclerosis? Circulation. 2006;113:2548-55.
67. Khera AV, Cuchel M, Llera-Moya MDL, et al. Cholesterol efflux capacity, high-density lipoprotein function, and atherosclerosis. N Engl J Med. 2011;364:127-35.
68. Lassel TS, Guerin M, Auboiron S, et al. Evidence for a cholesteryl ester donor activity of LDL particles during alimentary lipemia in normolipidemic subjects. Atherosclerosis. 1999;147:41-8.
69. Connelly PW. The role of hepatic lipase in lipoprotein metabolism. Clin Chim Acta. 1999;286:243-55.
70. Barter P. Managing diabetic dyslipidaemia—beyond LDL-C: HDL-C and triglycerides. Atheroscler Suppl. 2006; 7(4):17-21.

71. Genest J, Libby P, Gotto AM Jr. Lipoprotein disorders and cardiovascular disease. In: Zipes DP, Libby P, Bonow RO, Braunwald E (Eds). Braunwald's Heart Disease: A Textbook of Cardiovascular Medicine, 7th edition. Philadelphia, PA: Elsevier Saunders; 2005. pp. 1013-34.
72. Barter PJ, Ballantyne CM, Carmena R, et al. Apo B versus cholesterol in estimating cardiovascular risk and in guiding therapy: report of the thirty-person/ten-country panel. J Intern Med. 2006;259(3):247-58.
73. Steinberg D. Atherogenesis in perspective: hypercholesterolemia and inflammation as partners in crime. Nat Med. 2002;8:1211-7.
74. Libby P. Act local, act global: inflammation and the multiplicity of "vulnerable" coronary plaques. J Am Coll Cardiol. 2005;45:1600-02.
75. Fraley AE, Tsimikas S. Clinical applications of circulating oxidized low-density lipoprotein biomarkers in cardiovascular disease. Curr Opin Lipidol. 2006;17:502-9.
76. Tsimikas S, Glass C, Steinberg D, et al. Lipoproteins, lipoprotein oxidation and atherogenesis. In: Chien KR (Ed). Molecular Basis of Cardiovascular Disease: A Companion to Braunwald's Heart Disease. Philadelphia: W.B. Saunders Company; 2004. pp. 385-413.
77. Navab M, Ananthramaiah GM, Reddy ST, et al. The oxidation hypothesis of atherogenesis: the role of oxidized phospholipids and HDL. J Lipid Res. 2004;45:993-1007.
78. Nishi K, Itabe H, Uno M, et al. Oxidized LDL in carotid plaques and plasma associates with plaque instability. Arterioscler Thromb Vasc Biol. 2002;22:1649-54.
79. Holvoet P, Harris TB, Tracy RP, et al. Association of high coronary heart disease risk status with circulating oxidized LDL in the well functioning elderly: findings from the health, aging, and body composition study. Arterioscler Thromb Vasc Biol. 2003;23:1444-8.
80. Tanaga K, Bujo H, Inoue M, et al. Increased circulating malondialdehyde modified LDL levels in patients with coronary artery diseases and their association with peak sizes of LDL particles. Arterioscler Thromb Vasc Biol. 2002;22:662-6.
81. Holvoet P, Kritchevsky SB, Tracy RP, et al. The metabolic syndrome, circulating oxidized LDL, and risk of myocardial infarction in well functioning elderly people in the health, aging, and body composition cohort. Diabetes. 2004;53:1068-73.
82. Rodenburg J, Vissers MN, Wiegman A, et al. Oxidized low-density lipoprotein in children with familial hypercholesterolemia and unaffected siblings: effect of pravastatin. J Am Coll Cardiol. 2006;47:1803-10.
83. Tsimikas S, Kiechl S, Willeit J, et al. Oxidized phospholipids predict the presence and progression of carotid and femoral atherosclerosis and symptomatic cardiovascular disease: five-year prospective results from the Bruneck Study. J Am Coll Cardiol. 2006;47:2219-28.
84. Brunzell JD, Davidson M, Furberg CD, et al. Lipoprotein management in patients with cardiometabolic risk: consensus statement from the American Diabetes Association and the American College of Cardiology Foundation. Diabetes Care. 2008;31(4):811-22.
85. Genest J, McPherson R, Frohlich J, et al. Canadian Cardiovascular Society/Canadian guidelines for the diagnosis and treatment of dyslipidemia and prevention of cardiovascular disease in the adult—2009 recommendations. Can J Cardiol. 2009;25(10):567-79.
86. NHANES Investigators. National Health and Nutrition Examination Survey (NHANES) 2005–2006 documentation, codebook, and frequencies triglyceride, LDL-cholesterol and Apolipoprotein (ApoB) (TRIGLY_D). Available from: http://www.cdc.gov/nchs/nhanes/nhanes2005-2006/TRIGLY_D.htm#Component_Description. [Accessed May 5, 2011].
87. Fodor G, Frohlich J, Genest J Jr, et al., for the Working Group on Hypercholesterolemia and Other Dyslipidemias. Recommendations for the management and treatment of dyslipidemia. Can Med Assoc J. 2000;162(10):1441-7.
88. National Cholesterol Education Program. Third Report of the Expert Panel on Detection, Evaluation, and Treatment of High Blood Cholesterol in Adults (Adult Treatment Panel III). Bethesda, MD: National Heart, Lung and Blood Institute; 2001.
89. Kingsbury KJ, Bondy G. Understanding the Essentials of Blood Lipid Metabolism. p. 7. Available from http://www.medscape.com/viewarticle/451762_5.
90. Alonso R, Andres E, Mata N, et al. Lipoprotein(a) levels in familial hypercholesterolemia: an important predictor of cardiovascular disease independent of the type of LDL receptor mutation. J Am Coll Cardiol. 2014;63(19):1982-9.

CHAPTER 4

Pathogenesis of Atherosclerosis

Sekhar Chakravarty

- Introduction
- Hemodynamic stress and hypertension
- Hyperlipidemia
- Role of inflammation
- Role of infection
- Role of growth factors
- Summary

INTRODUCTION

The prevalence of mortality and morbidity due to clinical effect of atherosclerosis is significantly high across the globe. This has prompted researchers to put their efforts on unveiling the exact mechanism underlying the process. Although significant progress has been made so far, we are yet to know exactly how it occurs. The theories of atherogenesis have evolved with time. In 19th century, Virchow proposed that atheroma was a response to hemodynamic injury leading to increased uptake of lipid from circulating blood. This was known as "lipid insudation theory." In the same century, another scientist, Rokitansky, suggested organization of a mural thrombus to be the initial event to form an atheromatous plaque. This theory was then known as "thrombogenic theory". Benditt and Benditt in 1973 considered proliferation of the intimal smooth muscle cells (SMC) to be the key feature of atherogenesis. They went on to postulate that atherosclerotic plaque was essentially a neoplastic process, by establishing "monoclonality" of the proliferating SMC present in the plaque.[1] Later, Ross and Glomset postulated that all the features of an atheromatous plaque could be explained by endothelial cell injury and it was subsequently known as "Response to injury theory."[2]

The present-day view about atherogenesis is basically a modification and further refinement of the response to injury theory. It is now considered that atherosclerosis is a chronic inflammatory and repair process of the arterial wall, which occurs in response to injury of the vascular endothelium due to a wide spectrum of atherogenic agents of diverse nature.[3]

Injury to the vascular endothelium is the initial and single most important event in the process of atherogenesis. Endothelial cell dysfunction in absence of morphological evidence of endothelial cell injury is sufficient to initiate the process. The factors responsible and their exact mechanism of causing such endothelial cell dysfunction are not fully understood. But a wide range of factors, such as hemodynamic stress due to turbulence in the flow of blood, persistent hyperlipidemia, homocystenemia, cigarette smoking, mediators of inflammation and even certain infections can cause endothelial cell dysfunction. However, hemodynamic stress and persistent hyperlipidemia remain the two most notable causes among all.

HEMODYNAMIC STRESS AND HYPERTENSION

The atheromatous lesions tend to occur in certain anatomical sites such as bifurcation point of arteries, ostia of pulsating arteries and posterior wall of aorta. There is usually turbulence in the flow of blood at these sites, which becomes more pronounced in hypertension. This leads to hemodynamic stress causing injury and/or dysfunction of the intimal endothelial cells. In experimental animals, it has been shown that local antiatherogenic products are produced less in the turbulent areas. Superoxide dismutase is one such endothelial antiatherogenic substance that is found to be less in the areas of atheromatous plaque.[4] Nonturbulent blood flow also augments production of nitric oxide that, in addition to its vasodilator action, acts as an anti-inflammatory agent, which suppresses expression of adhesion molecules. These evidences illustrate the importance of hemodynamic stress in the cellular events of atherosclerosis.

HYPERLIPIDEMIA

Hyperlipidemia is considered the single most important risk factor for atherosclerosis. This has been supported by many epidemiological, experimental and clinical studies. Epidemiological evidences show significant correlation between plasma cholesterol and low-density lipids (LDL) level with severity of atherosclerosis. Lowering plasma cholesterol by drug or by diet restriction reduces risk of cardiovascular disease and also slows down the progression of atherosclerosis. The fibro-fatty atheromatous plaques are chiefly composed of cholesterol and esters of cholesterol. Diabetes mellitus, which is frequently associated with hyperlipidemia, promotes atherosclerosis at an early age. In experimental animals, artificially produced deficiencies of LDL receptors or Apolipoproteins cause accelerated atherosclerosis.[6]

Mechanism

Long-standing hyperlipidemia can contribute to atherogenesis in the following ways:

1. Hyperlipidemia may cause increased production of oxygen-free radicals, which in turn can cause direct injury to the vascular endothelium and accelerate nitric oxide decay, thereby reducing its vasodilator activity.
2. In prolonged hyperlipidemia, lipoproteins, particularly LDL is accumulated in the intima. The accumulated LDL is oxidized by the oxygen-free radicals generated locally. The oxidized LDL is then taken up by the macrophages. The ingestion of LDL is facilitated by the presence of a scavenger receptor over the surface of macrophages.[5] Lipid, in course of time, is released from the foam cell and becomes extracellular. This extracellular lipid starts accumulating in the intima. In addition, oxidized LDL is directly cytotoxic to the endothelial cell and can cause endothelial cell dysfunction.[6] Finally, oxidized LDL can also stimulate endothelial cells and macrophages to release a wide spectrum of cytokines, including growth factors.[7]

ROLE OF INFLAMMATION

Dysfunctional endothelial cells express adhesion molecules such as vascular cell adhesion molecule 1 (VCAM-I). These molecules promote adhesion of inflammatory cells particularly monocytes and T lymphocytes to the intimal surface.[8] After adhesion, these cells migrate into the intima under the influence of locally produced chemokines. The monocytes are transformed into macrophages that engulf oxidized LDL to form foam cells as discussed earlier. Oxidized LDL in turn stimulates macrophages and tumor necrosis factor production, which further increases leukocyte adhesion and recruitment of additional mononuclear cells. Activated macrophages produce more reactive oxygen species, leading to augmented LDL oxidization. They also elaborate growth factors that stimulate smooth muscle proliferation.

There is also recruitment of T lymphocytes in the intima. The activated T cells also elaborate gamma interferon and other inflammatory cytokines. They in turn stimulate macrophages, endothelial cells and SMCs. But it is not clear how the T cells accumulate over the intima. Possible mechanisms include response to some kind of antigen-like bacteria, virus, heat-shock protein (HSP) or nonspecific accumulation by inflammation process.[9]

ROLE OF INFECTION

In recent years, fascinating evidences have been accumulating, which contribute infection as the triggering event in atherogenesis. Different organisms such as *Chlamydia, pneumococcus*, cytomegalovirus and herpes virus have been demonstrated in the atheromatous plaques but not in normal intima.[10] Higher level of *Chlamydia pneumoniae* antibody has also been found in the blood of persons suffering from atherosclerosis in comparison to their normal counterparts and the level of antibody correlated with the degree of atherosclerosis.[7]

One possible hypothesis is that the immune response mounted against the organisms may cross-react with the host proteins in the form of molecular mimicry. One such group of protein is HSP, which is expressed by the cells of atheromatous plaque as well as secreted by various organisms such as *Chlamydia* and *Helicobacter pylori*. Further, purified anti-HSP antibody can recognize and cause lysis of the dysfunctional human endothelial cells and macrophages in vitro. There has been exacerbation of atherosclerosis in animals immunized with anti-HSP antibody.[11]

ROLE OF GROWTH FACTORS

One of the major features of atherosclerosis is proliferation of intimal SMCs and deposition of new extracellular matrix (ECM), leading to focal thickening of intima. These changes are believed to occur due to liberation of various growth factors, such as platelet-derived growth factor, fibroblast growth factor and transforming growth factor beta. In the early stages of atherosclerosis, there is upregulation of expression of growth factors and their receptors over the endothelial surface, while they are expressed at very low level normally. The growth factors are derived from vascular endothelial cells, SMCs as well as cells like T lymphocytes, macrophages and platelets that infiltrate the intima in atherosclerosis.[12]

SUMMARY

To summarize, the sequence of events in the evolution of atherogenesis may be as follows.

Fatty streaks are earliest lesions. In the presence of hyperlipidemia, hypertension and other atherogenic agents as discussed above, there is vascular endothelial cell dysfunction leading to insudation of lipid in the endothelium. Simultaneously, there is egress of blood monocyte and lymphocyte into the intima through overexpression of various adhesion factors brought about by different agents. The blood monocytes are converted to tissue macrophages in the intima.

The lipid entered inside the intima undergoes oxidation and the oxidized lipid is engulfed by the macrophages via scavenger receptor to form foam cell. Apoptosis of foam cell liberates lipid into the ECM. Liberation of various cytokines by endothelial cells, macrophages and lymphocytes stimulates subendothelial SMCs to migrate into the intima. On stimulation by the chemical mediators, the SMCs undergo proliferation and start synthesizing ECM. Thus, through interaction of various risk factors acting upon the vascular endothelium, a fibro-fatty atheromatous plaque is formed at some preferential site. The plaque thus formed has a fibrous cap retaining a central core of lipid-laden cells and fat debris. Over a period of time, the intimal plaque encroaches on vascular lumen and causes degeneration of the underlying media. Central fatty core may subsequently be calcified and the disruption of the fibrous cap can predispose to thrombus formation and acute vascular occlusion.

REFERENCES

1. Benditt EP, Benditt JM. Evidence for a monoclonal origin of human atherocletrotic plaques. Proc. Nat Acad Sci. 1973;70:1753-6.
2. Ross R, Glomset J, Harker L. Response to injury and atherogenesis. Am J Pathol. 1977;86(3):675-84.
3. Ross R. Atherosclerosis: an inflammatory disease. N Engl J Med. 1999;940:115-27.
4. Ross R. The pathogenesis of atherosclerosis: an update. N Engl J Med. 1986;314:488-500.
5. Steinbrecher UP, Lougheed M, Kwan DM. Recognition of oxidized low-density lipoprotein by the scavenger receptor of macrophages results from derivatization of apolipoprotein B by products of fatty acid peroxidation. J Biol Chem. 1989;264:15216-23.
6. Hessler JR, Robertson AL, Chisholm G. LDL-induced cytotoxicity and its inhibition by HDL in human vascular smooth muscle and endothelial cells in culture. Atherosclerosis. 1979;32:213-29.
7. Frostegard J, Ulfgren AK, Nyberg P et al. Cytokine expression in advanced human atherosclerotic plaques: dominance of pro-inflammatory (Th1) and macrophage-stimulating cytokines. Atherosclerosis. 1999;145:33-43.
8. Lindner V, Lappi DA, Baird A, et al. Role of basic fibroblast growth factor in vascular lesion formation. Circ Res. 1991;68:106-13.
9. Chui B. Multiple infections in carotid atherosclerotic plaque. Am Heart J. 1999;138(5):8534.
10. Libby F, Hanssen GK. Involvement of immune system in human atherogenesis: Current knowledge and unanswered questions. Lab Inves. 1991;64(1):5.
11. Gupta S et al. Elevated Chlamydia pneumoniae antibodies, cardiovascular events and azithromycin in male survivors of myocardial infarction. Circulation. 1997;96:404-07.
12. Raines EW, Ross R. Biology of atherosclerotic plaque formation: possible role of growth factors in lesion development and the potential impact of soy. J Nutr. 1995;125:624S-630S.

HDL Metabolism, Mutation and Targeting

Aijaz H. Mansoor and Tapan Ghose

- Introduction
- Classification of HDLs
- Biochemical impact of HDL on atherosclerosis
- Clinical impact of HDL on atherosclerosis
- HDL mutation
- HDL targeting
- Small molecule cholesteryl ester transfer protein inhibitors
- Conclusion

INTRODUCTION

Human serum lipoproteins are soluble complexes of proteins (apolipoproteins) and lipids. High-density lipoprotein (HDL) is the smallest and densest of plasma lipoproteins (Fig. 5.1). High-density lipoprotein isolated by ultracentrifugation is defined as the lipoprotein with density in the range 1.063–1.21 g/mL. The HDLs in human plasma are heterogeneous in terms of particle density, size, shape, surface charge and composition.[1] The functions of the different HDL subpopulations remain largely unknown. High-density lipoprotein particles are either spherical or discoidal.[2] Most of the particles are spherical and consist of a fatty core [mainly cholesteryl esters (CEs) with a small amount of triglyceride] surrounded by an outer layer of phospholipids, free (nonesterified) cholesterol and apolipoproteins. Discoidal HDL particles are in minority and are a nascent form of HDLs that usually exist only for a limited period in the circulation before being rapidly converted into the spherical form.

CLASSIFICATION OF HIGH-DENSITY LIPOPROTEINS

High-density lipoproteins are classified[3] based on size, charge, apolipoprotein composition and separation by hydrated density. Density gradient ultracentrifugation separates HDL into large spherical HDL2, small, dense, spherical HDL3 and very HDL. Gradient gel electrophoresis separates HDL into HDL2a, HDL2b, HDL3a, HDL3b and HDL3c. Two-dimensional gel electrophoresis separates HDL particles into the lipid-poor pre-b1, pre-b2, mature CE-containing a-HDL (a1–a4) and pre-b2 lipoproteins. Based on the apolipoprotein composition, HDL particles include two major particles, lipoprotein (Lp) A-I (which is lipid-free HDL

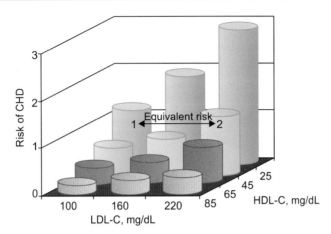

Figure 5.1: Structure of high-density lipoprotein

and represents 70% of total HDL protein) and LpA-II (about 20% of the total) and two minor lipoprotein particles, LpE and LpE:A-I. The concentration of ApoA-II in normal individuals is approximately 1.0 g/L, making it one of the most abundant proteins in human plasma. Virtually all of the ApoA-II resides in A-I/A-II HDLs in most people, whereas ApoA-I is distributed equally between A-I HDLs and A-I/A-II HDLs. A small proportion of the ApoA-I exists in a lipid-free or lipid-poor form. Some HDL particles also contain other minor apolipoproteins such as ApoA-IV, ApoA-V, ApoC-I, ApoC-II, ApoC-III, ApoD, ApoJ and ApoL. High-density lipoproteins also transport several additional proteins, including paraoxonase, cholesteryl ester transfer protein (CETP), lecithin:cholesterol acyltransferase (LCAT) and phospholipid transfer protein.

BIOCHEMICAL IMPACT OF HIGH-DENSITY LIPOPROTEINON ATHEROSCLEROSIS

For excess cholesterol entering the circulation, the liver is the major route of elimination. The transfer of cholesterol to the liver from peripheral tissues is termed reverse cholesterol transport (RCT) and, in a state of homeostasis, it balances that, which enters the circulation and is not consumed peripherally (Fig. 5.2). It is now recognized that the cholesterol in HDL is derived directly from the liver, as well as being incorporated into it from periphery in the course of RCT: a significant proportion of cholesterol entering the circulation from hepatocytes does so, not in very LDL, but directly through a transporter channel, the adenosine triphosphate (ATP)-binding cassette A1 (ABCA1), and, once in the circulation, it is taken up by small newly secreted HDL particles.[4] This is a major source of high-density lipoprotein-cholesterol (HDL-C). In analphalipoproteinemia (Tangier disease), for example, in which ABCA1 is mutated, HDL-C levels are virtually nonexistent because the small newly secreted HDL particles cannot receive sufficient cholesterol to grow to the point where they are large enough to avoid filtration through the glomerulus and subsequent catabolism by the renal tubular cells.[5] Pre-beta-HDL can stimulate the hydrolysis of intracellular CEs in peripheral tissues and the passage of free cholesterol, thus liberated, across the cell membrane where it can be incorporated into the surface of HDL molecules.[6,7] The free cholesterol is then re-esterified by LCAT, an enzyme present on HDL. The

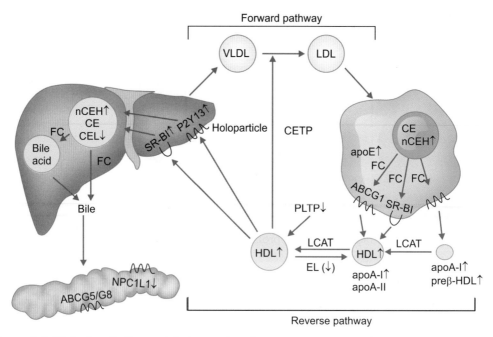

Figure 5.2: High-density lipoprotein forward and reverse transport pathway

intensely hydrophobic CE thus produced is then packed into the core of the HDL away from the surface aqueous interface. Once incorporated into HDL particles, CE can also undoubtedly be off-loaded to hepatocytes as the particles pass along the hepatic sinusoids through, for example, the scavenger receptor-B1, thus completing RCT. Two inherited disorders that virtually eliminate HDL, analphalipoproteinemia and LCAT deficiency, are not associated with any marked tendency to atherosclerosis.[8] Arguing that pathways other than the simple uptake of CE directly from HDL by the liver can also perform RCT. Several explanations have been ascribed for the beneficial effects of HDL-C on atherogenesis, particularly its role on RCT.[9] This process involves the transport of excessive cholesterol from foam macrophages in the arterial wall to HDL-C particles and onto the feces via the liver and bile. The large HDL2 particles promote cholesterol transport through the ATP cassette-binding transporter ABCG1 pathway, whereas the smaller HDL3 particles more efficiently enhance cholesterol efflux through the ABCA1 pathway.[7] In addition to their ability to reverse transport cholesterol from peripheral tissues back to the liver, HDLs display pleiotropic effects (Table 5.1), including antioxidant, antiapoptotic, anti-inflammatory, anti-infectious and antithrombotic properties that account for their protective action on endothelial cells. Vasodilatation via production of nitric oxide is also a hallmark of HDL action on those cells.[10]

CLINICAL IMPACT OF HIGH-DENSITY LIPOPROTEINMANIPULATION

High-density lipoprotein-cholesterols (HDL-C) are regarded as important parameters in the risk stratification by Framingham Risk Score. The normal HDL level is ≥ 40 mg/dL. High-density lipoprotein less than 40 mg/dL is regarded as low and HDL-C ≥ 60 mg is

Table 5.1: Important protective properties of high-density lipoprotein

Promotion of cholesterol efflux from macrophages in artery wall

Inhibition of oxidation

Inhibition of vascular inflammation

Binding of lipopolysaccharide

Promotion of endothelial repair

Stimulation of NO production by endothelium

Inhibition of synthesis of platelet-activating factor by endothelial cells

Promotion of angiogenesis

regarded as high; Low HDL is a major risk factor and high HDL ≥ 60 mg is considered as a negative risk factor and removes one risk factor form the total count. Intensive LDL lowering with statins (even in the presence of significant atherosclerosis) reduces the risk of major atherosclerotic cardiovascular events by approximately 40–50%.[3,11] This means that 50–60% of risk remains, and this is referred to as residual risk. Strategies to reduce this residual risk include increasing HDL-C levels because increased HDL-C is associated with favorable outcomes in atherosclerotic cardiovascular disease,12,13 and HDL-C is reported to be the strongest predictor of coronary heart disease (CHD) risk reduction in a review of 17 prospective, randomized lipid trials of >44,000 patients.[14] Every change of 10 mg/dL in the HDL-C level is associated with a 50% change in risk (based on the elderly cohort of the Framingham Heart Study).[15] For every 1 mg/dL increase in HDL-C, there is a 2% decrease in the risk of CHD in men and a 3% decrease in women, according to one meta-analysis.[16] The protective effect of HDL on atherosclerosis is suggested by the observation in humans that plasma HDL-C concentrations above 75 mg/dL (1.9 mmol/L) are associated with prolonged life (called the longevity syndrome) and relative freedom from CHD.[17] The Framingham Heart Study showed that, as HDL-C decreases, it contributes significantly to CHD risk at all levels of LDL-C (Fig. 5.3).[18] HDL-C is also a predictor of cardiovascular events at 5 years even when LDL-C is <70 mg/dL. An analysis of the Prospective Study of Pravastatin in the Elderly at Risk data indicated further that a specific subgroup received most of the benefit, that is, those with an HDL-C of <1.15 mmol/L (<45 mg/dL) or an LDL-C/HDL-C ratio >3.3.[19] In such individuals, the risk reduction for coronary events was 33% rather than the 19% seen in the whole cohort. Focusing on this subgroup reduces the number needed to treat to prevent 1 coronary event from 40 to 17. However, efforts to increase HDL-C with pharmacotherapy have not yet been shown to be associated with better outcomes, particularly in patients in whom significant risk reduction has already been achieved by lowering LDL levels with statin therapy.[20,21] The quest for HDL-increasing agents that have incremental, improved, cardiovascular outcomes is currently ongoing, and this is supported by post hoc analysis that suggests that HDL-C levels predict cardiovascular events in patients on statin therapy even when LDL-C levels are <70 mg/dL.[22] In the Third National Health and Nutrition Examination Survey, low HDL-C was reported in 35% of men (<40 mg/dL) and 39% of women (<50 mg/dL).[23] Therefore, the inverse relationship between HDL-C levels and atherosclerotic cardiovascular disease makes strategies to increase HDL a worthwhile investigative effort.

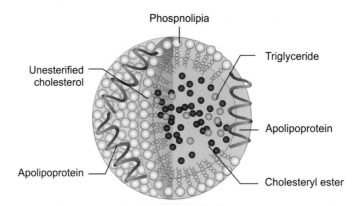

Figure 5.3: Low high-density lipoprotein-cholesterol is associated with increased coronary heart disease risk at all levels of low-density lipoprotein-cholesterol: based on data from The Framingham Study

Despite the substantial body of evidence of an inverse relationship between levels of HDL-C and cardiovascular risk presented above,24 low levels of HDL-C have not been established as causative of this relationship or with the development of atherosclerosis. The argument for lack of causality for low levels of HDL-C comes from Mendelian randomization analyses and the difficulty in demonstrating improved outcomes with therapies to raise HDL-C. The absence of premature CHD in individuals with rare disorders such as Tangier disease, who have very low levels of HDL-C but not the predicted increase cardiovascular disease, provides some further support for the lack of association. If HDL-C is found not to be causally associated with CHD, it is possible that other attributes of HDL could be causal. For instance, it is possible that some component of the HDL particle or one of its functions may protect against CHD events or atherosclerosis.[25,26]

HIGH-DENSITY LIPOPROTEIN MUTATIONS

Severe genetic abnormalities of HDL metabolism have been discovered in humans:

1. Dyslipidemia associated with low HDL level.
2. Dyslipidemia associated with high HDL level.

Dyslipidemia Associated with Low High-Density Lipoprotein

ApoA-I Variants

Discovery of ApoA-I Milano is an important milestone. This is a naturally occurring mutated variant (cysteine is substituted at position 173 for arginine) of ApoA-I discovered by Dr Cesare Sirtori in Milan. He reported that 3.5% of the population in a village (Limone Sul Garda) in Northern Italy carries this mutation. They had low HDL and high triglycerides, yet they were free of cardiovascular disease. A secondary prevention trial of ApoA-I Milano infusion in patients with acute coronary syndrome (ACS) had shown regression of human atherosclerosis. In total, 57 patients were randomized. Overall, 47 patients completed the protocol. Patients received 5 weekly infusions of placebo or phospholipids ApoA-I Milano complex (Apo-AI Milano) at 15 or 45 mg/kg. Intravascular ultrasound was performed within 2 weeks following ACS and after 5 weekly treatments. Mean percent atheroma volume decreased by 1.06% (+3.17%) in the active group (confidence interval = 1.53–0.34%, P = 0.02) compared with baseline. In the placebo arm, there were 0.14% increases (P = 0.97) in atheroma volume. Majority apo A-I variants are associated with decreased plasma HDL (hypoalphalipoproteinemia), hypertriglyceridemia, and/or defective LCAT (lecethin cholesterol acyl trensferase) activation. The first reported apo A-I variant associated with amyloidosis was apo A-II$_{IOWA}$ found in an Iowa kindred with British ancestry. Phenotypic expression was peripheral neuropathy, peptic ulcer disease, nephropathy, and death from renal failure.

ATP-Binding CassetteA1

Mutation in the ABCA1 transporter prevents synthesis of normal alpha HDL and cholesterol efflux. These individuals have Tangier disease characterized by orange tonsils, low LDL, low HDL and increased CVD risk.

Lecithin: Cholesterol Acyltransferase Deficiency

Cholesteryl ester transfer protein deficiency is an autosomal recessive disorder caused by the mutations of the LCAT gene located on chromosome 16q22. Lecithin:cholesterol acyltransferase reduction due to gene mutation results in partial or complete LCAT deficiency. This deficiency is characterized by cloudy corneas, low LDL, very high HDL, target cell hemolytic anemia and proteinuria with renal failure without risk of CVD. Partial LCAT deficiency is called fish eye disease because of appearance of the eye, which results from progressive corneal opacification.

Dyslipidemia Associated with High High-Density Lipoprotein

Cholesteryl Ester Transfer Protein Deficiency

Cholesteryl ester transfer protein deficiency phenotype is characterized by very high HDL, polydisperse LDL and normal triglycerides. High level of HDL is due to decreased catabolism of ApoA-I and ApoA-II. Further research is required to answer the question whether homozygotes with CETP deficiency have an increased risk of CVD.

Hepatic Lipase Deficiency

Complete deficiency of this enzyme is associated with increased levels of large HDL and decreased catabolism. Partial deficiency has normal HDL and normal HDL metabolism.

Familial Hyperalphalipoproteinemia

This phenotype has been reported to have very high HDL and ApoA-I levels and normal ApoA-II levels. This is associated with longevity. The cause of high HDL is due to higher synthesis of ApoA-I, ApoA-II production being normal.

HIGH-DENSITY LIPOPROTEIN TARGETING

Lifestyle and Dietary Approaches

Lifestyle changes associated with increased HDL are (i) quitting smoking, (ii) weight loss, (iii) increasing physical activity, (iv) regular aerobic exercise and (v) dietary changes.

Quitting smoking may increase HDL-C by up to 10%. Weight loss has a linear relationship with HDL level increment. For every 2.7 kg (6 lb) weight loss, HDL increases by 1mg/dL (0.03mmol/L). Regular physical exercises increase HDL concentration by 5%. At least 30minutes of brisk walking on most of the days of the week (>150 minutes per week) is associated with positive impact on HDL level. Familial Aggregation of Blood Lipid Response to Exercise Training in the Health, Risk Factors, Exercise Training, and Genetics (HERITAGE) study showed that exercise increased the HDL in particular in the individuals with low HDL, high triglyceride and abdominal obesity (metabolic syndrome). Duration of exercise is more important rather than the intensity brisk walking, running, cycling, swimming and playing basketball, which are the common form of isotonic physical exercises generally recommended. Exercise increases both HDL2 and HDL3 subfractions. Increased level of lipoprotein lipase activity associated with exercise is the mechanism of the HDL increment.

Dietary modification can increase HDL-C. Total dietary fat should not be >25–35% of the total calorie/day. Saturated fat should be <7%/day. Monounsaturated and polyunsaturated fats found in olive oil, peanut oil and canola oil increase HDL. Nuts and fish contain omega-3 fatty acids, which increase HDL-C.

Smoke dietary products and dietary supplements have a favorable impact on lipid level, including HDL-C. They are whole grains such as oat bran, oat meal and whole wheat products; nuts like walnut, almonds and Brazil nuts; plant sterols like beta sitosterol and sitostanol (found in margarine spread) and omega-3 fatty acids such as fatty fish, fish oil supplements, flaxseeds and flaxseed oil.

Moderate intake of alcohol increases HDL level. Up to one drink in women and two drinks in men are associated with favorable impact on HDL level. Alcohol should not be started to increase HDL levels. Recent subanalysis of INTERHERT study showed that alcohol may not protect Asians from the first acute myocardial infarction (MI).

Therapeutic Agents Raising High-Density Lipoprotein

Statins

Statins have been shown to increase HDL-C levels by about 5–10%, with the largest increases occurring usually in those with a low HDL-C and increased triglycerides.[27] Pretreatment HDL-C levels were the strongest predictor of statin-induced increase in HDL-C: the lower the pretreatment HDL-C level, the greater the increase in HDL-C after statin therapy.

Niacin

Niacin (or vitamin B3) was shown to reduce serum cholesterol levels[28] and, until recently, was considered promising for risk reduction because it increases HDL-C levels by as much as 15–35% in a dose-dependent manner, and also lowers LDL-C and triglycerides. A more recent study, the Atherothrombosis Intervention in Metabolic Syndrome with Low HDL/High Triglycerides: Impact on Global Health Outcomes trial, suggests that increasing HDL levels with niacin therapy may not have incremental outcome benefit to patients with baseline LDL-C levels below 70 mg/dL due to statin treatment.[29] This study was designed with 85% power to show a 25% reduction in the primary end point (a composite of the first event of death from CHD, hospitalization for an ACS, nonfatal MI, ischemic stroke or symptom-driven coronary or cerebral revascularization), with the addition of 1.5–2 g of niacin per day in patients > 45 years of age with known cardiovascular disease and dyslipidemia. Despite attaining desirable levels of HDL-C (an increase of 25%), LDL-C (a decrease of 12%) and triglycerides (a decrease of 29%) with niacin therapy, there was no reduction in the incidence of the primary composite end point, and it did not show any clinical benefit overall or in a major subgroup. The data and safety monitoring board stopped the clinical trial prematurely because the boundary for futility had been crossed, and an unexpectedly higher number of ischemic strokes were observed in patients assigned to niacin. These results do not support the addition of niacin to statin therapy in patients who have achieved LDL goals. In addition, the possible risk of increased risk of ischemic stroke with niacin and the flushing side effects of niacin make it particularly unattractive for routine risk reduction. However, niacin may have a role in statin-intolerant patients. Heart Protection Study2-Treatment of HDL to Reduce the Incidence of Vascular Events, a large clinical trial, evaluated the role of niacin and concluded that adding extended-release (ER) niacin/laropiprant to current standard treatment did not produce worthwhile reductions in the risk of heart attacks, strokes and bypass surgery. The study also found that using ER niacin/laropiprant did cause significant side effects.[30]

Cholesteryl Ester Transfer Protein

Human plasma contains a CETP that promotes the transfer of CEs from HDLs to other lipoprotein particles (including LDLs).[31] It follows that inhibition of CETP has the potential to retain cholesterol in the HDL fraction and thus increases the concentration of HDL-C while decreasing its concentration in potentially atherogenic, non-HDL particles. Cholesteryl ester transfer protein is a hydrophobic glycoprotein that is synthesized in several tissues but mainly in the liver.[32] It promotes bidirectional transfers of CEs and triglyceride between all plasma lipoprotein particles.[33]

Inhibition of CETP results in increased HDL-C levels (including ApoA-I levels) and some reductions in LDL-C levels (including ApoB levels). Agents belonging to this class include torcetrapib, dalcetrapib, anacetrapib and evacetrapib (Table 5.2).

Table 5.2: Cholesteryl ester transfer protein inhibitors

	Dalcetrapib	Torcetrapib	Anacetrapib	Evacetrapib
Chemical class	Benzenethiol	3,5-bis(CF_3) phenyl	3,5-bis(CF_3) phenyl	3,5-bis(CF_3) phenyl
Effect on CETP	Modulation (selective inhibition)	Complete inhibition	Complete inhibition	No data
Heterotypic CE transfer	Block	Block	Block	No data
Homotypic CE transfer	No effect	Block	Block	No data
RCT (fecal elimination of neutral sterols and bile acids)	Increase	Slight increase	No change	No data
Clinical stage	Phase III	Termination	Phase III	Phase II
Clinical data				
HDL increase	31%	72%	138%	132%

	Dalcetrapib	Torcetrapib	Anacetrapib	Evacetrapib
LDL decrease	No change	25%	36%	40%
Aldosterone levels	No change	Increase	No change	No change
Blood pressure	No change	Increase	No change	No change
Vascular inflammation	Reduction (PET/CT)	No data	No data	No data
Plaque progression	Reduction (MRI)	No data	No data	No data
Safety	Safe	Increased cardiovascular events and death	Safe	Safe

CF_3, trifluoromethyl; CETP, cholesteryl ester transfer protein; CE, cholesteryl ester; RCT, reverse cholesterol transport; HDL, high-density lipoprotein; LDL, low-density lipoprotein; PET, positron emission tomography; CT, computed tomography; MRI, magnetic resonance imaging.

SMALL MOLECULE CHOLESTERYL ESTER TRANSFER PROTEIN INHIBITORS

Torcetrapib

Torcetrapib development was halted after it was found to be associated with increased cardiovascular events, overall mortality, blood pressure, circulating aldosterone levels and altered serum electrolytes.[34] These adverse effects have been attributed to off-target effects on the renin–angiotensin–aldosterone axis unrelated to CETP inhibition.[35]

Dalcetrapib

Dal-OUTCOMES (ClinicalTrials.gov Identifier: NCT00658515) was a phase III, multicenter, randomized, double-blind, placebo-controlled clinical trial designed to test the hypothesis that CETP inhibition with dalcetrapib reduces cardiovascular morbidity and mortality in patients with recent ACS.[36] More than 15,000 patients, all of whom were treated with statins to achieve recommended levels of LDL-C, were randomized to receive dalcetrapib at a daily dose of 600 mg or matching placebo. The primary outcome was timed to first occurrence of a composite cardiovascular end point that included CHD death, nonfatal acute MI, unstable angina requiring hospital admission, resuscitated cardiac arrest or atherothrombotic stroke. The trial was initially planned to continue untill 1600 primary end point events have had occured with an anticipated reporting in 2013. However, it was announced in early May 2012 that the trial had been terminated on the basis of futility.

It is important to stress that the dal-OUTCOMES trial was not terminated on the basis of safety. As was found in the extensive phase II program with dalcetrapib, there was no evidence that dalcetrapib shared any of the off-target adverse effects observed with torcetrapib. The two most obvious explanations for the failure of dalcetrapib are that: (i) the increase in

HDL-C concentration induced by dalcetrapib is not accompanied by an enhancement of the protective functions of HDL or (ii) the inverse relationship between HDL-C concentration and cardiovascular risk observed in population studies is an epiphenomenon rather than being reflective of an ability of HDL to protect against cardiovascular disease.

Anacetrapib

The CETP inhibitors, anacetrapib and evacetrapib, not only more than double the level of HDL-C but also reduce the level of LDL-C by >30%.[37] This provides a powerful motivation for conducting cardiovascular clinical outcome trials with these agents. It has no effect on blood pressure, aldosterone or serum electrolytes in humans,[37] and does not stimulate the synthesis of aldosterone in adrenal cortical cells growing in tissue culture.[38] Furthermore, HDLs isolated from people taking anacetrapib have a normal or enhanced functionality.

Safety of Anacetrapib in Humans

The DEFINE study[37,39] was a randomized, double-blind, placebo-controlled 18-month trial designed to assess the lipid efficacy and safety profile of anacetrapib in patients (n = 1623) with manifest or at high risk of developing CHD. All participants were taking a statin to achieve optimal levels of LDL-C before being randomized to receive anacetrapib (100 mg/day) or matching placebo. By 24 weeks, the LDL-C level had been reduced from 81 to 45 mg/dL in the anacetrapib group, as compared with a reduction from 82 to 77 mg/dL in the placebo group, a 40% reduction with anacetrapib beyond that seen with placebo. The HDL-C level increased from 41 mg/dL at baseline to 101 mg/dL in the anacetrapib group, as compared with an increase from 40 to 46 mg/dL in the placebo group, an increase of 138% with anacetrapib beyond that seen with placebo. Treatment with anacetrapib had no effect on blood pressure or on electrolyte or aldosterone levels. Prespecified adjudicated cardiovascular events occurred in 16 patients treated with anacetrapib (2.0%) and 21 patients receiving placebo (2.6%, P = 0.40). The prespecified Bayesian analysis indicated that this event distribution provided a predictive probability of 94% that anacetrapib would not be associated with the increase in cardiovascular events seen with torcetrapib. Significantly fewer patients in the anacetrapib group than in the placebo group underwent revascularization (8 vs. 28, P = 0.001). It was concluded that treatment with anacetrapib had robust favorable effects on levels of LDL-C, and HDL-C had an acceptable side effect profile and, within the limits of the power of this study, did not result in the adverse cardiovascular effects observed with torcetrapib.

Effects of Anacetrapib on Clinical Cardiovascular Outcomes in Humans

Randomized EValuation of the Effects of Anacetrapib through Lipid-modification (ClinicalTrials.gov number, NCT01252953)[40] is a phase III trial designed to determine whether treatment with anacetrapib given at a daily dose of 100 mg reduces the risk of a composite end point (coronary death, MI or coronary revascularization) in patients with circulatory problems who have their LDL-C optimally treated with a statin. It is planned to randomize 30,000 subjects to anacetrapib 100 mg daily or matching placebo with a predicted follow-up of about 5 years. This study will include men and women with a history of MI, cerebrovascular atherosclerotic disease, peripheral arterial disease or diabetes mellitus with other evidence of symptomatic CHD. This study is ongoing.

Evacetrapib

Evacetrapib (LY2484595), a novel benzazepine compound, is a potent and selective inhibitor of CETP. This compound appears similar to anacetrapib and is under study.[41]

CONCLUSION

In summary, HDL particles possess multiple antiatherothrombotic properties. Low levels of HDL-C remain an important predictor of CHD events. Newer and more potent CETP inhibitors are under active evaluation in large randomized controlled trials. Nonpharmacological methods (lifestyle changes) remain at present the mainstay of raising HDL-C. Failure of HDL-raising drug torcetrapib to decrease the clinical events in spite of markedly raising HDL-C poses an important question "whether low HDL is the cause or simply a marker for atherosclerotic CVD?"

REFERENCES

1. Camont M, Chapman MJ, Kontush A. Biological activities of HDL subpopulations and their relevance to cardiovascular disease. Trends Mol Med. 2011;17(10):594-603.
2. Rye KA, Clay MA, Barter PJ. Remodelling of high density lipoproteins by plasma factors. Atherosclerosis. 1999;145(2):227-38.
3. Baliga RR. HDL–cholesterol: perfection is the enemy of good? Med Clin North Am. 2012;96:27-37.
4. Charlton-Menys V, Durrington PN. Human cholesterol metabolism and therapeutic molecules. Exp Physiol. 2008;93:27-42.
5. Schaefer EJ, Santos RD, Asztalos BF. Marked HDL deficiency and premature coronary heart disease. Curr Opin Lipidol. 2010;21:289-97. http://dx.doi.org/10.1097/MOL.0b013e32833c1ef6.
6. Rader DJ, Alexander ET, Weibel GL, et al. The role of reverse cholesterol transport in animals and humans and relationship to atherosclerosis. J Lipid Res. 2009;50(suppl):S189-94. http://dx.doi.org/10.1194/jlr. R800088-JLR200.
7. Chapman MJ, Le GW, Guerin M, et al. Cholesteryl ester transfer protein: at the heart of the action of lipid-modulating therapy with statins, fibrates, niacin, and cholesteryl ester transfer protein inhibitors. Eur Heart J. 2010;31:149-64. http://dx.doi.org/10.1093/eurheartj/ehp399.
8. Durrington PN. Hyperlipidaemia Diagnosis and Management, 3rd edition. London: Hodder Arnold; 2008.
9. Tabet F, Rye KA. High-density lipoproteins, inflammation and oxidative stress. Clin Sci (Lond). 2009;116:87-98. http://dx.doi.org/10.1042/CS20080106.
10. Hafiane A, Genest J. Review Article. HDL, Atherosclerosis, and Emerging Therapies. Cholesterol. Volume 2013, Article ID 891403, 18 pages, Hindawi Publishing Corporation.
11. Baigent C, Blackwell L, Emberson J, et al. Efficacy and safety of more intensive lowering of LDL cholesterol: a meta-analysis of data from 170,000 participants in 26 randomised trials. Lancet. 2010;376(9753):1670-81.
12. Castelli WP, Garrison RJ, Wilson PW, et al. Incidence of coronary heart disease and lipoprotein cholesterol levels. The Framingham Study. JAMA. 1986;256(20):2835-8.
13. Gordon T, Castelli WP, Hjortland MC, et al. High density lipoprotein as a protective factor against coronary heart disease. The Framingham Study. Am J Med. 1977;62(5):707-14.
14. Alsheikh-Ali AA, Abjourjaily HM, Stanek E, et al. Increases in HDL-Cholesterol Are the Strongest Predictors of Risk Reduction in Lipid Intervention Trials. New Orleans, LA: American Heart Association Scientific Sessions; 2004.

15. Kannel WB. High-density lipoproteins: epidemiologic profile and risks of coronary artery disease. Am J Cardiol. 1983;52(4):9B-12B.
16. Gordon DJ, Probstfield JL, Garrison RJ, et al. High-density lipoprotein cholesterol and cardiovascular disease. Four prospective American studies. Circulation. 1989;79(1):8-15.
17. Glueck CJ, Gartside P, Fallat RW, et al. Longevity syndromes: familial hypobeta and familial hyperalphalipoproteinemia. J Lab Clin Med. 1976;88:941.
18. Castelli WP. Cholesterol and lipids in the risk of coronary artery disease—the Framingham Heart Study. Can J Cardiol. 1988;4(Suppl A):5A-10A.
19. Packard CJ, Ford I, Robertson M, et al. Plasma lipoproteins and apolipoproteins as predictors of cardiovascular risk and treatment benefit in the PROspective Study of Pravastatin in the Elderly at Risk (PROSPER). Circulation. 2005;112(20):3058-65.
20. Nicholls SJ, Ballantyne CM, Barter PJ, et al. Effect of two intensive statin regimens on progression of coronary disease. N Engl J Med. 2011;365(22):2078-87.
21. Baliga RR, Cannon CP. Dyslipidemia. Oxford (UK): Oxford University Press; 2011.
22. Barter P, Gotto AM, LaRosa JC, et al. HDL cholesterol, very low levels of LDL cholesterol, and cardiovascular events. N Engl J Med. 2007;357(13):1301-10.
23. Ford ES, Giles WH, Dietz WH. Prevalence of the metabolic syndrome among US adults: findings from the third National Health and Nutrition Examination Survey. JAMA. 2002;287(3):356-9.
24. Gordon DJ, Rifkind BM. High-density lipoprotein—the clinical implications of recent studies. N Engl J Med. 1989;321:1311.
25. Mackey RH, Greenland P, Goff DC Jr, et al. High-density lipoprotein cholesterol and particle concentrations, carotid atherosclerosis, and coronary events: MESA (multi-ethnic study of atherosclerosis). J Am Coll Cardiol. 2012;60:508.
26. Voight BF, Peloso GM, Orho-Melander M, et al. Plasma HDL cholesterol and risk of myocardial infarction: a Mendelian randomisation study. Lancet. 2012;380:572.
27. Barter PJ, Brandrup-Wognsen G, Palmer MK, et al. Effect of statins on HDL-C: a complex process unrelated to changes in LDL-C: analysis of the VOYAGER database. J Lipid Res. 2010;51(6):1546-53.
28. Giugliano RP. Niacin at 56 years of age–time for an early retirement? N Engl J Med. 2011;365(24):2318-20.
29. Boden WE, Probstfield JL, Anderson T, et al. Niacin in patients with low HDL cholesterol levels receiving intensive statin therapy. N Engl J Med. 2011;365(24):2255-67.
30. Gouni-Berthold I, Berthold HK. The role of Niacin in lipid-lowering treatment: are we aiming too high? Curr Pharm Des. 2013;19(17):3094-106.
31. Tall AR. Plasma cholesteryl ester transfer protein. J Lipid Res. 1993;34:1255-74.
32. Drayna D, Jarnagin AS, McLean J, Henzel W, Kohr W, Fielding C, Lawn R. Cloning and sequencing of human cholesteryl ester transfer protein cDNA. Nature. 1987;327:632-4.
33. Barter PJ, Hopkins GJ, Calvert GD. Transfers and exchanges of esterified cholesterol between plasma lipoproteins. Biochem J. 1982;208:1-7.
34. Barter PJ, Caulfield M, Eriksson M, et al. Effects of torcetrapib in patients at high risk for coronary events. N Engl J Med. 2007;357(21):2109-22.
35. Vergeer M, Bots ML, van Leuven SI, et al. Cholesteryl ester transfer protein inhibitor torcetrapib and off-target toxicity: a pooled analysis of the rating atherosclerotic disease change by imaging with a new CETP inhibitor (RADIANCE) trials. Circulation.2008;118:2515-22. http://dx.doi.org/10.1161/CIRCULATIONAHA.108.772665.
36. Schwartz GG, Olsson AG, Abt M, et al. dal-OUTCOMES Investigators. Effects of dalcetrapib in patients with a recent acute coronary syndrome. N Engl J Med. 2012;367(22):2089-99.
37. Cannon CP, Shah S, Dansky HM, et al. Safety of anacetrapib in patients with or at high risk for coronary heart disease. N Engl J Med. 2010;363:2406-15.
38. Forrest MJ, Bloomfield D, Briscoe RJ, et al. Torcetrapib-induced blood pressure elevation is independent of CETP inhibition and is accompanied by increased circulating levels of aldosterone. Br J Pharmacol. 2008;154:1465-73.

39. Chapman MJ, Le Goff W, Guerin M, et al. Cholesteryl ester transfer protein: at the heart of the action of lipid-modulating therapy with statins, fibrates, niacin, and cholesteryl ester transfer protein inhibitors. Eur HeartJ. 2010;1(2):149-64.
40. Clinical trial.gov. REVEAL: randomized evaluation of the effects of anacetrapib through lipid-modification, 2010, http://clinicaltrials.gov/ct2/show/NCT01252953.
41. A Study of Evacetrapib in High-Risk Vascular Disease (ACCELERATE) http://clinicaltrials.gov/show/NCT01687998.

Clinical Approach to Lipid Disorders

Dheeraj Deo Bhatt and Tapan Ghose

- Introduction
- Primary lipid disorders
- Secondary lipid disorders
- Clinical features of dyslipidemias
- Investigations
- Treatment
- Conclusion

INTRODUCTION

Dyslipidemia is a common problem observed in medical practice. It is detected in a variety of clinical settings, ranging from asymptomatic individuals in preventive health check up to patients with established vascular diseases. It is a challenging task to correctly diagnose and treat dyslipidemia, because the same lipid level may be normal for one individual and abnormal for another. Identifying primary dyslipidemia is important because it helps screening other affected people in a family. Correctly identifying a secondary dyslipidemia is also important as it helps us to treat the primary reason for the abnormal lipid profile. In this chapter, we will discuss when to suspect lipid disorders and how to approach a patient with lipid disorder.

The lipid disorders can be broadly classified into the following two categories:

1. Primary lipid disorders
2. Secondary lipid disorders

It is important to note that many of these disorders are not clearly primary or secondary but are of mixed etiology. Moreover, the primary lipoprotein disorders present themselves only when they occur in the setting of a secondary cause of dyslipidemia, such as drug, alcohol, diabetes or pregnancy. Therefore, we should repeat the lipid profile test after appropriate modification of the secondary risk factors of dyslipidemia before labeling a person as having a primary dyslipidemia.

PRIMARY LIPID DISORDERS

As the name suggests, these disorders are primarily due to abnormalities in the lipoprotein synthesis and its metabolism. They are less common than secondary lipid disorders. The

Table 6.1: Types of hyperlipidemias

Fredrickson type	I	IIa	IIb	III	IV	V
Elevated lipoprotein	Chylomicron	LDL	LDL/VLDL	IDL	VLDL/Chylomicron	VLDL

LDL, low-density lipoprotein; VLDL, very low-density lipoprotein.

Table 6.2: List of some primary dyslipidemias with their genetic or molecular defect

Familial hypercholesterolemia	LDL receptor defect
Familial combined hyperlipidemia	Exact cause unknown, possible genetic heterogeneity. High Apo B nuclear factors (USF1, TCF7L2, HNF4alfa)
Familial dysbetalipoproteinemia	Apo E gene mutation
Familial hypertriglyceridemia	Exact cause unknown (inactivating mutation of lipoprotein lipase)
Chylomicronemia	Lipoprotein lipase deficiency, Apo CII deficiency
Tangier's disease	ABCA1 mutation
Abetalipoproteinemia	Microsomal triglyceride transfer protein defect

Apo B, apolipoprotein B; Apo E, apolipoprotein E; Apo CII, apolipoprotein CII; LDL, low-density lipoprotein.

traditional classification system of these disorders was based on the electrophoresis pattern first described in 1965 by Fredrickson and Lees (Table 6.1).[1]

It classifies lipoprotein disorders according to the type of lipoprotein that accumulates in the blood. However, a limitation of this classification is that it does not give information regarding the exact pathogenesis of the disorders. It does not represent actual diagnoses or address the source of dyslipidemia as primary or secondary. Moreover, this classification scheme does not include high-density lipoprotein cholesterol (HDL-C), which has important prognostic implications. Therefore, an alternative way to classify them is by identifying each disorder by its biochemical or genetic defect (Table 6.2).

Familial Hypercholesterolemia

Familial hypercholesterolemia (FH) is a disorder of low-density lipoprotein (LDL) metabolism and is inherited in autosomal dominant fashion. It falls under type IIa category in Fredrickson's classification. It is because of the mutation of the LDL receptor that leads to defective uptake and degradation of LDL. The homozygous form is rare but the heterozygous form is relatively common (1:500) in the general population. FH is presented with premature coronary artery disease (CAD), tendon xanthomas, xanthelasma and premature arcus cornea. The mean age for the onset of cardiovascular disease (CVD) in men with heterozygous FH is 42–46 years and in women it is 51–52 years. In patients with homozygous FH, the mean age at the time of diagnosis of CVD is 20 years.[2-4]

Table 6.3: Screening for Familial Hypercholesterolemia (FH)[6,7]

1. Universal screening for elevated serum cholesterol is recommended. FH should be suspected when untreated, fasting LDL-C or non-HDL-C levels are at or above the following:
   - Adults (>20 years): LDL-C >190 mg/dL or non-HDL-C >220 mg/dL.
   - Children, adolescents and young adults (<20 years): LDL-C >160 mg/dL or non-HDL-C >190 mg/dL.
2. For all individuals with these levels, a family history of high cholesterol and heart disease in first-degree relatives should be collected. The likelihood of FH is higher in individuals with a positive family history of hypercholesterolemia or of premature CHD (onset in men before age 55 years and women before age 65 years).
3. Cholesterol screening should be considered beginning at age 2 for children with a family history of premature CVD or elevated cholesterol. All individuals should be screened by age 20.
4. Although not present in many individuals with FH, the following physical findings should prompt the clinician to strongly suspect FH and obtain necessary lipid measurements if not already available:
   - Tendon xanthomas at any age (most common in Achilles tendon and finger extensor tendons, but can also occur in patellar and triceps tendons).
   - Arcus corneae in a patient under age 45.
   - Tuberous xanthomas or xanthelasma in a patient under age 20–25.
5. At the LDL-C levels listed below, the probability of FH is approximately 80% in the setting of general population screening. These LDL-C levels should prompt the clinician to strongly consider a diagnosis of FH and obtain further family information:
   - LDL-C >250 mg/dL in a patient aged 30 or above;
   - LDL-C >220 mg/dL for patients aged 20–29;
   - LDL-C >190 mg/dL in patients under age 2.

CHD, coronary heart disease; CVD, cardiovascular disease; FH, familial hypercholesterolemia; HDL-C, high-density lipoprotein cholesterol; LDL-C, low-density lipoprotein cholesterol.

When left untreated, patients with heterozygous FH typically have two- to threefold higher levels of plasma LDL-cholesterol (LDL-C) compared with healthy individual (about 200–400 mg/dL), whereas those with homozygous FH have six- to tenfold higher LDL-C than normal (>600 mg/dL).[5] Once we have identified a patient as having FH, we can screen other family members of the index patient for this disorder. The National Lipid Association therefore advocates screening for the diagnosis of FH (Table 6.3).[6,7]

Familial Combined Hyperlipidemia

Familial combined hyperlipidemia (FCH) is a common metabolic disorder. It falls under type IIb according to Fredrickson's classification. In the general population, its estimated prevalence is 0.5–2.0%. It is common in patients affected by coronary diseases (10%) and among acute myocardial infarct survivors aged <60 (11.3%).[8]

Genetic heterogeneity probably underlies this disorder. Though the exact genetic cause has not been identified, variations in the activity or the expression of various nuclear factors

(USF1, TCF7L2 and HNF4alfa) have a major role in the pathophysiology of FCH. These nuclear factors regulate the expression of multiple genes involved in the metabolism of lipids or carbohydrates.[9]

It is defined by (a) increase in cholesterolemia and/or triglyceridemia in at least two members of the same family, (b) intraindividual and intrafamilial variability of the lipid phenotype and (c) increased risk of premature coronary heart disease (CHD).[10] The cutoff for elevated triglyceride (TG) and LDL is >90–95th centile for the population.

Sometimes metabolic syndrome (MS) might have a similar lipid profile to FCH. The following are the major difference between FCH and MS.[11,12]

- Apolipoprotein B (ApoB) is constantly high in FCH, but not in MS. High plasma level of ApoB (125 mg/dL) is one of the best diagnostic and prognostic factors for FCH in adults.
- LDL-C values are usually normal or rather low in MS.
- The lipid phenotype is more variable in FCH (both in individuals and families). The marked variability of lipid profile, not explained by diet or body-weight variations, might represent the best diagnostic criterion to reduce the overlapping between MS and FCH.
- The inheritance of the disorder is much more evident in FCH, and lifestyle is much less relevant on FCH clinical manifestation and prognosis than on MS.
- Earlier age of onset of clinical and laboratory manifestation in FCH than in MS.
- Low-grade inflammation (high plasma level of high-sensitivity C-reactive protein (hsCRP) and adhesion molecules) or procoagulative conditions (high plasma level of fibrinogen and plasminogen activator inhibitor-1 (PAI-1)) have been more frequently associated with MS.

Familial Dysbetalipoproteinemia

It is a type III disorder under Fredrickson's classification, characterized by symmetric elevation of TG and cholesterol levels with an elevated very low-density lipoprotein (VLDL)-to-TG ratio (>0.3).[13] It is an autosomal recessive condition occurring at a frequency of 1/10,000 in the general population. The molecular defect is in the ApoE gene. Patients present with premature CAD. Tuberous or tuberoeruptive xanthomas can occur. Planar xanthomas of the palmar creases are pathognomonic of this condition.

Many homozygotes have normal lipid profile with dyslipidemia occurring only in the presence of secondary causes, such as diabetes or obesity.

Familial Hypertriglyceridemia

Familial hypertriglyceridemia (FHTG) is a common inherited disorder, thought to be autosomal dominant, which affects about 1% of the population. These patients are heterozygous for inactivating mutations of the LPL gene. The serum lipoprotein pattern fits into type IV and type V of Fredrickson's classification. It is characterized by an increased TG synthesis, which results in very large TG-enriched VLDL particles, secreted in normal numbers. It is associated with moderate elevations in the serum TG concentration (200–500 mg/dL). Affected people have elevated VLDL levels, but low levels of LDL-C and HDL-C are generally asymptomatic unless very severe hypertriglyceridemia develops. Secondary causes of dyslipidemia can exacerbate this syndrome. It is generally not associated with atherosclerotic vascular disease (ASVD).[15] It is often accompanied by insulin resistance, obesity, hyperglycemia, hypertension and hyperuricemia.

Chylomicronemia Syndrome

It is a syndrome characterized by severe hypertriglyceridemia and excessive accumulation of chylomicrons in the plasma. It is a rare disorder occurring at a frequency of 1/1,000,000 in the general population. It occurs because of a primary lipoprotein disorder in the clearance of TG from the serum-like LpL or ApoC II deficiency, or the presence of inhibitors of lipoprotein lipase.[16] More commonly familial hypertriglyceridemia or familial combined hyperlipidemia may develop chylomicronemia syndrome in the presence of secondary factors, such as alcohol, obesity, drugs or diabetes. Clinical findings include eruptive xanthomas, lipemia retinalis, pancreatitis and hepatosplenomegaly.

Tangier's Disease

Described initially by Fredrickson and his colleagues, Tangier's disease manifests clinically with hepatosplenomegaly, peripheral neuropathy and tonsils of unusual size and orange coloration.[17] Unlike other lipid disorders where the lipoproteins are high in the serum, this disease is characterized by abnormally low serum HDL-C. It is caused by mutation of ABCA1 gene that encodes for a cellular transporter, which facilitates efflux of unesterified cholesterol and phospholipids from cells to ApoA1.[18] They also have low levels of LDL-C and slightly increased risk of premature CAD, but the association is not robust.

Abetalipoproteinemia

It is a rare autosomal recessive disorder caused due to mutation in the gene encoding for TG microsomal triglyceride transfer protein. This protein is required to transfer lipids to nascent chylomicron or VLDL. Therefore, the patients have very low levels of VLDL and LDL and chylomicrons with no detectable ApoB in the plasma.[19] They present in early childhood with diarrhea, failure to thrive and fat malabsorption. Most clinical manifestations are due to lack of fat-soluble vitamins such as retinopathy and neuropathy.

SECONDARY LIPID DISORDERS

Secondary lipid disorders are the most common cause of abnormal lipid profiles in the general population. Therefore, epidemiologically they are much more important than primary dyslipidemias. We frequently encounter patients in this group of disorders during our daily clinical practice.

Common causes of secondary dyslipidemia are as follows:

- Hypothyroidism
- Obesity
- Diabetes mellitus
- Renal diseases
- Liver diseases
- Smoking
- Drugs
- Alcohol

Hypothyroidism

Hypothyroidism is a common cause of dyslipidemia. A survey of patients in a lipid disorder clinic revealed that approximately 5% had hypothyroidism.[20] In this condition the activity of hepatic lipase is decreased leading to increase in VLDL remnant. The decreased clearance of TGs and LDL-C from the blood leads to dyslipidemia. The severity of the lipid abnormalities increases in a graded fashion with the severity of the hypothyroidism.[21]

Obesity

Obesity is a well-recognized secondary cause of hypertriglyceridemia.[22] Excessive adiposity impairs TG clearance (underutilization), resulting in hypertriglyceridemia. Obesity is also associated with a number of deleterious changes in lipid metabolism, including high serum concentrations of total cholesterol (TC), LDL, VLDL and TGs and a reduction in serum HDL.[22] Loss of body fat can reduce hypercholesterolemia and hypertriglyceridemia.[23]

Diabetes Mellitus

The most common setting of secondary hypertriglyceridemia is MS and type 2 diabetes mellitus. Insulin resistance and hyperinsulinemia cause excess TG production and increase in free fatty acid. Clinical disorders related to insulin resistance, including diabetes mellitus, increase the risk for hypertriglyceridemia.[24,25] Insulin resistance leads to decreased TG clearance as well as its increased release from adipocytes, which in turn elevates its levels in the blood. The increase in large VLDL particles in type 2 diabetes initiates a sequence of events that generates atherogenic remnants, small dense LDL and small dense HDL particles.[26] Elevation of TG or low HDL-C is seen in about half of subjects with type 2 diabetes.[27]

Renal Diseases

Marked hyperlipidemia may occur in the nephrotic syndrome, primarily due to high serum TC and LDL-C concentrations. Increased hepatic production of lipoproteins, induced in part by the fall in plasma oncotic pressure, is the major abnormality, but diminished lipid catabolism may play a contributory role. Higher levels of proteinuria are correlated with more severe hyperlipidemia.

Chronic kidney disease typically causes elevation of TG and lowering of HDL-C, thereby leading to increased non-HDL-C. The elevation of TG is caused by both increased production and impaired removal of TRLs due to changes in regulatory enzymes and proteins. End-stage renal disease patients have prolonged catabolic rate of LDL. Therefore, TC, LDL-C and lipoprotein(a) (Lp(a)) have been found to be elevated. Moreover, there is increase of small and dense LDL particles.[28]

Liver Diseases

Patients with nonalcoholic fatty liver disease have elevated TG, small dense LDL and low HDL levels. The mechanism is not clear but is thought to be related to overproduction of VLDL from the liver and its decreased clearance from the circulation.[29]

Chronic hepatitis C-related liver disease may cause decrease in LDL-C. Hepatitis C virus (HCV) replication could decrease intrahepatic cholesterol synthesis. The decrease in available intracellular cholesterol may also lead to an increase in LDL receptors and intrahepatic LDL. This increase in LDL uptake may account for the decreased serum LDL levels in HCV.[30]

Smoking

Smokers have significantly higher serum cholesterol, TG and LDL levels.[31] It leads to decrease in HDL levels. Cessation of smoking leads to elevation of HDL levels.[32] The mechanisms responsible for HDL levels are not clearly known. The TG/HDL abnormalities have been suggested to be related to insulin resistance.[33]

Drugs

Cardiac medications, such as diuretics, beta blockers, bile-acid sequestrants, can cause hypertriglyceridemia. selective serotonin re uptake inhibitors (SSRI) and antipsychotic medications, such as sertraline, clozapine, quetiapine, risperidone, can also cause raised TG. Glucocorticoid therapy causes weight gain and exacerbates insulin resistance, leading to increases in TC, VLDL and TG and in the size and density of LDL particles.[33] Oral estrogen increases VLDL production.

Calcineurin inhibitors increase the activity of hepatic lipase, decrease LPL and bind the LDL receptors resulting in reduced clearance of atherogenic lipoproteins.[34] Alcohol abuse is an important common cause of hypertriglyceridemia.

CLINICAL FEATURES OF DYSLIPIDEMIAS

We will now focus on specific clinical features that need to be looked for in patients with suspected dyslipidemias during history and physical examination.

History

Symptoms related to dyslipidemia usually present in the form of:

- Myocardial infarction (MI)/angina
- Stroke/transient ischemic attack (TIA)
- Peripheral vascular disease
- Pancreatitis (hypertriglyceridemia)
- Skin lesions or ocular lesions

Family History

It is important to enquire about first-degree relatives with history of dyslipidemia, premature MI or other vascular diseases. Family history of premature CAD (first-degree relative with CAD at <55 years for male and <65 years for female) should alert us to the possibility of various familial dyslipidemias, such as FH, FCH and familial dysbetalipoproteinemia.

Family history of premature CAD in the first decade of life suggests homozygous hypercholesterolemia. The clinical diagnosis of FH is most likely when two or more first-degree relatives are found to have elevated LDL-C. Once we identify a person with FH, we have to screen other family members (cascade screening). In cascade screening, all first-degree relatives of a patient diagnosed with FH undergo lipid screening for evidence of FH. The probability of detecting FH in first-degree relatives of these patients is 50%; the probability in second-degree relatives is 25% and the probability in third-degree relatives is 12.5%.

History to Rule Out Secondary Causes

Since secondary causes of lipid disorders are much more common than the primary lipoprotein disorders, one must meticulously rule out these causes in the history. Does the patient have symptoms of nephrotic syndrome or chronic kidney disease? Is there a history of liver disease? Or is there a history of hypothyroidism or diabetes?

Dietary History

Taking dietary history is important because it can point to the presence of acquired lipid disorder. One should try to judge from the dietary history whether an individual is taking high amount of saturated fat (high intake of red meat, ghee and butter). Is the intake of cholesterol high (high intake of egg yolk)? Is the intake of fruit and vegetable adequate? History of alcohol intake and its quantification is important. Similarly, history of a sedentary lifestyle will also indicate predisposition to acquired lipid disorders.

Drug History

Drug history is crucial. Thiazides, cyclosporine and glucocorticoids may increase LDL and TG levels. Alcohol can increase serum VLDL concentrations. Similarly, presence of stress, sepsis and pregnancy may cause elevation of VLDL.

Sometimes we can suspect primary lipid disorders on the basis of history. History of residence in a particular geographic area or a particular ethnic community can sometimes help. Some populations, such as French Canadians and Dutch Afrikaners, are at a higher risk for FH owing to an increased prevalence of heterozygous FH-associated mutations in the LDL receptor gene, *LDLR*, in these founder populations.

History of pancreatitis may suggest the presence of rare primary lipoprotein disorders of ApoCII or lipoprotein lipase deficiency. It may also suggest the coexistence of mixed primary and secondary lipid disorders. FH and FCH in the presence of secondary disorders can cause pancreatitis due to elevated TGs.

Some primary lipid metabolism disorders have characteristic history and therefore it is important to ask for these questions, especially when a young patient with suspected lipid disorder presents to us. Episodes of hemolysis occurring in the presence of hypercholesterolemia suggest the rare disorder of sitosterolemia. A child presenting with failure to thrive and fat malabsorption may point towards abetalipoproteinemia. Ataxia, pigmentary retinopathy and intermittent peripheral neuropathy in the presence of low HDL suggest Tangier's disease.

Physical Examination

Important aspects of physical examination in a suspected case with dyslipidemia include measurement of blood pressure, examination of peripheral pulse, measurement of height, weight, visceral obesity and examination of eyes and skin.

Table 6.4: The National Cholesterol Education Program definition for metabolic syndrome

Definition	Abdominal obesity (cm)	Fasting blood glucose (mg/dL)	Hypertension (mmHg)	High TG (mg/dL)	Low HDL (mg/dL)
IDF	Male >90 Female >80 (obligatory criteria)	>100	>130/85	>150	Male <40 Female <50
ATP III	Male >102 Female >88	>100	>130/85	>150	Male <40 Female <50

ATP III, Adult Treatment Panel III; IDF, International Diabetes Federation; HDL, high-density lipoprotein; TG, triglyceride.

Measuring Parameters of Obesity

Several large population-based studies have shown that there is correlation between parameters of obesity and abnormal lipid profiles.[33,34]

Body mass index (BMI) is a measure of overall obesity. However, BMI has certain limitations. It does not account for the frame size and muscularity of a person. Moreover, some studies have identified higher BMI as being a protective factor from mortality from CVD, the so-called obesity paradox.[35] Therefore, there has been a shift from measuring index of general obesity (BMI) to indices of abdominal obesity (skinfold thickness, abdominal circumference, waist-hip ratio or waist-height ratios) as markers of risk factors for CVD.

Some studies have reported positive[36] while others have reported negative association[37] between abnormal lipid profile and fat distribution. Overall, the waist circumference has shown the most consistent and generally the strongest association with risk factors of CAD, including abnormal lipid profile.[38]

Therefore, measurement of waist circumference is part of the criteria for diagnosis of MS. The presence of MS identifies people with high risk of CAD. The underlying pathophysiology is thought to be insulin resistance. Its definition includes both abdominal adiposity and dyslipidemia.

The National Cholesterol Education Program, Adult Treatment Panel III (NCEP, ATP III) and International Diabetes Federation (IDF) have defined MS as outlined in Table 6.4.

NCEP, ATP III recommends that three out of five clinical and/or biochemical abnormalities should be present to satisfy this labeling, and the definition of the IDF requires abdominal obesity as an obligatory criterion and the presence of at least two other abnormal criteria. As these criteria for the MS were based on risk prediction in the non-Asian Indian populations, they may not apply to Asian Indians. The Indian consensus document for defining MS has modified the IDF definition by making the criteria of abdominal obesity as nonobligatory.[39]

Eye Examination

Arcus cornealis is the deposition of lipid in the cornea (see Fig. 6.1). The lipid is deposited near the corneoscleral limbus, but separated from the limbus by a lipid-free zone called the

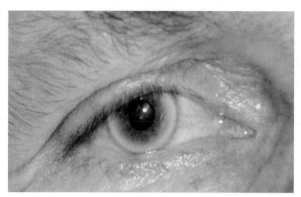

Figure 6.1: Arcus cornealis

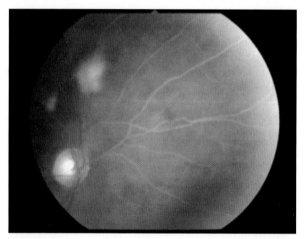

Figure 6.2: Lipemia retinalis[44]

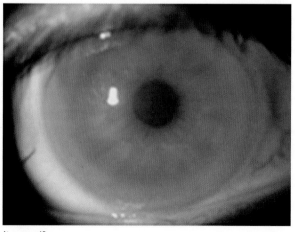

Figure 6.3: Fish Eye disease[45]

lucid interval of Vogt. Arcus formation usually begins at the superior and inferior poles of the cornea and often progresses to form a complete ring without visual impairment. Its prevalence increases with age and is also higher in smokers. Corneal arcus was first suggested as a cardiac risk factor by Virchow in 1852.[40] However, it does not appear to have an independent prognostic indicator for CAD.[41] If it is found in young (<50 years) patients it should indicate lipid screening.[42]

Lipemia retinalis may be seen in severe hypertriglyceridemia (Fig. 6.2). Creamy white appearance of retinal vessels occurs when triglyceride value reaches >2000 mg/dL. The fundus changes are thought to be due to high value of circulating chylomicrons in blood and the effect is due to dispersion of light caused by these chylomicrons. It most commonly occurs in type 1 hyperlipoproteinemia.[43,44]

Rare disorders of HDL and corneal opacity: In familial LCAT (lecithin cholesterol acyl transferase) deficiency, there is complete deficiency of LCAT whereas in fish eye disease there is a partial deficiency. Both are autosomal recessive disorders caused by mutations of the LCAT located on chromosome 16q22. Its deficiency causes accumulation of unesterified cholesterol in certain body tissues. Familial form causes corneal opacities, hemolytic anemia and renal failure. However, fish eye disease only causes corneal opacity. They do not have risk for premature atherosclerosis (Fig. 6.3).

Vascular System Examination

All peripheral pulses should be palpated because lipid deposition in atherosclerotic lesions can cause narrowing of vessels. Routine auscultation to look for carotid and renal bruit can help identify narrowed vessels due to atherosclerosis.

Ankle brachial index <0.8 is used to diagnose peripheral vascular disease. It is measured by taking the ratio of systolic blood pressure in the ankle and the arm.

Skin Examination

Abnormal deposition of lipids in the skin and subcutaneous tissue is called xanthoma and are important clues to underlying lipid disorder. Various types of xanthomas have been described.

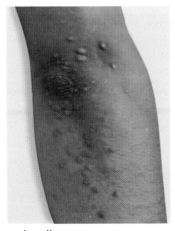

Figure 6.4: Eruptive xanthoma on the elbow

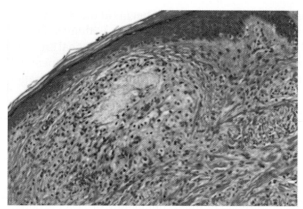

Figure 6.5: Histopathology showing extracellular lipid deposition

The most consistent relationship of dyslipidemia has been found with tendon xanthomas, which are part of diagnostic criteria for familial hypercholesterolemia.

Eruptive Xanthomas

Figures 6.4 and 6.5, respectively, show eruptive xanthoma on the elbow and histopathology showing extracellular lipid deposition.[45] These are crops of yellow papules with erythematous base occurring on pressure points of extensor surfaces (buttocks and extremities). They are asymptomatic and may enlarge with time. They occur with severe hypertriglyceridemia of any cause. They are most commonly encountered in uncontrolled diabetes and are associated with hypertriglyceridemia. They regress with fall in TG levels.

Tuberous Xanthomas

Tuberous xanthomas present a spectrum that ranges from small inflammatory lesions (tuberoeruptive xanthomas) to large nodular lesions. They often form by coalescence of

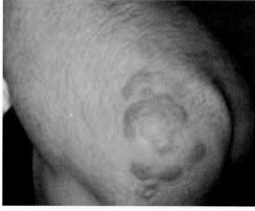

Figure 6.6: Tuberous xanthoma of the elbow[47]

smaller lesions. They occur in the presence of raised TG and cholesterol levels usually on dorsal aspects of large joints or on the hands. They are firm painless yellow-red nodules that may coalesce to form multilobulated lesions. They are most commonly found on the extensor surfaces of the elbows and knees. Tuberous xanthomas are characterized by the presence of vacuolated macrophages in dermis. These macrophages are filled with lipid droplets that are arranged in a multinodular pattern. Tuberous xanthomas are most commonly seen in homozygous FH, but are also found in severe heterozygous FH (Fig. 6.6).

Apart from hyperlipidemia they are also seen in hepatic cholestasis, cerebrotendinous xanthoma and β-sitosterolemia. With treatment of the underlying hyperlipidemia, there is usually slow resolution over many months.

Tendon Xanthomas

In tendinous xanthoma, lesions of varying size develop in ligaments, fasciae and tendon over a period of decades. They are most commonly found in the Achilles tendon or the extensor tendons of the hand. On histopathology the appearances are similar to those seen in tuberous xanthomas, except for the different tissue substrates. On physical examination there is nodularity of the tendon surface or thickening of the tendon that moves with the tendon (Fig. 6.7).

Apart from FH, they have also been reported in cerebrotendinous xanthoma (caused by a mutation in the sterol 27-hydroxylase gene), β-sitosterolemia, familial hyperlipoproteinemia (type III) and hepatic cholestasis.

Tendinous xanthomas form an important criteria of clinical diagnosis of FH. Although not present in many individuals with FH, the following physical findings should prompt the clinician to strongly suspect FH and obtain necessary lipid measurements, if not already available.

Tendon xanthomas at any age (most common in Achilles tendon and finger extensor tendons but can also occur in patellar and triceps tendons).

Arcus corneae in patients aged <45 years.

Tuberous xanthomas or xanthelasma in patients aged <20 years.

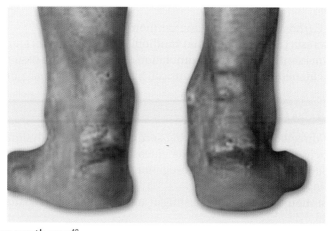

Figure 6.7: Tendon xanthoma[48]

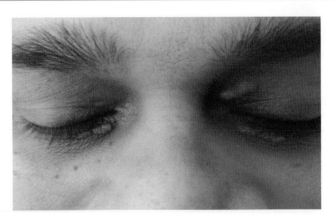

Figure 6.8: Xanthelasma

Planar Xanthomas

Planar xanthomas are yellow macules or orange plaques, which can further be classified on the basis of their location in xanthelasmas, intertriginous xanthomas, xanthoma striatum palmaris and diffuse (generalized) plane xanthomas. A further variant, planar xanthoma of cholestasis, is sometimes recognized (Fig. 6.8).

If found in the palmar creases, they are called palmar crease xanthomas and are diagnostic of dysbetalipoproteinemia. Interdigital xanthomata and planar xanthomas in skin creases are observed in homozygous FH and occasionally in dysbetalipoproteinemia. Xanthelasmas occur on the eyelids and are least specific for the presence of lipid disorders. Lipid levels are normal in approximately 50% of affected individuals, although in young people there is a higher incidence of hyperlipidemia.

Differential Diagnosis of Xanthomas

Although xanthomas are present in hyperlipidemia, these skin manifestations can also occur in the absence of dyslipidemia.

- Primary biliary cirrhosis (tuberous/plane xanthomas)
- Plasma cell dyscrasia (normolipemic flat xanthomas on upper trunk and face)
- Cerebrotendinous xanthomatosis (accumulation of cholestanol in tissues)
- Normolipemic cutaneous non-Langerhans cell histiocytosis (palmar xanthoma)

INVESTIGATION

Investigations are directed toward identifying secondary causes of dyslipidemia. Therefore, fasting plasma glucose, postprandial plasma glucose, thyroid, renal and liver function tests need to be done. Similarly, appropriate investigations to rule out other secondary causes need to be done according to the clinical setting.

Lipid profile test should be done after fasting of at least 10–12 hours so that the TG levels are not overestimated.

Most laboratories directly measure TC, TG and HDL and then estimate the LDL-C using the Friedewald equation:

LDL cholesterol = Total cholesterol – HDL cholesterol – TG/5

This equation holds true if the level of TG is <400 mg/dL.

Direct method of LDL measurement should be used whenever available. The evidence showing that reducing TC and LDL-C can prevent CVD is strong and compelling, based on results from multiple randomized controlled trials. TC and LDL-C levels therefore continue to constitute the primary targets of therapy.[48] The TC to HDL-C ratio having the highest predictive value for future CAD is usually calculated.

The ratio of ApoA to ApoB also has prognostic implication for risk stratification. Measurement of ApoB is not recommended for routine risk stratification. The major disadvantages of ApoB are that it is not included in algorithms for calculation of global risk, and it has not been a predefined treatment target in controlled trials. Recent data from a meta-analysis by the Emerging Risk Factor Collaboration[49] indicate that ApoB does not provide any benefit beyond non-HDL-C or traditional lipid ratios. Likewise, ApoB provided no benefit beyond traditional lipid markers in people with diabetes in the Fenofibrate Intervention and Event Lowering in Diabetes (FIELD) study.[50] In contrast, in another meta-analysis of LDL-C, non-HDL-C and ApoB, the latter was superior as a marker of CV risk.[51]

Non-HDL-C is used as an estimation of the total number of atherogenic particles in plasma [VLDL + intermediate-density lipoprotein (IDL) + LDL] and relates well to ApoB levels. Non-HDL-C is easily calculated from TC minus HDL-C. Non-HDL-C can provide a better risk estimation compared with LDL-C, particularly in hypertryglyceridemia in diabetes mellitus, the MS or chronic kidney disease. This is supported by a recent meta-analysis including 14 statin trials, seven fibrate trials and six nicotinic acid trials.[52] However, this approach of treating dyslipidemia with respect to certain target levels of LDL and non-HDL-C has been done away with in recent guidelines.

Plasma Lp(a) is not recommended for risk screening in the general population; however, Lp(a) measurement should be considered in people with high CVD risk.

Apolipoprotein A1 (Apo A1) is the major protein of HDL and provides a good estimate of HDL concentration. Plasma ApoA1 of 120 mg/dL for men and 140 mg/dL for women approximately correspond to what is considered as low for HDL-C. Again, ApoA1 measurement is not indicated routinely.

Determination of small dense LDL may be regarded as an emerging risk factor that may be used in the future,[55] but is not currently recommended for risk stratification. Atherogenic lipid triad consists of the co-existence of VLDL remnants manifested as mildly elevated TGs, increased small dense LDL particles and reduced HDL-C levels. However, clinical trial evidence is limited on the effectiveness and safety of intervening in this pattern to reduce CVD risk; therefore, this pattern or its components must be regarded as optional targets of CVD prevention.[50]

TREATMENT

Recently, after a long wait, the ACC/AHA has published guidelines for the management of dyslipidemia.[56] The following discussion is largely based on these guidelines.

The ATP IV guidelines have emphasized as in the previous guidelines that lifestyle modification is the foundation of all primary and secondary prevention efforts. It is pertinent to note that secondary causes of dyslipidemia have to be ruled out before starting statin therapy and individuals with TG >500 mg/dL need to be treated with lipid-lowering agents, especially fibrates.

However, the focus of the current guidelines is identification of statin benefit groups. The current guidelines have proposed identifying those subgroups who have been found to have established benefits from statin therapy. For this we have to ask four simple questions.

1. Is there a history of heart disease or stroke? (this is secondary prevention)
2. Is the LDL-C >190 mg/dL? (assume the patient has FH)
3. Is the patient diabetic, 40–75 year with an LDL of 70–189 mg/dL? Is the patient's 10 year global risk score ≥7.5%?

If the answer to any of the above questions is yes, then the patient requires statin—high-intensity statin (LDL reduction of 50%) for the first two groups and moderate intensity statin (LDL reduction of 30–50%) for the last two. If age is >75 years, we have to use moderate intensity statin. If a diabetic 40–75 years has >7.5% risk, then we have to prescribe high-intensity statin.

Usual high-intensity statin would be atorvastatin 40–80 mg and rosuvastatin 20–40 mg. Usual moderate intensity statin would be atorvastatin 10–20 mg, rosuvastatin 5–10 mg and simvastatin 20–40 mg.

People with established vascular disease fall under the statin benefit group. This has been termed ASCVD (atherosclerotic cardiovascular disease) and has been used in the guidelines to include acute coronary syndromes, history of MI, stable or unstable angina, coronary or other arterial revascularization, stroke, TIA or peripheral arterial disease presumed to be of atherosclerotic origin. To guide therapy for primary prevention, the ATP IV guideline has used

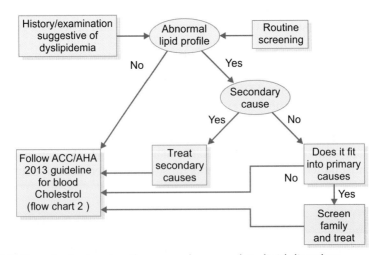

Flowchart 6.1: Flowcharts showing the general approach to lipid disorders

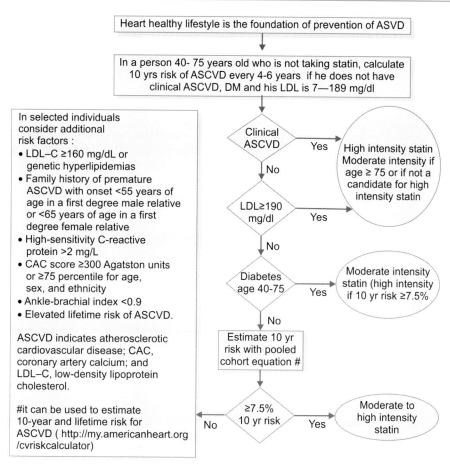

Heart healthy lifestyle is the foundation of prevention of ASVD

In a person 40- 75 years old who is not taking statin, calculate 10 yrs risk of ASCVD every 4-6 years if he does not have clinical ASCVD, DM and his LDL is 7—189 mg/dl

In selected individuals consider additional risk factors :
- LDL–C ≥160 mg/dL or genetic hyperlipidemias
- Family history of premature ASCVD with onset <55 years of age in a first degree male relative or <65 years of age in a first degree female relative
- High-sensitivity C-reactive protein >2 mg/L
- CAC score ≥300 Agatston units or ≥75 percentile for age, sex, and ethnicity
- Ankle-brachial index <0.9
- Elevated lifetime risk of ASCVD.

ASCVD indicates atherosclerotic cardiovascular disease; CAC, coronary artery calcium; and LDL–C, low-density lipoprotein cholesterol.

#it can be used to estimate 10-year and lifetime risk for ASCVD (http://my.americanheart.org /cvriskcalculator)

Clinical ASCVD — Yes → High intensity statin Moderate intensity if age ≥ 75 or if not a candidate for high intensity statin

No ↓

LDL≥190 mg/dl — Yes →

No ↓

Diabetes age 40-75 — Yes → Moderate intensity statin (high intensity if 10 yr risk ≥7.5%)

No ↓

Estimate 10 yr risk with pooled cohort equation #

↓

≥7.5% 10 yr risk — Yes → Moderate to high intensity statin

No ←

Flowchart 6.2: Approach to lipid disorders

Source: Stone NJ, Robinson J, Lichtenstein AH, et al. 2013 ACC/AHA guideline on the treatment of blood cholesterol to reduce atherosclerotic cardiovascular risk in adults: a report of the American College of Cardiology/American Heart Association Task Force on Practice Guidelines. Circulation[55]

the pooled Cohort equation. It gives the estimated 10-year or "hard" ASCVD risk that includes the first occurrence of nonfatal MI, CHD death, and nonfatal and fatal stroke.

The guideline mentions that if there is still lack of clarity on whether to start lipid-lowering therapy for primary prevention after risk stratification then the following variables have to be evaluated. Coronary calcium score, LDL-C >160 mg/dL or genetic dyslipidemia, family history of premature CAD, ankle brachial index <0.9 and hsCRP >2 mg/L. This might be especially true when we are considering a person who is <40 years of age or has a strong family history of CAD or is extremely obese and physically inactive. These variables are not adequately represented in the risk calculations; therefore, risk might be underestimated in these situations. A modified flowchart adapted from ATP IV guidelines is shown in Flowcharts 6.1 and 6.2.

CONCLUSION

History and physical examination if performed meticulously can provide clues to the underlying lipid disorder. Our emphasis during preliminary history and physical examination should be to rule out possible secondary causes of dyslipidemia as they are the most common causes of abnormal lipid profile. If secondary causes can be identified, then these should be treated first before trying to treat the abnormal lipid level.

We should also have a high index of suspicion for the presence of primary lipid disorders and consider them in the appropriate clinical setting. Some primary lipid disorders are relatively common and some are very rare but their identification is important as they have different prognosis and their management varies accordingly. Once abnormal lipid profile has been identified, the further treatment depends on the level of abnormality, associated ASCVD, diabetes or 10 year or lifetime risk for ASCVD as given by the pooled cohort equation.

REFERENCES

1. Fredrickson DS, Lees RS. A system for phenotyping hyperlipoproteinemia. Circulation. 1965;31:321-7.
2. Kolansky DM, Cuchel M, Clark BJ, et al. Longitudinal evaluation and assessment of cardiovascular disease in patients with homozygous familial hypercholesterolemia. Am J Cardiol. 2008;102(11):1438-43.
3. Alonso R, Mata N, Castillo S, et al. Cardiovascular disease in familial hypercholesterolaemia: influence of low-density lipoprotein receptor mutation type and classic risk factors. Atherosclerosis. 2008;200(2):315-21.
4. Jansen AC, van Aalst-Cohen ES, Tanck MW, et al. The contribution of classical risk factors to cardiovascular disease in familial hypercholesterolaemia: data in 2400 patients. J Intern Med. 2004;256(6):482-90.
5. Liyanage KE, Hooper AJ, Defesche JC, et al. High-resolution melting analysis for detection of familial ligand-defective apolipoprotein B-100 mutations. Ann Clin Biochem. 2008;45(Pt 2):170-76.
6. Hopkins PN, Toth PP, Ballantyne CM, et al. Familial hypercholesterolemias: prevalence, genetics, diagnosis and screening recommendations from the National Lipid Association Expert Panel on Familial Hypercholesterolemia. J Clin Lipidol. 2011;5(3 Suppl):S9-S17.
7. Goldberg AC, Hopkins PN, Toth PP, et al. Familial hypercholesterolemia: screening, diagnosis and management of pediatric and adult patients: clinical guidance from the National Lipid Association Expert Panel on Familial Hypercholesterolemia. J Clin Lipidol. 2011;5(3 Suppl):S1-S8.
8. Gaddi A, Galetti C, Pauciullo P, et al. On behalf of the Committee of experts of the Atherosclerosis and Dysmetabolic Disorders Study Group. Familial combined hyperlipoproteinemia: expert panel position on diagnostic criteria for clinical practice. Nutr Metab Cardiovasc Dis. 1999;9:304-11.
9. Aguilar-Salinas C, Gómez-Díaz R, Tusié-Luna MT. Fifty years studying hyperlipidemias: the case of familial combined hyperlipidemia. [Article in Spanish] Invest Clin. 2010;51(2):145-58.
10. Sniderman AD, Castro CM, Ribalta J, et al A proposal to redefine familial combined hyperlipidaemia—third workshop on FCH held in Barcelona from 3 to 5 May 2001, during the scientific sessions of the European Society for Clinical Investigation. Eur J Clin Invest. 2002;32(2):71-3.
11. de Graaf J, van der VG, Stalenhoef AF. Diagnostic criteria in relation to the pathogenesis of familial combined hyperlipidemia. Semin Vasc Med. 2004;4:229-40.
12. Gaddi A, Cicero AF, Odoo FO, et al. Atherosclerosis and Metabolic Diseases Study Group. Practical guidelines for familial combined hyperlipidemia diagnosis: an up-date. Vasc Health Risk Manag. 2007;3(6):877-86.
13. Fredrickson DS, Morganroth J, Levy RI. Type III hyperlipoproteinemia: analysis of two contemporary deficiencies. Ann Intern Med. 1975;82:150-7.

14. Berglund L, Brunzell JD, Goldberg AC, et al. Evaluation and treatment of hypertriglyceridemia: an endocrine society clinical practice guideline. J Clin Endocrinol Metab. 2012;97(9):2969.
15. Austin MA, McKnight B, Edwards KL, et al. Cardiovascular disease mortality in familial forms of hypertriglyceridemia: a 20-year prospective study. Circulation. 2000;101:2777-82.
16. Santamarina-Fojo S. The familial chylomicronemia syndrome. Endocrinol Metab Clin North Am. 1998;27(3):551-67.
17. Fredrickson DS. The inheritance of high density lipoprotein deficiency (Tangier disease). J Clin Invest. 1964;43:228-36.
18. Brooks-Wilson A, Marcil M, Clee SM, et al. Mutations in ABC1 in Tangier disease and familial high-density lipoprotein deficiency. Nat Genet. 1999;22:336-45.
19. Zamel R, Khan R, Rebecca L, et al. Abetalipoproteinemia: two case reports and literature review. Orphanet J Rare Dis. 2008,3:19.
20. Tsimihodimos V, Bairaktari E, Tzallas C, et al. The incidence of thyroid function abnormalities in patients attending an outpatient lipid clinic. Thyroid. 1999;9:365-8.
21. Canaris GJ, Manowitz NR, Mayor G, et al. The Colorado thyroid disease prevalence study. Arch Intern Med. 2000;160:526-34.
22. Hubert HB, Feinleib M, McNamara PM, et al. Obesity as an independent risk factor for cardiovascular disease: a 26-year follow-up of participants in the Framingham Heart Study. Circulation. 1983;67:968-77.
23. Katzel LI, Coon PJ, Rogus E, et al. Persistence of low HDL-C levels after weight reduction in older men with small LDL particles. Arterioscler Thromb Vasc Biol. 1995;15:299-305.
24. Zavaroni I, Dall'Aglio E, Alpi O, et al. Evidence for an independent relationship between plasma insulin and concentration of high density lipoprotein cholesterol and triglyceride. Atherosclerosis. 1985;55:259-66.
25. Goldberg IJ. Clinical review diabetic dyslipidemia: causes and consequences. J Clin Endocrinol Metab. 2001;86:965-71.
26. Adiels M, Olofsson S-O, Taskinen M-R, et al. Overproduction of very low-density lipoproteins is the hallmark of the dyslipidaemia in the metabolic syndrome. Arterioscler Thromb Vasc Biol. 2008;28:1225-36.
27. Scott R, O'Brien R, Fulcher G, et al. Effects of fenofibrate treatment on cardiovascular disease risk in 9,795 individuals with type 2 diabetes and various components of the metabolic syndrome. Diab Care. 2009;32:493-8.
28. Kwan BC, Kronenberg F, Beddhu S, et al. Lipoprotein metabolism and lipid management in chronic kidney disease. J Am Soc Nephrol. 2007;18(4):1246-61.
29. Chatrath H, Vuppalanchi R, Chalasani N. Dyslipidemia in patients with nonalcoholic fatty liver disease. Semin Liver Dis. 2012;32(1):22-9.
30. Monazahian, M, Bohme, I, Bonk, S, et al. Low density lipoprotein receptor as a candidate receptor for hepatitis C virus. J Med Virol. 1999;57:223-9.
31. Craig WY, Palomaki GE, Haddow JE. Cigarette smoking and serum lipid and lipoprotein concentrations. An analysis of published data. BMJ. 1989;298:784-8.
32. Gepner AD, Megan E, Piper ME, Johnson HM. Effects of smoking and smoking cessation on lipids and lipoproteins: outcomes from a randomized clinical trial. Am Heart J. 2011;161(1):145-51.
33. Reaven G, Tsao PS. Insulin resistance and compensatory hyperinsulinemia. The key player between cigarette smoking and cardio-vascular disease. J Am Coll Cardiol. 2003;41:1044-7.
34. Hilbrands LB, Dermacker PN, Hoitsma AJ, et al. The effects of cyclosporine and prednisone on serum lipid and (apo)lipoprotein levels in renal transplant recipients. J Am Soc Nephrol. 1995;5:2073-81.
35. Peiris AN, Hennes MI, Evans DJ, et al. Relationship of anthropometric measurements of body fat distribution to metabolic profile in premenopausal women. Acta Med Scand Suppl. 1988;723:179-88.

36. Pouliot M, Després JP, Lemieux S, et al. Waist circumference and abdominal sagittal diameter: best simple anthropometric indexes of abdominal visceral adipose tissue accumulation and related cardiovascular risk in men and women. Am J Cardiol. 1994;73:460-8.

37. Corral AR, Montori VM, Somers VK, et al. Association of bodyweight with total mortality and with cardiovascular events in coronary artery disease: a systematic review of cohort studies. Lancet. 2000;368:666-78.

38. Freedman DS, Srinivasan SR, Harsha DW, et al. Relationship of body fat patterning to lipid and lipoprotein concentrations in children and adolescents: the Bogalusa Heart Study. Am J Clin Nutr. 1989;50:930-9.

39. Becque MD, Hattori KH, Katch VL, et al. Relationship of fat patterning to coronary artery disease risk in obese adolescents. Am J Phys Anthropol. 1986;71:423-9.

40. Sangi H, Mueller WH. Which measure of body fat distribution is best for epidemiologic research among adolescents. Am J Epidemiol. 1991;133:870-83.

41. Misra A, Chowbey P, Makkar BM, et al. Consensus statement for diagnosis of obesity, abdominal obesity and the metabolic syndrome for Asian Indians and recommendations for physical activity, medical and surgical management. J Assoc Physicians India. 2009;57:163-70.

42. Virchow V. Uber parenchymatose entzundum. Virchows Arch Pathol Anat. 1852;4:261.

43. Fernandez AB, Keyes MJ, Pencina M, et al. Relation of corneal arcus to cardiovascular disease (from the Framingham Heart Study Data Set). Am J Cardiol. 2009;103(1):64-6.

44. Shanoff HM, Little JA. Studies of male survivors of myocardial infarction due to "essential" atherosclerosis III corneal arcus: incidence and relation to serum lipids and lipoproteins. CMAJ. 1964;91:835-9.

45. Rymarz E, Matysik-Woźniak A, Baltaziak L, et al. Lipemia retinalis—an unusual cause of visual acuity deterioration. Med Sci Monit. 2012;18(8):CS72-75.

46. Kettritz R, Elitok S, Koepke M, et al. The case: the eyes have it! Kidney Int. 2009;76:465-6.

47. Digby M, Belli R, McGraw T, et al. Eruptive xanthomas as a cutaneous manifestation of hypertriglyceridemia: a case report. J Clin Aesthet Dermatol. 2011;4(1):44-6.

48. AMY SEINFELD Image: Tuberous Xanthomas. University of Miami. www.consultant live.com

49. Image tendon xanthoma http://clinicalexamskills.blogspot.in/2010/10/lipids-and-skin.html

50. ESC/EAS Guidelines for the Management of Dyslipidaemias. The task force for the management of dyslipidaemias of the European Society of Cardiology (ESC) and the European Atherosclerosis Society (EAS). Eur Heart J. 2011;32:1769-1818.

51. Di Angelantonio E, Sarwar N, Perry P, et al. The emerging risk factors collaboration. Major lipids, apolipoproteins, and risk of vascular disease. JAMA. 2009;302;1993-2000.

52. Taskinen MR, Barter PJ, Ehnholm C, et al. on behalf of the FIELD Study Investigators. Ability of traditional lipid ratios and apolipoprotein ratios to predict cardiovascular risk in people with type 2 diabetes. Diabetologia. 2010;53:1846-55.

53. Sniderman AD, Williams K, Contois JH, et al. Meta-analysis of LDL-C, non-HDL-C and apo B as markers of cardiovascular risk. Circ Cardiovasc Qual Outcomes. 2011;4:337-45.

54. Robinson JG, Wang S, Smith BJ, et al. Meta-analysis of the relationship between non-high-density lipoprotein cholesterol reduction and coronary heart disease risk. J Am Coll Cardiol. 2009;53:316-22.

55. Packard CJ. Small dense low-density lipoprotein and its role as an independent predictor of cardiovascular disease. Curr Opin Lipidol. 2006;17:412-7.

56. Stone NJ, Robinson J, Lichtenstein AH, et al. 2013 ACC/AHA guideline on the treatment of blood cholesterol to reduce atherosclerotic cardiovascular risk in adults: a report of the American College of Cardiology/American Heart Association Task Force on Practice Guidelines. Circulation (online).

Lipoprotein(a) and Atherosclerosis

D. Dev

- Introduction
- Structure of lipoprotein(a)
- Plasma level of lipoprotein(a)
- Lipoprotein(a) and atherosclerosis
- How lipoprotein(a) causes atherosclerosis?
- Difficulties in lipoprotein(a) estimation and standardization
- Effect of pharmacological and nonpharmacological intervention on lipoprotein(a)
- Clinical implications of Lp(a)
- Future needs

INTRODUCTION

Lipoprotein(a) [Lp(a)], also known as lipoprotein little a, was identified by Berg[1] in the year 1963. Several retrospective clinical studies and some prospective studies could establish a positive direct association of Lp(a) with atherosclerotic diseases, and this molecule is considered as an emerging risk factor for coronary heart disease (CHD).

STRUCTURE OF LIPOPROTEIN(A)

The challenging molecule Lp(a) has a complex structure in which apolipoprotein(B) [apo(B)] of low-density lipoprotein (LDL), the bad cholesterol, is attached to a glycoprotein moiety apolipoprotein(a) [apo(a)] by a single disulfide bond.[2] The glycoprotein apo(a) is synthesized and secreted from the liver. Lipoprotein(a) contains apo(B) and apo(a) in a 1:1 molar ratio. It is responsible for both atherosclerosis and thrombosis. Apolipoprotein(B) of LDL present in the Lp(a) is responsible for atherosclerosis, and the glycoprotein apo(a) of Lp(a) is responsible for thrombosis. Apolipoprotein(a) contains repeated kringle motifs that are similar to the sequence found in proenzyme plasminogen. McLean et al.[3] reported that the sequence of human apo(a) bears a striking similarity to serine protease zymogen plasminogen.

PLASMA LEVEL OF LIPOPROTEIN(A)

In the human population, plasma concentration of Lp(a) in blood is variable because of the difference in Lp(a) production rather than its catabolism.[4] The production of apo(a) in Lp(a) is under strong genetic control for which Lp(a) is relatively resistant to pharmacologic intervention.[5-7] Several different isoforms of apo(a) are responsible for variation in the concentration of Lp(a). An inverse correlation has been established between plasma Lp(a) concentration and apo(a) isoform size;[8] however, this relationship is not absolute; there are marked differences in this relation in different ethnic groups, for example, in blacks, there is greater Lp(a) concentration with midsize apo(a) isoform compared with whites.[9]

LIPOPROTEIN(A) AND ATHEROSCLEROSIS

Lipoprotein(a) is classified as an emerging lipid risk factor for cardiovascular disease (CVD).[10] Plasma concentration of Lp(a) >30 mg/dL has been identified as a risk factor for atherosclerotic diseases like peripheral vascular disease,[11,12] ischemic stroke,[13,14] aortic aneurysm[15] and premature CHD.[16,17]

The clinical significance of Lp(a) in CHD has been confirmed in several retrospective case-control studies.[6,7,16] In all these studies, the plasma concentration of Lp(a) was high in the patients with existing CHD compared with match control. The results were conflicting ranging from a strong positive association between Lp(a) and CHD[18,19] to weak association[20] to no association.[21,22] However, majority of the prospective studies established increased level of plasma Lp(a) as a predictor of CHD. Meta-analysis of 12 prospective studies between 1991 and 1997 indicated plasma Lp(a) as an independent risk factor in both men and women, and there was a dose–and there was a dosetor in 1991 es esLp(a) concentration and CHD risk.[23]

A recent meta-analysis of 27 prospective studies[24] indicates that in the general population, individuals with Lp(a) concentration in top third of baseline measurement are at approximately 70% increased risk for CHD compared with individuals in bottom third. The concentration of Lp(a) has a strong association with the events at baseline, but its predictive value reduces when LDL concentration was reduced below 100 mg/dL.[25] The recent prospective epidemiological study of myocardial infarction (PRIME) study. It is found that increased level of Lp(a) increases the risk of myocardial infarction and angina, and the effect is more pronounced in males with high LDL level.[26]

In a women high Lth study,[27] it was found that extremely high Lp(a) levels (>90th percentile) increased the risk in women with high LDL level.

HOW LIPOPROTEIN(A) CAUSES ATHEROSCLEROSIS?

Although several studies could establish a positive association between Lp(a) and atherosclerosis, the mechanism how Lp(a) cause atherosclerosis is poorly understood. It is documented that deposition of Lp(a) in the arterial wall is proportional to the Lp(a) concentration in blood.[28] Accumulation of Lp(a) in the arterial wall indicates a direct causative role of Lp(a) for atherosclerotic lesion initiation or lesion progression or both. Many in vitro and animal model studies postulated both proatherosclerotic and prothrombotic effect of Lp(a). Apolipoprotein(a) portion of Lp(a) is responsible for prothrombotic effect and apo(B) portion of LDL present in Lp(a) is for proatherosclerotic effect.

Prothrombotic effect of lipoprotein is due to the ability of (i) apo(a) to interfere with the activation of plasminogen to plasmin,[29] (ii) Lp(a) to alter the architecture of fibrin clot, thereby decreasing the susceptibility to breakdown,[30] (iii) Lp(a) to inactivate the tissue factor pathway inhibitor[31] and (iv) Lp(a) to hasten platelet aggregation.[32]

Pro-atherosclerotic effect Lp(a) is due to the following reasons: (i) Lp(a) can stimulate migration and proliferation of arterial smooth muscle cell,[33] (ii) increase the endothelial cell permeability and the deposition of LDL in the arterial wall,[34] (iii) increase endothelin, a cell adhesion molecule[35] and (iv) also act as a carrier of oxidized phospholipids.[36]

Human atherosclerotic lesion shows an association of Lp(a) deposition with the area of calcification.[37] An immunologic and proinflammatory property of Lp(a) is also proposed.[38]

DIFFICULTIES IN LIPOPROTEIN(A) ESTIMATION AND STANDARDIZATION

To explore the predictive value of Lp(a), methods of its measurement must be accurate. Different immunologic methods of estimation of Lp(a) are enzyme-linked immunosorbent assay, nephelometry and immunoturbidity. Drawback of the immunologic methods is that the antibody used in the type of assay will not possess the same immunoreactivity per particle if apo(a) isoforms are not same.

To bypass the problems of immunologic methods of estimation of Lp(a), quantification of Lp(a) was tried by measuring cholesterol content by ultracentrifugation or by lectin affinity chromatography.

Now, standardization of different methods of estimation of Lp(a) is in progress.[39,40]

EFFECT OF PHARMACOLOGICAL AND NONPHARMACOLOGICAL INTERVENTIONS ON LIPOPROTEIN(A)

Lipoprotein(a) is relatively resistant to the commonly used pharmacologic and nonpharmacologic interventions used to reduce plasma lipid concentrations due to gene encoding the apo(a) portion of it. However, some pharmacologic agents alone or in combination with other agents are capable to reduce the plasma Lp(a) concentrations. High dose of niacin[41] is reported to be effective in lowering plasma Lp(a). Other agents like L-carnitine in a dose 2 g/day[42] and ascorbic acid in combination with L-lysine monohydrochloride[43] are capable to reduce plasma Lp(a) concentrations. In a small study,[44] aspirin was found to be effective in lowering Lp(a).

Hormones can reduce plasma Lp(a) concentrations; these are androgens, such as danazol[45] and tibolone,[46] and estrogen and tamoxifan.[47]

The effect of the commonly used lipid-lowering agent, statin, on Lp(a) is variable. In patients receiving simvastatin[48] and atorvastatin,[49] an increase in Lp(a) concentrations was reported. Rosuvastatin or atorvastatin when used with niacin can reduce the serum Lp(a) concentration.[50]

Although Lp(a) is resistant to the nonpharmacologic interventions like exercise and diet modification, in one study,[51] a low caloric diet with concomitant weight reduction caused significant reduction in Lp(a) concentrations in obese women with high baseline Lp(a) concentrations.

CLINICAL IMPLICATIONS OF LIPOPROTEIN(A)

The 2012 American Association of Clinical Endocrinologists guidelines have concluded that the risk associated with elevated Lp(a) varies between ethnic groups. The guideline endorses Lp(a) as a major cardiovascular (CV) risk factor independently of triglyceride, LDL cholesterol, and HDL testing for Lp(a) is not generally recommended, although it may provide useful information to ascribe risk in white patients with coronary artery disease (CAD) or in those with an unexplained family history of early CAD.

The 2011 European Society of Cardiovascular/European Atherosclerosis Society (EAS) guidelines state that Lp(a) might not be a target for risk screening in the general population, yet it should be considered in individuals with elevated CV risk or a family history of premature vascular diseases.

Emerging Risk Factors Collaboration focusing on low- to intermediate-risk populations showed that Lp(a) slightly improves CVD prediction in addition to HDL cholesterol and total cholesterol.

European Atherosclerosis Society (The EAS) Consensus Panel recommends screening individuals at intermediate and high CVD risk, including familial hypercholesterolemia and hyper-Lp(a), and in patients with a family history of premature CVD and a ≥ 3% 10-year fatal CVD risk according to the EAS guidelines.

FUTURE NEEDS

A suitable and standardized method of estimation of Lp(a) is to be developed to reduce the false positive (high risk) and false negative (low risk) group. The development standardized method is also needed to compare the result of different studies. An effective Lp(a)-lowering agent is the need of future.

REFERENCES

1. Berg K. A new serum type system in man: the Lp system. Acta Pathol Microbiol Scand. 1963;59:362-82.
2. Koschinsky ML, Cote GP, Gabel B, et al. Identification of the cysteine residue in apolipoprotein(a) that mediates extracellular coupling with apolipoprotein-B-100. J Biol Chem. 1993;268:19819-25.
3. McLean JW, Tomlinsion JE, Kuang WJ, et al. cDNA sequence of human apolipoprotein(a) is homologous to plasminogen. Nature. 1987;330:132-7.
4. Reader DJ, Cain W, Ikewaki K, et al. The inverse association of plasma lipoprotein(a) concentration with apolipoprotein(a) isoform size is not due to differences in Lp(a) catabolism but to difference in production rate. J Clin Invest. 1994;93:2758-63.
5. Angelin B. Therapy for lowering lipoprotein(a) levels. Curr Opin Lipidol. 1997;8:337-41.
6. Anuurad E, Boffa MB, Koschinsky ML, et al. Lipoprotein(a): a unique risk factor for cardiovascular disease. Clin Lab Med. 2006;26:751-72.
7. Marcovina SM, Koschinsky ML, Albers JJ, et al. Report of the National Heart Lung and Blood Institute Workshop on Lipoprotein(a) and Cardiovascular Disease: recent advances and future directions. Clin Chem. 2003;49:1785-96.
8. Utermann G, Menzel HJ, Kraft HG, et al. Lp(a) glycoprotein phenotypes. Inheritance and relation to Lp(a) Lipoprotein concentrations in plasma. J Clin Invest. 1987;80:458-65.
9. Marcovina SM, Albers JJ, Wijsman E, et al. Differences in Lp(a) concentrations and apo(a) polymorphs between black and white Americans. J Lipid Res. 1996;37:2569-89.
10. Expert Panel on Detection, Evaluation and High Blood Cholesterol in Adults. Executive Summary of the Third Report of The National Cholesterol Education Programme (NCEP). JAMA. 2001; 285:2486-97.
11. Aboyans V, Criqui MH, Denenberg JO, et al. Risk factors for progression of peripheral arterial disease in large and small vessels. Circulation. 2006;113:2623-39.

12. Cheng SW, Ting AC, Wong J. Lipoprotein(a) and its relationship to risk factors and severity of atherosclerotic peripheral vascular disease. Eur Vasc Endovasc Surg. 1997;14:17-23.

13. Ohira T,Schreiner PJ, Morrisett JD, et al. Lipoprotein(a) and incidence of ischemic stroke: the Atherosclerosis Risk in Communities (ARIC) study. Stroke. 2006;37:1407-12.

14. Peng DQ, Zhao SP, Wang JL. Lipoprotein(a) and apolipoprotein E epsilon 4 as independent risk factors for ischemic stroke. J Cardiovasc Risk. 1999;6:1-6.

15. Jones GT, van Rij AM, Cole J, et al. Plasma lipoprotein(a) indicates risk for 4 distinct forms of vascular disease. Clin Chem. 2007;53:679-85.

16. Koschinsky ML. Lipoprotein(a) and atherosclerosis: new perspective on the mechanism of action of an enigmatic lipoprotein. Curr Atheroscler Rep. 2005;7:389-95.

17. Genest J Jr, Jenner JL, McNamara JR, et al. Prevalence of lipoprotein(a){Lp(a)} excess in coronary artery disease. Am J Cardiol. 1991;67:1039-145.

18. Assmann G, Srchulte H, von Eckardstein A. Hypertriglyceridemia and elevated lipoprotein(a) are risk factors for major coronary events in middle aged men. Am J Cardiol. 1996;77:1179-84.

19. Wald NJ, Law M, Watt HC, et al. Apolipoproteins and ischemic heart disease: implication for screening. Lancet. 1994;343:75-9.

20. Schaefer EJ, Lamon-Fava S, Jenner JL, et al. Lipoprotein(a) levels and risk of coronary heart disease in men. The lipid research clinics coronary primary prevention trial. JAMA. 1996;271:999-1003.

21. Jauhininen M, Koskinen P, Ehnholm C, et al. Lipoprotein(a) and coronary heart disease risk: a nested case-control study of the Helsinki Heart Study participants. Atherosclerosis. 1991;89:59-67.

22. Ridker PM, Hennekens CH, Stampfer MJ. A prospective study of lipoprotein(a) and the risk of myocardial infarction. JAMA. 1993;270:2195-9.

23. Craig WY, Neveux LM, Palomaki GE, et al. Lipoprotein(a) as a risk factor for ischemic heart disease. Meta-analysis of prospective studies. Clin Chem. 1998;44:2301-06.

24. Danesh J, Collins R, Peto R. Lipoprotein(a) and coronary heart disease. Meta-analysis of prospective studies. Circulation. 2000;102:1082-5.

25. Maher VM, Brown BG, Marcovina SM, et al. Effects of lowering elevated LDL cholesterol on the cardiovascular risk of lipoprotein(a). J Am Med Assoc. 1995;274:1771-4.

26. Luc G, Bard JM, Arveiler D, et al. Lipoprotein(a) as a predictor of coronary heart disease: the PRIME study. Atherosclerosis. 2002;163:377-84.

27. Suk Danik J, Rifai N, Buring JE, et al. Lipoprotein(a) measured with an assay independent of apolipoprotein(a) isoform size and risk of future cardiovascular events among initially healthy women. JAMA. 2006;296:1363-70.

28. Rath M, Niendorf A, Reblin T, et al. Detection and quantification of lipoprotein(a) in the arterial wall of 107 coronary bypass patients. Atherosclerosis. 1989;9:579-92.

29. Marcovina SM, Koschinsky ML. Evaluation of lipoprotein(a) as aprothrombotic factor: progress from bench to bed side. Curr Opin Lipidol. 2003;14:361-6.

30. Undas A, Stnepien E, Tracz W, et al. Lipoprotein(a) as a modifier of fibrin clot permeability and susceptibility to lysis. J Thromb Haemost. 2006;4:973-5.

31. Caplice NM, Panetta C, Peterson TE, et al. Lipoprotein(a) binds and inactivates tissue factor pathway inhibitor: a novel link between lipoprotein and thrombosis. Blood. 2001;98:2980-7.

32. Rand ML, Sangrar W, Hancock MA, et al. Apolipoprotein(a) enhances platelet responses to the thrombin receptor-activating peptide SFLLRN. Arterioscler Thromb Vasc Biol. 1998;18:1393-9.

33. O.998;18:, Boffa MB, Hancock MA, et al. Stimulation of vascular smooth muscle cell proliferation and migration by apolipoprotein(a) is dependent on inhibition of transforming growth factor-beta activation and on the presence of kringle IV type 9. J Biol Chem. 2004;279:55187-95.

34. Kronenberg F, Kronenberg MF, Kiechl S, et al. Role of lipoprotein(a) and apolipoprotein(a) phenotype in atherogenesis: prospective result from the Bruneck study. Circulation. 1999;100:1154-60.

35. Allen S, Khan S, Tam S-P, et al: Expression of adhesion molecules by Lp(a): a potential novel mechanism for its atherogenicity. FASEB J. 1998;12:1765-76.

36. Tsimimkas S, Bergmark C, Beyer RW, et al. Temporal increase in plasma markers of oxidized low-density lipoprotein strongly reflect the presence of acute coronary syndromes. J Am Coll Cardiol. 2003;41:360-70.

37. Sun H, Unoki H, Wang X, et al. Lipoprotein(a) enhances advanced atherosclerosis and vascular calcification in WHHL transgenic rabbits expressing human apolipoprotein(a). J Biol Chem. 2002;277:47486-92.

38. Edelstein C, Pfaffinger D, Hinman J, et al. Lysine physphatidylcholine adducts in kringle V impart unique immunological and protein pro-inflammatory properties to human apolipoprotein(a). J Biol Chem. 2003;278:52841-7.

39. Tate JR, Berg K, Couderc R, et al. International Federation of Clinical Chemistry and Laboratory Medicine (IFCC) standardization project for measurement of Lipoprotein(a). Phase 2: selection and properties of a proposed secondary reference material for lipoprotein(a). Clin Chem Lab Med. 1999;37:949-58.

40. Dati F, Tate JR, Marcovina SM, et al. First WHO/IFCC International Reference Reagent for Lipoprotein(a) for immunoassay-Lp(a) SRM 2B. Clin Chem Lab Med. 2004;42:670-76.

41. Crouse JR III. New developments in the use of niacin of treatment of hyperlipidemia: new considerations in the use of an old drug. Coron Artery Dis. 1996;7:321-6.

42. Sirtori CR, Calabresi L, Ferrara S, et al. L-carnitine reduces the plasma lipoprotein(a) level in patient with hyper Lp(a). Nutr Metab Cardiovasc Dis. 2000;10:247-51.

43. Dalessandri KM. Multiple method for reduction of lipoprotein(a). Atherosclerosis. 2002;163:409-10.

44. Akaike M, Azuma H, Kagawa A, et al. Effect of Aspirin treatment on serum concentration of lipoprotein(a) in patients with atherosclerotic diseases. Clin Chem. 2002;48:1454-9.

45. Crook D, Sidhu M, Seed M, et al. Lipoprotein(a) levels are reduced by danazol, an anabolic steroid. Atherosclerosis. 1992;92:41-7.

46. Rymer J, Crook D, Sidhu M, et al. Effect of tibolone on serum concentration of lipoprotein(a) in postmenopausal women. Acta Endocrinol. 1993;128:259-62.

47. Shewmon DA, Stock JL, Rosen CJ, et al. Tamoxifen and estrogen lower circulating lipoprotein(a) concentration s in healthy postmenopausal women. Atherioscler Thromb. 1994;14:1586-93.

48. Plenge JK, Hernandez TL, Weil KM, et al. Simvastatin lowers C-reactive protein within 14 days: an effect independent of low density lipoprotein cholesterol reduction. Circulation. 2002;106:1447-52.

49. Dujovne CA, Harris WS, Altman R, et al. Effect of atorvastatin on hemorheologci-hemostatic parameters and serum fibrinogen levels in hyperlipidemic patients. Am J Cardiol. 2000;85:350-53.

50. McKenney JM, Jones PH, Bays HE, et al. Comparative effects on lipid levels of combination therapy with statin and extended–Comparative effects on lipid levels of combination therapy . Atherosclerosis. 2007;192:432-7.

51. Kiortsis DN, Tzotzas T, Giral P, et al. Changes in lipoprotein(a) levels and hormonal correlations during weight reduction programme. Nutr Metab Cardiovasc Dis. 2001;11:153-7.

CHAPTER 8

Guideline for the Management of Dyslipidemias

Supertiksh Yadav and Tapan Ghose

- Introduction
- Identification of individuals at risk
- Risk stratification
- Current guidelines
- Monitoring
- Which statin to be used
- Non-statin drugs
- Lifestyle modification
- Future directions
- Conclusion

INTRODUCTION

Abnormal lipids are one of the most important predisposing factors for the development of cardiovascular diseases (CVDs). As CVDs are one of the leading causes of mortality and morbidity in both developed and developing world, there are many guidelines published by different societies all over the world for the management of lipids. Management of abnormal lipids not only includes drug therapy but also identification and stratification of individuals at risk. Our further discussion will be based mainly on the guidelines given by American College of Cardiology/American Heart Association (ACC/AHA),[1] National Institute for Health and Care Excellence (NICE) guidelines[2] and Canadian Cardiovascular Society for the diagnosis and treatment of dyslipidemia for the prevention of CVD in the adult.[3]

IDENTIFICATION OF INDIVIDUALS AT RISK[3]

The following individuals are at an increased risk of cardiovascular (CV) events and merit further evaluation:

- Men ≥40 years of age and women ≥50 years of age or postmenopausal
- All patients with the following conditions, regardless of age:
  - Diabetes
  - Hypertension
  - Current cigarette smoking
  - Obesity (body mass index >27)
  - Family history of premature coronary artery disease

- Family history of hyperlipidemia
- Inflammatory diseases
- Chronic kidney diseases
- Evidence of atherosclerosis or abdominal aneurysm
- Human immunodeficiency virus infection
- Clinical manifestations of hyperlipidemias
- Erectile dysfunction
- Chronic obstructive pulmonary disease
- Children with a family history of hypercholesterolemia or chylomicronemia

How to Screen[3]

- *For all:* history and examination, low-density lipoprotein (LDL), high-density lipoprotein (HDL), triglyceride (TG), non-HDL (will be calculated from profile), glucose and epidermal growth factor receptor (eGFR)
- *Optional:* apoB (instead of standard lipid panel), urine albumin creatinine ratio (if eGFR <60, hypertension and diabetes) and high-sensitivity C-reactive protein (hs-CRP)
- If the Framingham risk score ≥5%, the investigations are repeated every year, otherwise every 3–5 years.

RISK STRATIFICATION

Once individuals at risk are identified, it is recommended that a CV risk assessment using the "10-year risk" method should be done. The most common 10-year risk assessment tools being used are the Framingham risk scoring model in the United States and QRISK2 scoring model in the United Kingdom.[2] These risk calculators are available online for risk calculation.

On the basis of calculated risk, patients can be divided into three risk categories:

1. Low risk: with a 10-year calculated risk of <10%
2. Intermediate risk: with a calculated risk of ≥10 and ≤20%
3. High risk: with a 10-year calculated risk of ≥20%

In recent ACC/AHA guidelines, the 10-year and lifetime risk for atherosclerotic cardiovascular disease (ASCVD) was calculated.[1] The ASCVD is defined as coronary death or nonfatal myocardial infarction (MI), or fatal or nonfatal stroke. The following are included in clinician ASCVD:

1. Acute coronary syndrome
2. Stable or unstable angina
3. History of MI
4. Coronary or peripheral revascularization
5. Stroke
6. Transient ischemic attack
7. Peripheral arterial disease due to atherosclerosis.

The information required to estimate ASCVD risk includes age, sex, race, total cholesterol, HDL cholesterol, systolic blood pressure, blood pressure-lowering medication use, diabetes status and smoking status.

Estimates of 10-year risk of ASCVD are based on data from multiple community-based populations. Primarily, they are applicable to African American and non-Hispanic white men and women at 40 through 79 years of age. For other ethnic groups, the guidelines recommend use of the equations for non-Hispanic whites. These estimates may potentially underestimate the risk for persons from some race/ethnic groups, especially American Indians, some Asian Americans (e.g., of South Asian ancestry) and some Hispanics (e.g., Puerto Ricans), and may overestimate the risk for others, including some Asian Americans (e.g., of East Asian ancestry) and some Hispanics (e.g., Mexican Americans).

The estimates of lifetime risk are most directly applicable to non-Hispanic whites. On the basis of this risk calculator, patients are divided into three categories: high risk (>10%), moderate risk (>7.5% to <10%) and low risk (<5%).

CURRENT GUIDELINES

All the previous guidelines published have got certain target levels of cholesterol to reach in different subgroups. But the most recent guidelines published from ACC/AHA group[1] have refrained from giving such targets to reach (target-based therapy). Instead, they have laid more stress on reduction in relation to the patient's basal LDL cholesterol level in different risk category groups (risk-based therapy). Salient features of current guidelines are as follows:

Cornerstones of these guidelines are risk stratification, lifestyle modification and drug treatment to modify blood cholesterol levels.

These guidelines have broadly stratified the patients into four groups according to their risk and drug therapy, i.e. high, moderate and low intensity, depending upon the reduction achieved in LDL levels. Key recommendations of these guidelines are as follows:

1. Healthy lifestyle habits to be encouraged in all individuals.
2. If a patient is having clinical ASCVD, then the patient should receive high-intensity statin therapy, provided the patient is <75 years of age, and there are no safety concerns for statin, otherwise use moderate-intensity statin (secondary prevention).
3. In patients without ASCVD but LDL levels ≥190 mg/dL, use high-intensity statin therapy to achieve >50% reduction in baseline LDL level. If the levels are not achieved, non-statin therapy can also be used. But secondary cause of hyperlipidemia should be ruled out before starting therapy (primary prevention).
4. In patients without ASCVD but with diabetes mellitus and LDL level between 70 and 189 mg/dL in the age group 40–75 years, moderate-intensity statin therapy is recommended. Consider high-intensity statin when 10-year ASCVD risk >7.5%.
5. In patients with LDL level 70–189 mg/dL, age 40–75 years with no diabetes and no clinical ASCVD, consider 10-year ASCVD score every 4–6 years.
6. If 10-year risk ≥7.5, consider moderate- to high-intensity statin and if 10-year risk is 5–7.5%, then consider moderate-intensity statin. In deciding the therapy, other factors like LDL ≥160 mg/dL, family history of premature ASCVD, hs-CRP ≥2.0 mg/dL, coronary artery calcium score ≥300 Agatston units and ankle brachial index <0.9 are considered.
7. In patients with LDL <190 mg/dL, age <40 years or >75 years and 10-year ASCVD risk <5%, statin therapy may be considered in selected individuals.
8. Statin therapy is not routinely recommended in patients with New York Health Association class II–IV heart failure and patients who are on maintenance hemodialysis.

MONITORING[1]

1. Assess adherence, response to therapy and adverse effects within 4–12 weeks of start and change of therapy.
2. Measure a fasting lipid profile and do not routinely measure liver function tests and creatine kinase unless symptomatic.
3. Screen and treat diabetes mellitus according to current guidelines.
4. Anticipated therapeutic response in high-intensity statin group is ≥50% reduction from baseline LDL level and in moderate-intensity group is between 30 and 50%.
5. If there is insufficient response to therapy, reinforce lifestyle modification, rule out secondary cause of hyperlipidemia and increase the statin dose to the maximum tolerated level.
6. Consider addition of non-statin treatment in selected high-risk individuals whose target levels are not achieved, such as patients with clinical ASCVD, LDL level ≥190 mg/dL and diabetics in the age group 40–75 years.

WHICH STATIN TO BE USED

Atorvastatin is the most preferred statin.[2]

1. High-intensity group[1] (target baseline LDL reduction >50%) = atorvastatin 40–80 mg, rosuvastatin 20–40 mg.
2. Moderate-intensity group[1] (target baseline LDL reduction 30–50%) = atorvastatin 20–40 mg, rosuvastatin 5–10 mg, pravastatin 40 mg, simvastatin 20–40 mg, lovastatin 20–40 mg, fluvastatin 40 mg twice daily.
3. Low-intensity group[1] (target baseline LDL reduction <30%) = simvastatin 10–20 mg, pravastatin 20 mg, lovastatin 10–20 mg.

NON-STATIN THERAPY FOR LIPID MANAGEMENT

Other drugs that can be used for dyslipidemia include fibrates, bile acid sequestrants (BAS), omega-3 fatty acids and cholesterol absorption inhibitor drugs like ezetimibe.

Fibrates

Do not routinely offer fibrates for the prevention of CVD to any of the following:[2]

1. People who are being treated for primary prevention
2. People who are being treated for secondary prevention
3. People with chronic kidney disease (CKD)
4. People with type 1 diabetes
5. People with type 2 diabetes.

Gemfibrozil should not be initiated in patients who are already on statin therapy because of an increased risk of muscle symptoms and rhabdomyolysis. However, fenofibrate may be used concomitantly with low- or moderate-intensity statin therapy when TGs are high (≥500 mg/dL). Risk versus benefit of combination therapy should be considered before initiation of combination therapy.

Renal status should be assessed before fenofibrate initiation, within 3 months after initiation and every 6 months thereafter. Assess renal safety with both a serum creatinine level and an eGFR based on creatinine.

- Fenofibrate should not be used if moderate or severe renal impairment, defined as eGFR <30 mL/min/1.73 m^2, is present.
- If eGFR is between 30 and 59 mL/min/1.73 m^2, the dose of fenofibrate should not exceed 54 mg/day.
- If during follow-up the eGFR decreases persistently to <30 mL/min/1.73 m^2, fenofibrate should be discontinued.[1]

Bile Acid Sequestrants

Do not routinely offer BAS for the prevention of CVD to any of the following:[2]

1. People who are being treated for primary prevention
2. People who are being treated for secondary prevention
3. People with CKD
4. People with type 1 diabetes
5. People with type 2 diabetes.

Bile acid sequestrants should not be used in individuals with baseline fasting TG levels ≥300 mg/dL or type III hyperlipoproteinemia. This may cause severe elevation of TG level. A fasting lipid profile should be obtained before BAS are initiated, 3 months after initiation and every 6–12 months thereafter.[1]

It is reasonable to use BAS with caution if baseline TG levels are 250–299 mg/dL. A fasting lipid panel should be obtained 4–6 weeks after initiation. If TGs exceed 400 mg/dL,[1] BAS are discontinued.

Nicotinic Acid (Niacin)

Do not routinely offer niacin for the prevention of CVD to any of the following:[2]

1. People who are being treated for primary prevention
2. People who are being treated for secondary prevention
3. People with CKD
4. People with type 1 diabetes
5. People with type 2 diabetes.

In the contemporary period of clinical practice, they have only a limited role. The statin intolerant group is a target.

Baseline hepatic transaminases, fasting blood glucose or hemoglobin (Hb) A1c and uric acid should be obtained before initiation of niacin and again during up-titration to a maintenance dose and every 6 months thereafter.[1]

Niacin should not be used if:[1]

- Hepatic transaminase levels are higher than two to three times upper limit of normal (ULN).
- Persistent severe cutaneous symptoms, persistent hyperglycemia, acute gout, or unexplained abdominal pain or gastrointestinal symptoms occur.
- New-onset atrial fibrillation or weight loss occurs.

The potential for ASCVD benefits and the potential for adverse effects should be reconsidered before reinitiation of niacin therapy.

The frequency and severity of adverse cutaneous symptoms can be reduced by severe means:

- Start niacin at a low dose and up-titrate to a higher dose slowly over a period of weeks as tolerated
- Always advise to take niacin with food or premedicate with aspirin 325 mg, 30 minutes before niacin dosing to alleviate cutaneous flush
- If an extended-release preparation is used, increase the dose of extended-release niacin from 500 mg to a maximum of 2,000 mg/day over 4–8 weeks
- If immediate-release niacin is chosen, start at a dose of 100 mg, three times daily and up-titrate to 3 g/day, divided into two or three doses.

Omega-3 Fatty Acids

The role of omega-3 fatty acids in lipid management is controversial. The AHA recommended individuals without documented CHD to include fish test two times a week to attain an average intake of omega-3 fatty acids up to 500 mg/day.[4]

For patients with established CHD, intake should be increased up to 1 g/day.

In patients with hypertriglyceridemia, recommendation is up to 2–4 g/day under supervision.

If eicosapentaenoic acid and/or docosahexaenoic acid are used for the management of severe hypertriglyceridemia, defined as TGs ≥500 mg/dL, it is reasonable to evaluate the patient for gastrointestinal disturbances, skin changes and bleeding.[1]

But recent NICE guidelines have not supported their use in the management of dyslipidemia.

Do not offer omega-3 fatty acid compounds for the prevention of CVD to any of the following:[2]

1. People who are being treated for primary prevention
2. People who are being treated for secondary prevention
3. People with CKD
4. People with type 1 diabetes
5. People with type 2 diabetes.

In view of divergent views on the role of omega-3 fatty acids, we suggest to increase omega-3 fatty acid uptake in diet from natural sources like fish, walnut and flaxseed oil.

Ezetimibe

People with primary hypercholesterolemia should be considered for ezetimibe in line with the use of ezetimibe for the treatment of primary (heterozygous familial and nonfamilial) hypercholesterolemia.[2]

It is reasonable to obtain baseline hepatic transaminases before initiation of ezetimibe. When ezetimibe is coadministered with a statin, monitor transaminase levels as clinically indicated and discontinue ezetimibe if persistent alanine aminotransferase elevations greater than or equal to three times ULN occur.[1]

LIFESTYLE MODIFICATIONS[3]

Cardioprotective Diet

- People at high risk of or with CVD should be advised to have a diet in which total fat intake is 30% or less of total energy intake, saturated fats are 10% or less of total energy intake and intake of dietary cholesterol is <300 mg/day. Saturated fats should be replaced by monounsaturated and polyunsaturated fats.
- People at high risk of or with CVD should be advised to take at least five portions of fruit and vegetables per day.
- People at high risk of or with CVD should be advised to consume at least two portions of fish per week, including a portion of oily fish that includes the following: mackerel, salmon, sardines, herring or hilsa. Pregnant women should be advised to limit their oily fish to no more than two portions per week.
- People should not routinely be recommended to take omega-3 fatty acid supplements for the primary prevention of CVD.

Plant Stanols and Sterols

- People should not routinely be recommended to take plant sterols and stanols for the primary prevention of CVD.

Physical Activity

- People at high risk of or with CVD should be encouraged to do 30 minutes of physical activity (brisk walking, cycling or swimming) a day, of at least moderate intensity, at least 5 days a week. For Asian Indians, this period extended to 45 minutes because of increased visceral obesity.
- People who are unable to perform moderate-intensity physical activity at least 5 days a week because of comorbidity, medical conditions or personal circumstances should be encouraged to exercise at their maximum safe capacity.
- Isotonic exercises are cardioprotective. Recommended types of physical activities are those that can be incorporated into everyday life, such as brisk walking, using stairs and cycling.
- People should be advised that bouts of physical activity of 10 minutes or more accumulated throughout the day, which are as effective as longer sessions.

Weight Management

- People at high risk of or with CVD who are overweight or obese should be offered appropriate advice and support to work toward achieving and maintaining a healthy weight, in line with "obesity."

Alcohol Consumption

- Alcohol consumption should be limited to up to 3–4 units a day for men and up to 2–3 units a day for women. People should avoid binge drinking.

Smoking Cessation

All people who smokes should be a advised to stop smoking.

FUTURE DIRECTIONS

In spite of the treatment with high-dose statin, some event still occur (residual risk). Blocking the LDL receptor degradation is one approach. Proliferator-activated receptor gamma blockers have shown success in diabetic dyslipidemias. They reduce LDL, TG and also HbA1c levels. These molecules are likely to be incorporated in the management in individual cases.

CONCLUSION

Management of abnormal lipids requires a holistic approach centered around the patient's clinical and biochemical parameters and total risk profile. Diet, exercise and drugs are the twice pronged approach to treatment. Statin group of drugs have a strong role in the secondary prevention of CV death and major adverse events. The patient should be regularly monitored for the effectiveness of therapy and adherence. Adherence to therapy is associated with the maximal benefit.

REFERENCES

1. Stone NJ, Robinson J, Lichtenstein AH, et al. 2013 ACC/AHA guideline on the treatment of blood cholesterol to reduce atherosclerotic cardiovascular risk in adults: a report of the American College of Cardiology/American Heart Association Task Force on practice guidelines. J Am Coll Cardiol. 2013;63(25 Pt B):2889-934.
2. National Institute for Health and Clinical Excellence. Lipid modification: cardiovascular risk assessment and the modification of blood lipids for the primary and secondary prevention of cardiovascular disease. London: NICE; 2008. www.nice.org.uk/CG67.
3. Anderson TJ, Grégoire J, Hegele RA, et al. 2012 Update of the Canadian Cardiovascular Society Guidelines for the diagnosis and treatment of dyslipidemia for the prevention of cardiovascular disease in the adult. Can J Cardiol. 2013;29:151-67.
4. Kris-Etherton PM, Harris WS, Appel LJ. Fish consumption, fish oil, omega-3 fatty acids and cardiovascular disease. Circulation. 2002;106:2747-57.

Diet in Dyslipidemia

Dipti Sharma

- Introduction
- Different nutrients
- Management of dyslipidemia
- Dietary modifications of cardiovascular protection
- Combination diets
- Stepwise approach to diet therapy
- Assessing response to therapeutic lifestyle changes
- Conclusion

INTRODUCTION

Human nutrition is the provision to ingest and utilize materials necessary for its survival. A human being can survive between 2 and 8 weeks without food, whereas survival without water is usually approximately for 4 days. Nutrients can be classified into two major groups: macronutrients and micronutrients.

Macronutrients are needed in large amounts. They are (i) carbohydrates, (ii) fats, (iii) proteins, (iv)water and (v) fibers. Micronutrients are required in small quantities. They are (i) minerals, (ii) vitamins, (iii) antioxidants and (iv) phytochemicals.

DIFFERENT NUTRIENTS

Carbohydrates supply 17 kJ (kilojoules) or 4 kcal of energy/g. Carbohydrates can be simple (monosaccharides that contain one sugar unit, e.g., glucose, fructose and galactose) or complex (polysaccharides that contain three or more sugar units, e.g., starch). Simple carbohydrates are absorbed rapidly and hence cause early and higher peak of blood glucose level (high glycemic index) than the complex carbohydrates (which are broken down to small units and cause delayed and lower peak level of plasma glucose (low glycemic index). Carbohydrates come from rice-, bread- and grain-based products.

Dietary fat contains fatty acids bonded to glycerol. Typically, they are found in triglycerides (three fatty acids bonded to one glycerol). Fats can be classified into saturated or unsaturated fats. All carbon atoms of the fatty acids are bonded to hydrogen atoms in saturated fats, whereas in unsaturated fats, some of the carbon atoms are not bonded to hydrogen atom and contain double bonds. Unsaturated fats may be monounsaturated (one double bond) or polyunsaturated (more than one double bond). Depending on the double bond location in the fatty acid chain, unsaturated fats may be further divided into omega-3 or omega-6 fatty acids. Unsaturated fats with transisomer bonds are called trans fats that result from cooking and industrial processing by the process of hydrogenation. Saturated fats are solid at room temperature (butter and ghee). Unsaturated fats are liquid at room temperature (mustard oil, olive oil and flaxseed oil). Essential fatty acids (EFAs) are the fatty acids that cannot be synthesized in human body and must be supplied from outside of body. They are α-linolenic acid (an omega-3 fatty acid) and linoleic acid (omega-6 fatty acid). Conditionally, EFAs are docosahexaenoic acid (DHA) (omega-3) and gamma linolenic (omega-6) acids. Fats provide 37 kJ (9kcal) energy/g.

Proteins are the building blocks of organisms. Muscle skin, hair and organs contain proteins. Amino acids are grouped together to form proteins. In other words, when proteins are digested by proteolytic enzymes, amino acids are liberated. The human body contains approximately 22 amino acids and about 10 of them are essential and must be included in the diet. Sources of proteins in the human diet are meat, tofu, soy products, grains, legumes, egg, fish, milk, cheese and curd.

Minerals are elements that are essential for humans. They are carbon, hydrogen, nitrogen and calcium. Calcium is required in a large quantity. The recommended daily allowance (RDA) of calcium is 1000 mg/dL of age 19–51 years. Overall, 99% of the calcium lies in bones and teeth. Some calcium is in free form and some is bound to proteins in the plasma. Some sources of calcium are milk products, turnip, mustard greens, tofu, cheese, milk, sardines, animal and fish bones and oysters. Magnesium (RDA for men at age >31 years is 420 mg/day) is required for both bodybuilding and enzyme function as it acts as a coenzyme in many biochemical reactions. Sources of magnesium are cereals, tofu, meat, milk, legumes, chocolate, green vegetables and apricot.

Phosphorus (RDA 700 mg/day) is another important mineral that is obtained from cheese, eggs, milk, meat, fish, poultry and whole grain cereals. Potassium (K+) is obtained from fruits and vegetables, fresh meat and dairy products, whereas sodium (Na+) is obtained from all of the food items and classical common salt (sodium chloride). Iron (RDA 8 mg/day for men, 18 mg/day for women) is required for hemoglobin synthesis.

Trace elements are those elements that are required in a minute quantity (<200 mg/day) for body functions. They are cobalt, chromium, copper, zinc, iodine, manganese, molybdenum, selenium and nickel. Thiamine (β1), riboflavin (β2), niacin (β3), pyridoxine (β6), cobalamin (β12), ascorbic acid (vitamin C) and vitamin A, D, E and K are the vitamins required for human health.

MANAGEMENT OF DYSLIPIDEMIA[1]

Therapeutic lifestyle changes (TLC), which was formerly called lifestyle modification, is the cornerstone in managing dyslipidemia. A multidimensional lifestyle modification approach is recommended to reduce the risk of coronary heart disease (CHD). Manipulation in the diet, regular isotonic physical exercise and drug therapy are the three pronged approaches to the management of cardiometabolic disorders.

Therapeutic lifestyle changes denote dietary modification, weight reduction, regular isotonic physical activity, cessation of smoking and alcohol restriction. They should precede or be initiated together with drug therapy and should be directed especially at individuals who are obese, who smoke and who seldom exercise. In the population without CHD or CHD risk equivalents (i.e., primary prevention of coronary artery disease), emphasis should be placed on lifestyle modification. Therapeutic lifestyle changes diet and other low-density lipoprotein (LDL)-lowering options reduce LDL cholesterol (LDL-C) by 24–37%.

DIETARY MODIFICATION FOR CARDIOVASCULAR PROTECTION

Impact of diet on human behavior and outcomes were described in ancient Indian literature (in SradhatrayaBibhag Yoga in Bhagavad Gita, 3500 BC) and during biblical times.

Dietary modifications that have been shown to be cardioprotective are (i) increased consumption of fruits and vegetables; (ii) consumption of whole grain; (iii) consumption of fish protein and fish oil; (iv) reduction in the amount of dairy products; (v) consumption of nuts, legumes and seeds and (vi) moderation in alcohol intake.

Fruits and Vegetables

Nurses' Health Study showed that consumption of fruits and vegetables >8 servings/day was associated with cardioprotection. Green leafy vegetable- and vitamin C-rich foods are most cardioprotective. Women Health Study and Physician Health study showed similar benefit. A physician health study ($N = 22,000$, follow-up period 12 years) showed that consumption of at least 2 servings of vegetables reduced CHD by 22% (relative risk 0.77, 95% confidence interval 0.60–0.98). Vasculoprotective effect of diet was shown in the reduction of myocardial infarction (MI), CHD mortality, stroke incidence and death from stroke.

Grains

These include wheat, brown rice, corn, oats, barley, rye, triticale, bulgur, sorghum and millet. Consumption of whole grain confers vascular protection. Whole grain supplies dietary fiber, minerals, vitamins and other micronutrients in addition to the calorie. Progression of carotid intima media thickness is reduced by consumption of whole grains. A meta-analysis of seven prospective cohort studies showed that consumption of whole grain (0.25 mg/dL, 2.5 servings/dL) is associated with 21% reduction in CVD events.

Dietary Supplements

Lipid level in the blood is altered by a number of dietary approaches or specific dietary supplements. Dietary modifications or supplements differ with respect to mechanism of action and to the degree and type of lipid lowering. Hence, the indications for a particular dietary supplement are influenced by the underlying lipid abnormality.

The characteristics and efficacy of the lipid-modifying dietary supplements or dietary components have been described in the following section.

Fish Oil and Omega-3 Fatty Acids[2,3,4]

Rich sources of omega-3 fatty acids are fatty fish, especially salmon. The plant sources are flaxseed and flaxseed oil, canola oil, soybean oil and nuts. Docosahexaenoic acid and eicosapentaenoic acid (EPA) are long-chain omega-3 fatty acids that have been used as supplements in statin refractory or statin-intolerant individuals.

Fish oil concentrate capsule administered at high doses (>6 g/day) can reduce levels of triglycerides through inhibition of the synthesis of very low-density lipoprotein-triglycerides and apolipoprotein B.

In hypertriglyceridemic subjects, fish oil supplement (at a dose of 15 g/day) in addition to regular exercise lowers triglyceride levels by approximately 50%. Since fish oil lowers plasma triglyceride concentration, which in turn determines the density of LDL, it is possible that fish oil will decrease the concentration of small dense LDL particles. Reduction in cholesterol ester transferase activity following fish oil therapy supports this hypothesis.

Several dietary intervention studies have also observed an increase in overall LDL particle size with 4 g purified DHA. In contrast, 2.5 g of omega-3 fatty acids daily for 2 months did not significantly change this fraction in patients with type 2 diabetes when compared with placebo. The pharmacological use of fish oil supplements should be restricted to patients with refractory hypertriglyceridemia, more so when statin therapy is not tolerated or desired by the patient. At present, it seems that both EPA and DHA have triglyceride-lowering properties.

Effective doses of omega-3 fatty acids range from 3 to 5 g/day, which can only be obtained consistently by supplementation. Consumption of fish reduced the incidence of MI, cardiac mortality, stroke and stroke mortality. A meta-analysis of 13 cohort studies has shown that fish consumption was associated with cardiac mortality benefit. Fish consumption 5 times/week reduced CHD mortality by 38%. Omega-3 fatty acids, particularly two linolenic acids, confer a cardioprotective effect.

Soy

Soy contains soy proteins and isoflavones. Isoflavones are micronutrients that have properties similar to estrogen. Soy is extracted from soybean.

When very large amount of soy protein, approximately 50 g, is substituted by other dietary proteins, LDL-C concentrations decrease by an average of 3%. No significant effect on high-density lipoprotein cholesterol (HDL-C), triglycerides or lipoprotein (a) is seen.

Apart from lipid effects, intake of soy proteins has other vascular benefits. The phytoestrogen genistein causes endothelium-dependent vasodilation with a similar potency to estradiol. This beneficial effect on endothelial function may be related to soy isoflavones.

Substituting soy protein by other proteins does not appear to have clinically important health benefits. Recommendations suggest that isoflavone supplements do not appear to be of benefit and should not be taken with a goal of improving lipids and cardiovascular risk.

Red Yeast Rice[5]

Red yeast rice is a fermented rice product that has been used in Chinese food. The product contains varying amounts of substances called monacolins that have 3-hydroxy-3-methylglutaryl-coenzyme A (HMG-CoA) reductase inhibitor activity. Other active ingredients in red yeast rice that may affect cholesterol lowering include sterols (β-sitosterol, campesterol, stigmasterol and sapogenin), isoflavones and monounsaturated fatty acids.

The efficacy of red yeast rice for cholesterol lowering was evaluated in a prospective, double-blind study. Red yeast at a dose of 2.4 g/day reduced total cholesterol and LDL-C with no effect on HDL-C. One of the monacolins in red yeast rice extract used in this study, monacolin K, is the active ingredient in the HMG-CoA reductase inhibitor lovastatin. Other studies have also found that red yeast rice lowers total cholesterol and LDL-C.

Plant Sterols[6,7]

Plant sterols are similar in chemical structure to cholesterol, differing in their side chain configuration. The mechanism by which they lower cholesterol is by inhibition of cholesterol absorption. However, the decrease in serum cholesterol is less than that expected by the degree of reduced absorption.

None of these products has been adequately studied for clinical end points. Local accumulation of plant sterols has been observed in patients with aortic valve lesions. By consuming 1.6–3 g/day of plant stanols or sterols found in enriched foods, LDL can be modestly lowered. This is a very important dietary modification in statin-intolerant patients.

Margarines

Cholesterol-lowering margarines enriched with plant sterols are available. Plants contain a number of sterols. Two saturated plant stanols, sitostanol and campestanol, are the main sterols present in supplements. Daily intake of 0.8–3 g of plant stanols and/or sterols in these margarines appears to lower serum cholesterol level. Responses to plant sterol ester-containing spreads may vary by ApoE genotype.

A number of studies have examined the efficacy of plant stanol- and sterol-enriched margarines for lowering cholesterol. Stanol-enriched margarine can also reduce cholesterol in patients receiving a stable dose of a statin drug. As an example, one series of 167 subjects with an LDL-C ≥130 mg/dL, in spite of at least 3 months of statin therapy, found that 5.1 g/day of plant stanol ester for 8 weeks reduced total cholesterol by 12% (vs. 5% for placebo) and LDL-C by 17% (vs. 7% for placebo).

Short-term studies have shown no adverse effects of consumption of margarines fortified with plant sterols/stanol esters.

There have been no studies demonstrating that consumption of these stanol ester-containing margarines influences the incidence of CHD. Concerns related to the accumulation of plant sterols do not apply to these products since stanol esters are not absorbed, unlike plant sterols; they protect against the potential accumulation associated with β-sitosterolemia.

Polyphenols

Polyphenols are substances found in plants and foods made from plants, such as tea, coffee, cocoa, olive oil and red wine that appear to have antioxidant effects. They also appear to have immunomodulatory and vasodilatory properties that could contribute to cardiovascular risk reduction. Polyphenols include flavonoids and flavonoid derivatives, lignans, phenolic acids and stilbenes.

A randomized crossover trial in 200 men compared the effects on serum lipids of virgin olive oil (high in polyphenols), refined olive oil (low in polyphenols) and a mixture of the two with intermediate polyphenol content. A dose–response was seen, where olive oil with higher amounts of polyphenols had greater effects on raising HDL-C and lowering oxidized LDL.

In addition to these lipid effects, a meta-analysis of randomized trials found consistent evidence that both acute and chronic chocolate and cocoa ingestion increase flow-mediated vasodilatation, reduce systolic and diastolic blood pressures and reduce serum insulin level.

Fiber[11]

Eating a diet that is high in fiber confers many health benefits. This includes a decreased risk of heart disease, stroke and type 2 diabetes. Most dietary fiber is not digested or absorbed, so it stays within the intestine where it modulates digestion of other foods and affects the consistency of excreta.

There are two types of fibers: soluble and insoluble fibers. Dietary fiber is the sum of all soluble and insoluble fibers.

Soluble fiber consists of a group of substances that is made of complex carbohydrates and dissolves in water. Examples of various foods that contain soluble fiber include fruits, oats, barley and legumes (peas and beans).

Insoluble fiber is obtained from plant cells' walls and it does not dissolve in water. Examples of various foods that contain insoluble fiber include wheat, rye and other grains. The traditional fiber that is used most often, wheat bran, is a type of insoluble fiber.

Certain soluble fibers (psyllium, pectin, wheat dextrin and oat products) have the capacity to reduce LDL-C in plasma when they are used as a supplement. In a meta-analysis, every gram increase in soluble fiber reduced LDL-C by an average of 2.2mg/dL. The molecular weight and amount of β-glucan in food products such as oats may alter the LDL-lowering effects. The addition of psyllium supplementation may result in small further reductions in LDL-C concentrations in patients receiving low-dose statin therapy.

Both the Third Report of the Expert Panel on Detection, Evaluation and Treatment of High Blood Cholesterol in Adults (ATP III) and the American Heart Association recommend soluble fiber as an optional dietary strategy to reduce cholesterol levels. The recommended amount of dietary fiber is 20–35 g/day.

Nuts[8]

Small randomized trials have shown that walnuts, which are rich in polyunsaturated fatty acids, have a beneficial effect on serum lipids. Walnut-rich diets cause a 4–12% reduction in serum total cholesterol and a 6–12% reduction in serum LDL-C.

Other trials demonstrated similar lipid-lowering effects with almonds and pistachios and other nuts. With a mean daily intake of 67 g of nuts, total cholesterol decreases by 10.9 mg/dL and LDL-C decreased by 10.2 mg/dL. A dose–response effect is seen, and different types of nuts had similar effects on lipid levels.

There is also evidence that increased nut intake is associated with improved cardiovascular outcomes.

Green Tea[9]

A meta-analysis of 14 randomized trials found that consumption of green tea beverages and extracts results in a statistically significant reduction in LDL-C (–2.19 mg/dL) but no statistically significant change in HDL-C. This small reduction in LDL-C is unlikely to be clinically important. Although not specifically related to lipid levels, an observational study from Japan found that consumption of green tea was inversely associated with all-cause mortality and cardiovascular mortality.

Alcohol

Moderation of alcohol intake (½ to 1/day for women and 1–2/day for men) is associated with cardioprotective effect. The benefit conferred by alcohol intake was shown to be related to increased HDLconcentration or genetic factors. In the recent INTERHEART study, moderate alcohol consumption was associated with prevention of first MI. However, this benefit was not shown in an Indian cohort of the same study.

COMBINATION DIET

Mediterranean Diet

A Mediterranean diet appears to reduce the risk of cardiovascular events. There is no single Mediterranean diet, but such diets are typically high in fruits, vegetables, whole grains, beans, nuts and seeds and include olive oil as an important source of fat; there are typically low-to-moderate amounts of fish, poultry and dairy products, and there is little red meat. It is uncertain whether the cardiovascular benefits of a Mediterranean diet are due to its lipid effects.

A large randomized trial ($N = 7447$) compared three diets in patients at high cardiovascular risk: a Mediterranean diet supplemented with olive oil, a Mediterranean diet supplemented with mixed nuts and advice to reduce dietary fat. The trial was stopped early after a median follow-up of 4.8 years. For the primary composite cardiovascular end point of MI, stroke and cardiovascular death, event rates were similar for the Mediterranean diets supplemented with olive oil and mixed nuts, and lower than for the control diet (8.1 and 8.0 events/1000 person-years respectively, vs. 11.2 events/1000 person-years). Even in patients with an acute coronary syndrome, adherence to a Mediterranean diet is associated with better prognosis and greater preservation of left ventricular systolic function.

Dietary Approaches to Stop Hypertension Diet

The Dietary Approaches to Stop Hypertension (DASH) diet is rich in fruits and vegetables, moderate in low-fat dairy products, low in animal protein and contains many plant sources of protein, including legumes and nuts. The DASH diet decreases LDL-C and has been shown to improve several lipid markers in type 2 diabetics. It may also decrease the risk of stroke and CHD.

STEPWISE APPROACH TO DIET THERAPY[10,12]

The guidelines are designed to assist individuals in achieving and maintaining a healthy dietary pattern that translates in the reduction and regression in the process of atherosclerosis in the various vascular territories in the human body.

Healthy Diet: Variation in Type and Source

- One should consume a variety of fruits and vegetables and grain products, including whole grains.
- Diet should include fat-free and/or low-fat dairy products, fish, legumes, poultry and lean meats.

Attain and Maintain an Ideal Body Weight Associated with Reduced Vascular Events

- Match intake of energy (calories) to overall energy needs; limit consumption of foods with a high caloric density and/or low nutritional quality, including those with a high content of sugars.
- Maintain a level of physical activity that achieves fitness and balances energy expenditure with energy intake; for weight reduction, expenditure should exceed intake.

Aim for a Healthy Blood Cholesterol and Lipoprotein Profile

- Limit the ingestion of foods with a high content of saturated fatty acids and cholesterol.
- Substitute grains and unsaturated fatty acids from vegetables, fish, legumes and nuts.

Achieve Desirable Blood Pressure

- Limit the intake of salt (sodium chloride) to <6 g/day.
- Limit alcohol consumption (no more than 1 drink/day for women and 2 drinks/day for men).

ASSESSING RESPONSE TO THERAPEUTIC LIFESTYLE CHANGES

The lipid profile should be measured 6–8 weeks after initiating lifestyle measures. Generally, TLC may reduce lipid levels (at best) up to 20%. Individuals who attain target lipid levels should continue these lifestyle changes lifelong to maintain these effects. They can be reassessed every 6 months with a full lipoprotein analysis. If, however, these levels are not achieved, patient compliance should be reassessed and TLC regimen intensified. They are then reassessed after 6–8 weeks. There is a genetically determined interindividual variability in the response to both dietary manipulation and exercise. Thus, poor response to TLC is not always due to noncompliance.

For individuals at low risk, failure to achieve a defined target value for LDL-C does not necessarily mean that dietary therapy should be replaced by drug therapy. Whatever reduction that is achieved will help lower the risk of CHD, especially with the concomitant adoption of a healthy lifestyle. Statin may be added at this juncture. When a decision has been made to start drug therapy, TLC must still be continued indefinitely because it provides substantial additive LDL-C-lowering effects.

CONCLUSION

Increasing evidence supports the benefits of maintaining normal plasma lipoprotein levels, body weight and blood pressure for reducing risk of cardiovascular events and reducing its progression and even regression. Dietary guidelines provide a means for achieving these goals while ensuring an overall balanced and nutritious dietary pattern. Adoption of these recommendations, together with other healthy practices such as regular physical exercise and smoking cessation, can contribute substantially to reducing the burden of cardiovascular disease in the general population. This low-cost intervention is the most effective high-yield intervention that is possible across to apply to every population group.

REFERENCES

1. Varady KA, Jones PJ. Combination diet and exercise interventions for the treatment of dyslipidemia: an effective preliminary strategy to lower cholesterol levels? J Nutr. 2005;135:1829.
2. Rissanen T, Voutilainen S, Nyyssönen K, et al. Fish oil-derived fatty acids, docosahexaenoic acid and docosapentaenoic acid, and the risk of acute coronary events: the Kuopio ischaemic heart disease risk factor study. Circulation. 2000;102:2677.

3. Harper CR, Jacobson TA. The fats of life: the role of omega-3 fatty acids in the prevention of coronary heart disease. Arch Intern Med. 2001;161:2185.
4. Sullivan DR, Sanders TA, Trayner IM, et al. Paradoxical elevation of LDLapoprotein B levels in hypertriglyceridaemic patients and normal subjects ingesting fish oil. Atherosclerosis. 1986;61:129.
5. Becker DJ, Gordon RY, Halbert SC, et al. Red yeast rice for dyslipidemia in statin-intolerant patients: a randomized trial. Ann Intern Med. 2009;150:830.
6. Chen JT, Wesley R, Shamburek RD, et al. Meta-analysis of natural therapies for hyperlipidemia: plant sterols and stanols versus policosanol. Pharmacotherapy. 2005;25:171.
7. MacDougall DE, Ntanios F, Vanstone CA. Dietary phytosterols as cholesterol-lowering agents in humans. Can J Physiol Pharmacol. 1997;75:217.
8. Sabaté J, Fraser GE, Burke K, et al. Effects of walnuts on serum lipid levels and blood pressure in normal men. N Engl J Med. 1993;328:603.
9. Kuriyama S, Shimazu T, Ohmori K, et al. Green tea consumption and mortality due to cardiovascular disease, cancer, and all causes in Japan: the Ohsaki study. JAMA. 2006;296:1255.
10. American Heart Association Nutrition Committee, Lichtenstein AH, Appel LJ, et al. Diet and lifestyle recommendations revision 2006: a scientific statement from the American Heart Association Nutrition Committee. Circulation. 2006;114:82.
11. Brown L, Rosner B, Willett WW, et al. Cholesterol-lowering effects of dietary fiber: a meta-analysis. Am J Clin Nutr. 1999;69:30.
12. National Cholesterol Education Program (NCEP) Expert Panel on Detection, Evaluation, and Treatment of High Blood Cholesterol in Adults (Adult Treatment Panel III). Third Report of the National Cholesterol Education Program (NCEP) Expert Panel on Detection, Evaluation, and Treatment of High Blood Cholesterol in Adults (Adult Treatment Panel III) final report. Circulation. 2002;106:3143.

Lifestyle Modifications for the Management of Dyslipidemia

SC Manchanda and Kushal Madan

- Introduction
- Role of physical exercise (PE)
- Effects of PE on HDL cholesterol
- Effects of PE on triglycerides
- Effects of PE on LDL cholesterol
- Role of smoking cessation on lipids
- Effect of alcohol on lipids
- Effect of yoga on lipids
- Conclusion

INTRODUCTION

Lifestyle modifications, including diet control, physical exercise (PE), tobacco cessation, moderate alcohol intake and stress management, are essential and are most important cost-effective methods to control dyslipidemia and for overall primary and secondary prevention of heart disease.

ROLE OF PHYSICAL EXERCISE

There is ample evidence that physical inactivity is an important risk factor for the development of coronary artery disease (CAD), hypertension, obesity, dyslipidemia and type II diabetes mellitus (T2DM).[1-3] Conversely, PE is associated with reduction in risk for CAD, T2DM, hypertension and obesity.[4] The benefit of PE on cardiovascular (CV) risk has been postulated to be multifactorial, including effects on thrombus, endothelial function, inflammation, autonomic nervous system, decrease in blood pressure, obesity, glucose metabolism, insulin resistance and effects on lipids.

Physical exercise has been documented to raise high-density lipoprotein cholesterol (HDL-C) but there is a wide variability in the HDL-C-raising effect of PE, probably due to differences in baseline characteristics and genetic factors. In addition, PE has been shown to reduce triglycerides (TGs) as well as improve the low-density lipoprotein cholesterol (LDL-C) particle size. In fact, the triad of elevated TG, low HDL and small dense LDL, often referred as been shown to reduce trig,"particle size. In fact, thmetabolic syndrome, which affects a large number of Indians and is associated with increased incidence of CV disease and T2DM. Thus, PE in Indian patients who are frequently affected with atherogenic dyslipidemia may prove to be especially important in reducing CV disease.

EFFECTS OF PHYSICAL EXERCISE ON HIGH-DENSITY LIPOPROTEIN CHOLESTEROL

Several cross-sectional and prospective cohort studies have shown that HDL-C values are higher in physically active people compared with less active counterparts.[5-7] Randomized clinical trials (RCT) addressing the effects of at least 12 weeks aerobic exercise on lipids, where diet was held constant, have also reported significant increase in HDL-C levels.[8-10] In the Health Risk Factors Exercise Training and Genetics (HERITAGE) Family Study,[11] the largest published interventional study, 675 normolipidemic subjects were given 20 weeks of supervised exercise and their HDL-C concentrations increased by 3.6 ± 11% in both males and females compared with baseline with significant individual variability.

The reasons for individual variability in HDL response to PE are not entirely clear. Data are inconsistent regarding whether greater benefit occurs with low versus normal to high baseline HDL.[12-14] However, subjects with high baseline TG and low HDL as seen in metabolic syndrome appear to show a significant increase in HDL levels (+ 4.9%),[13] suggesting that effect of HDL from PE may be linked to baseline TG levels. Another issue is whether effect of PE on HDL levels is dependent on the amount or intensity of PE. Kraus et al.[8] found that high amount/high-intensity exercise significantly increased HDL-C by 8.8% ($P < 0.02$). High-density lipoprotein particle size and diameter also increased suggesting a more beneficial effect on HDL_2 fraction on this lipoprotein. However, other studies have not shown a consistent relationship between the intensity of exercise and increase in HDL-C.[15,16] The HERITAGE Family Study[11,17] also suggests that genetics may play a key role in response of HDL-C to exercise. The possible heritable factors suggested include apolipoprotein E, cholesteryl ester transfer protein genotype and lipoprotein lipase genotype.[18-20]

EFFECTS OF PHYSICAL EXERCISE ON TRIGLYCERIDES

Physical exercise has a consistent favorable effect on serum TG levels, especially in patients with disorders of TG–HDL axis. Observational studies have shown an inverse association between PE and TG levels.[5] However, the results from clinical trials have been mixed depending upon the subset of patients studied.[21] It appears that PE affects TG more significantly in men compared with women.[5,11] A subset analysis of 200 men in the HERITAGE Family Study[13] showed that 20 weeks of exercise reduced TG by 15%, especially in subjects with abnormalities of TG–HDL axis. In another randomized trial of 111 sedentary overweight adults with dyslipidemia, TG reduced from 10% to 26% in the PE group compared with 18% increase in the nonexercising control group.[8] A recent meta-analysis in the overweight/obese children and adolescents shows that PE decreases TG in these subjects.[21]

EFFECTS OF PHYSICAL EXERCISE ON LOW-DENSITY LIPOPROTEIN CHOLESTEROL

Low-density lipoprotein is the most important lipid predictor of CV events. Although LDL can be reduced by low-fat diet, PE alone has shown no significant effect on LDL as reported in several systemic reviews.[5,15,21] One review noted that the subset of studies that showed reduction in LDL by PE also showed significant reduction in body fat and weight.[10] A recent meta-analysis of RCT on the effects of aerobic exercise on lipids in adults with type II diabetes suggests that

Table 10.1: Recommendation of physical activity and exercise

Age group	Activity
5–17 years	Daily > 60 minutes of vigorous intensity exercise, e.g., cycling and jogging
18–64 years	Weekly > 150 minutes of moderate intensity exercise every week, e.g., brisk walking Or > 75 minutes of vigorous intensity aerobic exercise throughout the week
65 years or more	Same as above. When they cannot perform these exercises, they should be advised to be physically active

overall aerobic exercise lowers LDL-C level in adults with T2DM.[22] However, additional controlled trials are needed in such subjects. Resistance training over longer periods may also reduce LDL-C.[23,24] Although the effects of PE on LDL are mixed, PE appears to increase the average size of LDL particle and reduce the number of small dense LDL.[8] This is of particular importance to Indians who have been reported to have increased small dense LDL, which is associated with CAD.

Thus, available evidence suggests that aerobic exercise can raise HDL-C modestly by 3–10%, lower TG by 15–25% and increase LDL particle size. Resistance training appears to lower LDL-C levels. Thus, atherogenic dyslipidemia found frequently in Indians can be favorably affected by regular PE.

The following recommendations are made as per World Health Organization'ganizationng recommendations are madeActivity for Health (2010) (Table 10.1):[23]

- Children and young people aged 5–17 years should accumulate at least 60 minutes of moderate-to-vigorous intensity exercise (such as jogging) daily.
- Adults aged 18gity exercise (d 5e made as per Wndians can be favo HDLo have insuch as brisk walking) PE throughout the week, or do at least 75 minutes of vigorous-intensity aerobic exercise throughout the week or an equivalent combination of moderate- and vigorous-intensity exercise.
- For adults aged 65 years and above, the recommended level of PE is similar to adults aged 18–64 years, but when adults of this age group cannot do the recommended amounts of exercise due to health conditions, they should be as physically active as their abilities and conditions may allow.

ROLE OF SMOKING CESSATION ON LIPIDS

Smoking intensity has been associated with small statistically significant increase in LDL-C and decrease in HDL-C.[24-26] Some studies have described small dense LDL particles among current smokers and improvements in lipids after smoking cessation, though these findings are less consistent.[27,28] A recent large RCT suggests that smoking cessation improved HDL-C, total HDL and large HDL particle especially in women in spite of increase in weight.[29] Increase in HDL may mediate part of reduced CV disease after smoking cessation.

Smokers should quit smoking cessation because it decreases the CV mortality and morbidity and also of beneficial effects on lipids. Though data on bidi smoking and chewable tobacco are not available, they should also be avoided.

EFFECT OF ALCOHOL ON LIPIDS

Moderate alcohol intake has been shown to reduce the risk of CAD by 40–70% compared with nondrinkers and heavy drinkers in several prospective cohort studies. A recent meta-analysis by Castelnuovo et al. of 34 studies has shown a similar effect.[30] Several factors such as antioxidant, antithrombotic, enhanced insulin sensitivity and increase in HDL have been hypothesized for this benefit. However, binge drinking and heavy drinking increase the CV mortality.[31] Heavy drinking has also been shown to be associated with metabolic syndrome through elevation of blood pressure and TGs in male patients with diabetes.[32]

Although moderate alcohol intake was protective against myocardial infarction in the entire study population from 52 countries in INTERHEART study,[3] it was not beneficial for Indians.[33] Similarly, a cross-sectional study by Roy et al.[34] among 4465 alcohol users in India showed that alcohol intake increased the risk for CAD in Indians.

Thus, in spite of the fact that moderate alcohol intake has shown cardioprotective effects and increase in HDL, it has been found to be harmful in Indian subjects. Hence, it should not be recommended in Indians. Heavy drinking can cause metabolic syndrome and increase TGs and blood pressure, so it should be completely avoided. In brief, alcohol intake in any form in Indians should be avoided.

EFFECT OF YOGA ON LIPIDS

Yoga is an ancient Indian and holistic technique that has been shown to control stress. It has also been shown to have several cardioprotective effects in several small studies like control of hypertension,[35] body weight, blood sugar and improvement in lipids.[36-38] Many controlled studies have demonstrated that yoga may be useful for regression of early[39,40] and advanced coronary atherosclerosis.[41-43] A recent controlled trial of secondary prevention in blacks showed that meditation (which is an essential component of yoga) reduced major adverse CV events (death, myocardial infarction, stroke) by 48%[44] over a 5.4 years average follow-up. These studies have also demonstrated a marked decrease in total cholesterol (TC), LDL-C and TG. One study in normal volunteers has shown an increase in HDL-C apart from decrease in TC, LDL-C and TG.[45] Two studies suggest that yoga may improve lipid profile in patients with end-stage renal disease.[46,47] Another recent Indian study has also demonstrated that regular yoga practice has a favorable effects on lipid in diabetic patients.[48] However, larger studies are needed to confirm the usefulness of yoga in control of dyslipidemia.

CONCLUSION

Therapeutic lifestyle changes encompassing dietary measures, PE, smoking cessation, moderation in alcohol intake form an integral part for the management of dyslipidemia. Evidence suggests that regular physical activity, particularly isotonic exercise of moderate-to-severe intensity and yoga, is very effective in the prevention and treatment of dyslipidemia. Physical exercise and yoga are the most cost-effective measures and public health interventions that can help control the global burden of CV epidemic.

REFERENCES

1. Hu FB, Li TY, Colditz GA, et al. Television watching and other sedentary behaviors in relation to risk of obesity and type 2 diabetes mellitus in women. JAMA. 2003;289:1785-91.
2. Jakes RW, Day NE, Khaw KT, et al. Television viewing and low participation in vigorous recreation are independently associated with obesity and markers of cardiovascular disease risk: EPIC-Norfolk population-based study. Eur J Clin Nutr. 2003;57:1089-96.
3. Yusuf S, Hawkin S, Ounpuu S, et al. Effect of potentially modifiable risk factors associated with myocardial infarction in 52 countries (the INTERHEART study): case control study. Lancet. 2004;364:937-52.
4. Thompson PD, Buchner D, Pina IL, et al. Exercise and physical activity in the prevention and treatment of atherosclerotic cardiovascular disease: a statement from the Council on Clinical Cardiology (Subcommittee on Exercise, Rehabilitation, and Prevention) and the Council on Nutrition, Physical Activity, and Metabolism (Subcommittee on Physical Activity). Circulation. 2003;107:3109-16.
5. Durstine JL, Grandjean PW, Davis PG, et al. Blood lipid and lipoprotein adaptations to exercise: a quantitative analysis. Sports Med. 2001;31:1033-62.
6. Wei M, Macera CA, Hornung CA, et al. Changes in lipids associated with change in regular exercise in free-living men. Clin Epidemiol. 1997;50:1137-42.
7. Skoumas J, Pitsavos C, Panagiotakos DB, et al. Physical activity, high density lipoprotein cholesterol and other lipids levels, in men and women from the ATTICA study. Lipids Health Dis. 2003;2:3.
8. Kraus WE, Houmard JA, Duscha BD, et al. Effects of the amount and intensity of exercise on plasma lipoproteins. N Engl J Med. 2002;347:1483-92.
9. Fahlman MM, Boardley D, Lambert CP, et al. Effects of endurance training and resistance training on plasma lipoprotein profiles in elderly women. J Gerontol A Biol Sci Med Sci. 2002;57:B54-60.
10. Furukawa F, Kazuma K, Kawa M, et al. Effects of an off-site walking program on energy expenditure, serum lipids, and glucose metabolism in middle-aged women. Biol Res Nurs. 2003;4:181-92.
11. Leon AS, Rice T, Mandel S, et al. Blood lipid response to 20 weeks of supervised exercise in a large biracial population: the HERITAGE Family Study. Metabolism. 2000;49:513-20.
12. Zmuda JM, Yurgalevitch SM, Flynn MM, et al. Exercise training has little effect on HDL levels and metabolism in men with initially low HDL cholesterol. Atherosclerosis. 1998;137:215-21.
13. Couillard C, Despres JP, Lamarche B, et al. Effects of endurance exercise training on plasma HDL cholesterol levels depend on levels of triglycerides: evidence from men of the Health, Risk Factors, Exercise Training and Genetics (HERITAGE) Family Study. Arterioscler Thromb Vasc Biol. 2001;21:1226-32.
14. Thompson PD, Rader DJ. Does exercise increase HDL cholesterol in those who need it the most? Arterioscler Thromb Vasc Biol. 2001;21:1097-8.
15. King AC, Haskell WL, Young DR, et al. Long-term effects of varying intensities and formats of physical activity on participation rates, fitness, and lipoproteins in men and women aged 50 to 65 years. Circulation. 1995;91:2596-604.
16. Crouse SF, O'Brien BC, Grandjean PW, et al. Training intensity, blood lipids, and apolipoproteins in men with high cholesterol. J Appl Physiol. 1997;82:270-7.
17. Leon AS, Gaskill SE, Rice T, et al. Variability in the response of HDL cholesterol to exercise training in the HERITAGE Family Study. Int J Sports Med. 2002;23:1-9.
18. Hagberg JM, Ferrell RE, Katzel LI, et al. Apolipoprotein E genotype and exercise training-induced increases in plasma high-density lipoprotein (HDL)- and HDL2-cholesterol levels in overweight men. Metabolism. 1999;48:943-5.
19. Wilund KR, Ferrell RE, Phares DA, et al. Changes in high-density lipoprotein-cholesterol subfractions with exercise training may be dependent on cholesteryl ester transfer protein (CETP) genotype. Metabolism. 2002;51:774-8.

20. Hagberg JM, Ferrell RE, Dengel DR, et al. Exercise training-induced blood pressure and plasma lipid improvements in hypertensives may be genotype dependent. Hypertension. 1999;34:18-23.

21. Kelley GA, Kelley KS. Aerobic exercise and lipids and lipoproteins in children and adolescents: a meta-analysis of randomized controlled trials. Atherosclerosis. 2007;191(2):447-53.

22. Kelley GA, Kelley KS. Effects of aerobic exercise on lipids and lipoproteins in adults with type 2 diabetes: a meta-analysis of randomized-controlled trials. Public Health. 2007;121(9):643-55.

23. Global Recommendations on Physical Activity for Health. World Health Organisation. 2010. Available from: whqlibdoc.who.int/publications/2010/9789241599979_eng.pdf.

24. Gossett LK, Johnson HM, Piper ME, et al. Smoking intensity and lipoprotein abnormalities in active smokers. J Clin Lipidol. 2009;3:372-8.

25. Campbell SC, Moffatt RJ, Stamford BA. Smoking and smoking cessation—the relationship between cardiovascular disease and lipoprotein metabolism: a review. Atherosclerosis. 2008;201:225-35.

26. Criqui MH, Wallace RB, Heiss G, et al. Cigarette smoking and plasma high-density lipoprotein cholesterol. The Lipid Research Clinics Program Prevalence Study. Circulation. 1980;62:IV70-76.

27. Griffin BA, Freeman DJ, Tait GW, et al. Role of plasma triglyceride in the regulation of plasma low density lipoprotein (LDL) subfractions: relative contribution of small, dense LDL to coronary heart disease risk. Atherosclerosis. 1994;106:241-53.

28. Urahama N, Iguchi G, Shimizu M, et al. Smoking and small, dense low-density lipoprotein particles: cross-sectional study. Nicotine Tob Res. 2008;10:1391-95.

29. Gepner AD, Piper ME, Johnson HM, et al. Effects of smoking and smoking cessation on lipids and lipoproteins: outcomes from a randomized clinical trial. Am Heart J. 2011;161(1):145-51.

30. Di Castelnuovo A, Costanzo S, Bagnardi V, et al. Alcohol dosing and total mortality in men and women: an updated meta-analysis of 34 prospective studies. Arch Intern Med. 2006;166:2437-45.

31. Roerecke, M, Rehm, J. Irregular heavy drinking occasions and risk of ischemic heart disease: a systematic review and meta-analysis. Am J Epidemiol. 2010;171:633-44.

32. Wakabayashi I. Association between alcohol drinking and metabolic syndrome in Japanese male workers with diabetes mellitus. J Atheroscler Thromb. 2011;18(8):684-92.

33. Joshi P, Islam S, Pais P, et al. Risk factors for early myocardial infarction in South Asians compared with individuals in other countries. JAMA. 2007;297:286-94.

34. Roy A, Prabhakaran D, Jeemon P, et al. Impact of alcohol on coronary heart disease in Indian men. Atherosclerosis. 2010;210(2):531-5.

35. Anderson JW, Liu C, Kryscio RJ. Blood pressure response to transcendental meditation: a meta-analysis. Am J Hypertens. 2008;21(3):310-6.

36. Raub JA. Psychophysiologic effects of Hatha Yoga on musculoskeletal and cardiopulmonary function: a literature review. J Altern Complement Med. 2002;8(6):797-812.

37. Schmidt T, Wijga A, Von Zur MHatha Yoga on musculoskeletal and cardiopulmonary function: a literature review. J Altern Complement Med. 2002;JAMA8;ve contribution of small, dense LDL to coronary Physiol Scand Suppl. 1997;640:158-62.

38. Mahajan AS, Reddy KS, Sachdeva U. Lipid profile of coronary risk subjects following yogic lifestyle intervention. Indian Heart J. 1999;51(1):37-40.

39. Mehrotra UC, Manchanda SC, Mohanty A, et al. Regression of carotid intimal thickness by yoga in metabolic syndrome. Indian Heart J. 2011;63:492.

40. Fields JZ, Walton KG, Schneider RH, et al. Effect of a multimodality natural medicine program on carotid atherosclerosis in older subjects: a pilot trial of Maharishi Vedic Medicine. Am J Cardiol. 2002;89(8):952-8.

41. Ornish D, Brown SE, Scherwitz LW, et al. Can lifestyle changes reverse coronary heart disease? The Lifestyle Heart Trial. Lancet. 1990;336(8708):129-33.

42. Manchanda SC, Narang R, Reddy KS, et al. Retardation of coronary atherosclerosis with yoga lifestyle intervention. J Assoc Physicians India. 2000;48(7):687-94.

43. Gupta SK, Sawhney RC, Rai L, et al. Regression of coronary atherosclerosis through healthy lifestyle in coronary artery disease patients—Mount Abu Open Heart Trial. Indian Heart J. 2011;63:461-9.

44. Schneider RH, Grim CE, Rainforth MV, et al. Stress reduction in the secondary prevention of cardio-vascular disease: randomized, controlled trial of transcendental meditation and health education in Blacks. Circ Cardiovasc Qual Outcomes. 2012;5(6):750-8.

45. Prasad KVV, Sunita M, Raju PS, et al. Impact of Pranayam and Yoga on lipid profile of normal healthy volunteers. J Ex Physiol. 2006;9:1.

46. Gordon L, McGrowder DA, Pena YT, et al. Effect of exercise therapy on lipid parameters in patients with end-stage renal disease on hemodialysis. J Lab Physicians. 2012;4(1):17-23.

47. Gordon LA, Morrison EY, McGrowder DA, et al. Effects of exercise therapy on lipid profile and oxidative stress indicators in patients with type 2 diabetes. BMC Complement Altern Med. 2008; 13(8):21.

48. Shantakumari N, Sequeira S, El Deeb R. Effects of a yoga intervention on lipid profiles of diabetes patients with dyslipidemia. Indian Heart J. 2013;65(2):127-31.

CHAPTER 11

Obesity, Weight Loss and Lipid Disorders

Harsh Wardhan and Kuntal Bhattacharyya

- Introduction
- Obesity and dyslipidemia
- Management
- Conclusion

INTRODUCTION

Obesity is a state of excess adipose tissue mass. Obesity is highly prevalent in the developed countries and gradually increasing in developing countries. The World Health Organization (WHO) has declared overweight as one of the top 10 risk conditions in the world. By 2015 approximately 2.3 billion adults will be overweight and >700 million will be obese. National Health and Nutrition Examination Survey declared that 66.3% of the adult population of the United States are overweight and 32% are obese.[1] According to the report of National Centre for Health Statistics, 16% of children and adolescents are overweight.[2] It is very difficult for an individual to restrain himself from overeating in current era. The increased intake of modern food and beverages as combined with dramatic decrease in physical activity is the main culprit for obesity epidemic. Physical labor at work was replaced by labor saving machine in most of the fields. Most of the leisure time activities are now passive like watching television, Internet and computer games instead of active movement. As a result, people are expending less energy daily at a time when they are eating more calories, leading to marked weight gain.[3]

Obesity is responsible for several health problems. It is associated with diabetes mellitus, dyslipidemia, hypertension and cardiovascular disease. Obesity increases the risk of nonalcoholic steatohepatitis, gall stones, sleep apnea, osteoarthritis and depression. Dyslipidemia is a common problem often coexists with obesity particularly in diabetics.

OBESITY AND DYSLIPIDEMIA

For the management of dyslipidemia, we should know the total fat burden and fat distribution pattern of a patient. Body mass index (BMI) in kg/m^2 can give the estimate of total fat burden. According to the WHO, BMI of 18.5–24.9 kg/m^2 is defined as normal, 25–29.9 kg/m^2 as overweight and >30 kg/m^2 as obese, with 30–34.9% defined as class 1 obesity, 35–39.9% as

Table 11.1: Classification of weight status and risk of disease

	BMI (kg/m2)	Obesity class	Risk of disease
Underweight	<18.5		
Healthy weight	18.5–24.9		
Overweight	25.0–29.9		Increased
Obesity	30.0–34.9	I	High
Obesity	35.0–39.9	II	Very high
Extreme obesity	40	III	Extremely high

Source: Adapted from National Institutes of Health, National Heart, Lung, and Blood Institute. Clinical Guidelines on the Identification, Evaluation, and Treatment of Overweight and Obesity in Adults. U.S. Department of Health and Human Services, Public Health Service; 1998.

class 2 and >40% as class 3 (Table 11.1).[4] Central fat distribution can be evaluated by measuring waist–hip ratio. A waist-to-hip ratio >1.0 in men and >0.85 in women is considered abnormally high.[5]

Excess abdominal fat, assessed by measurement of waist circumference or waist-to-hip ratio, is independently associated with higher risk of diabetes mellitus and cardiovascular disease. Measurement of the waist circumference is a surrogate for visceral adipose tissue and should be performed in the horizontal plane above the iliac crest. Cut points that define higher risk for men and women based on ethnicity have been proposed by the International Diabetes Federation (Table 11.2)

Table 11.2: Ethnic-specific values for waist circumference

Ethnic group	Waist circumference
Europeans	
Men	>94 cm (37 in)
Women	>80 cm (31.5 in)
South Asians and Chinese	
Men	>90 cm (35 in)
Women	>80 cm (31.5 in)
Japanese	
Men	>85 cm (33.5 in)
Women	>90 cm (35 in)
Ethnic south and central Americans	Use south Asian recommendations until more specific data are available.
Sub-Saharan Africans	Use European data until more specific data are available.
Eastern Mediterranean and Middle East (Arab) populations	Use European data until more specific data are available.

Source: From KGMM Alberti et al. for the IDF Epidemiology Task Force Consensus Group. The metabolic syndrome—a new worldwide definition. Lancet. 2005;366:1059.

Table 11.3: Weight loss therapy: a guide to selecting treatment

	BMI category				
Treatment	25–26.9	27–29.9	30–35	35–39.9	40
Diet, exercise, behavioral therapy	With comorbidities	With comorbidities	+	+	+
Pharmacotherapy		With comorbidities	+	+	+
Surgery				With comorbidities	+

Source: From National Heart, Lung, and Blood Institute, North American Association for the Study of Obesity (2000).
BMI, body mass index.

MANAGEMENT

Physical Fitness

The primary goal of treatment is to improve obesity-related comorbid conditions and reduce the risk of developing future comorbidities. The modality and aggressiveness of treatment are determined by the patient's risk status, expectations and available resources. Depending on BMI risk category, therapy for obesity always begins with lifestyle management and may include pharmacotherapy or surgery (Table 11.3). Setting an initial weight-loss goal of 10% over 6 months is a realistic target. This weight-loss goal is associated with significant improvement in dyslipidemia.

Before starting a weight-loss program, a careful preliminary assessment has to be made. Obesity care involves attention to three essential elements of lifestyle: dietary habits, physical activity and behavior modification. A history of previous weight-loss attempts and the reason why they failed should be taken. Losing weight is a difficult and time-consuming process. The patient has to be appropriately motivated. Behavior modification is focused mainly on changing eating habits, increasing physical activity, altering attitudes and developing support systems. Motivation can be increased by describing to the patient the health risks of obesity. Initially, the patient and the physician need to set an achievable goal. [6]It is wise to begin with a modest goal of 10% because this can be achieved by a motivated person who is well managed. Many recent guidelines have suggested a loss of about 10% from baseline weight.[7,8]If the patient is successful to achieve this goal, then maintenance at this lower weight for a time is better. If the patient continues to follow the guidelines successfully, then further weight loss can be attempted.

Behavioral Therapy

Not only maladaptive eating but environmental, social and genetic factors are also responsible for obesity. Behavioral change has broadened to include changes in physical activity, the environment and the social setting of an individual attempting to lose weight.[9] The aim of behavioral therapy is to change behavior by means of small, achievable steps and to mainly focus on diet and exercise. Specific behavioral therapies include self-monitoring, stress management, stimulus control, problem solving, contingency management, cognitive restructuring and social support.[10]

Self-monitoring consists of observing and recording various aspects of behavior, such as food intake, physical activity and medication use faithfully and truthfully. Stimulus control is working at identifying what social or environmental cues lead to undesirable behavior. Once identified, a sustained effort is made to eliminate, change or avoid these cues. Stimulus control is closely tied to stress management. Learning to identify these causes and trying to change or avoid them are an important aim of behavior modification. Contingency management involves the application of rewards for moving to appropriate behavior patterns for weight loss and maintenance. This contingency management is often done with the use of contracts, whereby the patient agrees to modify a certain behavior (increase exercise bouts, decrease alcohol, decrease fried foods etc.) in return for which a reward is negotiated. Social support can be helpful in achieving success. Relapse prevention is an important component of behavioral therapy.[10] It is very important to individualize behavioral change. Management of stress is very important to correct a particular dysfunctional eating. After weight loss, maintenance of reduced weight is another difficult issue. To prevent regain in weight, the same effort at diet and physical activity needs to be continued.[11]

Diet

Most of the obese persons consume a very high amount of calories, and this must be reduced. Diet modification is a key component of a weight-loss program. A calorie-deficit diet helps in not only significant weight loss but also improvement in dyslipidemia.[12] Fat should be decreased and total calories reduced. Sugar should be discouraged. High-fiber foods such as fruits and vegetables should be encouraged. Alcohol should be eliminated or drastically curtailed. One should target at a deficit of about 1000 kcal/day; this would translate to about 1 kg of weight loss per week. Low-calorie formula diet in place of one or two meals per day gives a good control of caloric intake and benefit can be observed if used for 12–16 weeks. The aim of weight loss is to lose fat without losing lean body mass. This is done by taking adequate high-quality protein (egg white, fish, poultry, low fat dairy products).The intake of protein should be at a level of 1–1.5 g/kg of ideal body weight. The ideal body weight for a person should be calculated using BMI of 25. The daily carbohydrate intake should include 20–30 g of fiber from fruits, vegetables, legumes and grains[13] (Tables 11.4 and 11.5). Adequate amounts of vitamins and minerals should be taken daily. About 0.5–1 kg/week weight loss is possible if daily calorie deficit of 500–1500 calories is practiced.[13] A low-calorie diet includes 800–1500 calories/day. A diet of 1200–1500 calories/day for men and one of 1000–1200 calories/day for women are usually about right, but they need to be individualized in relation to original intake and physical activity. These types of diets can cause a 10% weight loss in 6 months, with 75% being fat and 25% lean body mass.[14].Very-low-calorie diets below 800 calories are not recommended. Usually, the weight loss plateaus after a period of 4–6 months. To prevent weight regain, reduced food intake and physical activity should be continued. The Revised Dietary Reference Intakes for Macronutrients released by the Institute of Medicine recommends 45–60% of calories from carbohydrate, 20–35% from fat and 10–35% from protein. The fiber intake should be 38 g for men, 25 g for women if age is above 50 years and 30 g for men and 21 g for women if age is <50. Atkins diet (low carbohydrate and

Table 11.4: Nutrient composition of therapeutic lifestyle changes in adult treatment panel III

Nutrient	Recommended intake
Saturated fat (lower trans fat)	<7% of total calories
Polyunsaturated fat	Up to 10% of total calorie
Monounsaturated fat	Up to 20% of total calories
Total fat	25–35% of total calories
Carbohydrate (emphasize complex sources)	50–60% of total calories
Fiber	20–30 g/day
Protein	Approximately 15% of total calories
Cholesterol	<200 mg/day
Total calories (energy)	Balance energy intake and output to maintain healthy body weight and prevent weight gain

Table 11.5: Cumulative low-density lipoprotein cholesterol reduction by dietary modification[3]

Dietary component	Dietary change	Approximate LDL reduction
Saturated fat	<7% of calories	8–10%
Trans fat	<1% of calories	1–2%
Dietary cholesterol	<200 mg/day	3–5%
Weight reduction	Lose 10 lb	5–8%
Soy protein		3–5%
Viscous fiber	5–10 g/day	3–5%
Plant sterol/stanol esters	2 g/day	6–15%
Cumulative estimate		24–37%

LDL, low-density lipoprotein.

high protein diet) increases high-density lipoprotein (HDL) level and decreases triglyceride (TG) level. Multiple studies showed that there is no significant difference in weight loss among different types of diets. Sustained adherence to a particular diet is the best predictor of weight-loss outcome.

Physical Activities

It is not only helpful in reducing weight but also for its maintenance. In a recent review by Wing, out of 13 trials only 2 trials showed more weight loss in patients who exercised in comparison to patients without exercise.[15] There has been less controversy as to whether exercise is helpful for weight maintenance. Pavlou et al. showed that individuals who maintained an exercise regimen maintained their weight loss, whereas those who abandoned the exercise regained their weight.[16] In the absence of a contraindication such as a cardiac, orthopedic or metabolic reason, exercise should always be encouraged. Initially, an effort is made simply to increase walking at a normal pace. The goal is to increase initially to 30 minutes/day and eventually to 60 minutes/day. The exercise can be done in bouts. The program needs to start slowly. Depending on the fitness, jogging, running, swimming etc. can be done. According to the National Weight Loss Registry, physical activity to expend 400 kcal/day is required to maintain weight loss.[17] Exercise has been shown to improve lipid profile. Regular exercise causes no or little changes in total cholesterol and low-density lipoprotein (LDL) level but increases HDL level and decreases TG level.

Drugs

Pharmacotherapy should be considered in patients of BMI >30 kg/m^2 or 27 kg/m^2 with concomitant obesity-related diseases and when diet and physical activity therapy have not been successful. Patient should not discontinue lifestyle modification program while on pharmacotherapy. If drug therapy is successful, it generally needs to be continued indefinitely.

Centrally Acting Drugs

By increasing satiety and reducing hunger, these agents help patients to reduce caloric intake. The target site for these drugs is hypothalamus. The mechanism of action is by augmenting neurotransmission of norepinephrine, serotonin and dopamine. *Sibutramine* functions as a serotonin and norepinephrine reuptake inhibitor. Sibutramine is not pharmacologically related to amphetamine and has no addictive potential. There is increased risk of nonfatal myocardial infarction and nonfatal stroke in patients with pre-existing cardiovascular disease. There is mild increase in heart rate by 4–6 bpm and diastolic blood pressure 2–3 mmHg. The other side effects are dry mouth, headache, constipation etc. In Sibutramine Trial in Obesity Reduction and Maintenance, 10 mg sibutramine was more effective than placebo to maintain reduced weight that was lost on a hypocaloric diet.[18] Phentermine is an adrenergic drug. It is effective both in continued use and intermittent use. Fenfluramine was banned because of serious adverse side effects related to heart valves and pulmonary fibrosis.[19]

Peripherally Acting Drugs

Orlistat is a synthetic hydrogenated derivative of naturally occurring lipase inhibitors, lipostatin. Orlistat is a potent slowly reversible inhibitor of pancreatic, gastric lipase and phospholipase A$_2$. The drug acts in the lumen of stomach and small gut by forming covalent bond with the active site of lipase. At therapeutic dose of 120 mg tid, orlistat blocks the digestion and absorption of 30% of dietary fat. The most common side effects of orlistat are gastrointestinal, such as fatty or oily stools and more frequent defecation. Another side effect is a slight reduction in fat-soluble vitamins. The European Multicentre Orlistat Group conducted a double-blind study in which 688 obese individuals (average BMI, 36 kg/m^2) were assigned to orlistat therapy or placebo for 1 year, in combination with a hypocaloric diet (minimum energy intake, 1000–1200 kcal/day). At the end of the first year of the study, the mean weight loss was 10.2% for the orlistat group and 6.1% for the placebo group.[20] A US study showed similar results. At the end of the first year, the participants taking orlistat had lost more weight than those taking placebo (8.76 ± 0.37 vs. 5.81 ± 0.67 kg). At the end of the second year, participants taking orlistat 120 mg tid regained less weight than those taking orlistat 60 mg tid or placebo (3.2 ± 0.45, 4.26 ± 0.57 and 5.63 ± 0.42 kg, respectively).[21] Weight loss with orlistat also helps in the treatment of comorbidities, including dyslipidemia.

Endocannabinoids

The endocannabinoid system in brain controls food intake and appetite mainly mediated by cannabinoid (CB1) receptor. Rimonabant, a selective CB1 receptor antagonist, suppresses appetite. Several large prospective trials have demonstrated the effectiveness of this drug as a weight-loss agent with concomitant improvement in cardiovascular risk factors. This drug is not approved by U. S. Food and Drug Administration because of increased side effects like seizure, depression and suicidal ideation.

Surgery for Weight Loss

Surgery for weight loss may be advised in patients who repeatedly fail to lose weight by diet, physical activity and pharmacotherapy. National Institutes of Health consensus conference guidelines suggest a BMI of 40 or greater in the absence of comorbidities and BMI of 35 or greater in the presence of comorbid conditions as appropriate for surgery.[22] Gastric banding and vertical-banded gastroplasty are restrictive procedures, reducing the ability to ingest food. Gastric bypass and biliopancreatic bypass are primarily malabsorptive. The weight loss is least with banding, next for vertical-banded gastroplasty, next for gastric bypass and most for biliopancreatic bypass. Biliopancreatic bypass is associated with adverse side effects like severe diarrhea and liver disease.

The Swedish Obese Subjects (SOS) study reported the result of surgery compared to medical therapy. The magnitude of weight loss was 23% ± 10% of excess weight in those undergoing vertical-banded gastroplasty and 33% ± 10% for those undergoing gastric bypass.[23,24] There was better control of glucose levels, lipids and blood pressure in the surgical group. The SOS study concluded that weight losses from baseline stabilized after 10 years at 25% for gastric bypass, 16% for vertical-banded gastroplasty and 14% for banding.[25]

Weight Maintenance

The calories requirement goes down after weight loss. Individuals require less energy to do the same physical task.[26] With weight reduction, the responsiveness of adipose tissue lipoprotein lipase to meals is enhanced.[27] A permanent restriction in caloric intake is required because a patient's total energy expenditure will decline after weight loss. The lifestyle changes learned during the weight-loss period need to be continued. If weight-loss drugs have been successful, without adverse effects, they should be continued under medical supervision.

Weight Loss and Its Effect on Lipids

The obesity-associated dyslipidemia has high TG, reduced HDL cholesterol and small dense LDL particles.[28,29] Weight loss is associated with significant beneficial effect on the lipid parameters. The TG level declines, HDL cholesterol level increases and small dense LDL particles size increases. The particles become less atherogenic.[30] In some individuals with obesity, the total cholesterol and LDL cholesterol levels may be increased.[31] Short-term studies have proven the value of therapeutic interventions. They are behavioral, low-calorie

Table 11.6: Summary of studies with diet and exercise on lipids.

S. No.	Study	Year	Clinical characteristics	Weight loss	Lipid changes
1.	Evaluation of the cholesterol lowering diet used in the Coronary Prevention Programme in controlling hypertriglyceridemia[33]	1972	$n = 140$ men, obesity = 90 triglyceridemia = 50, low saturated fat, reduced calorie diet, moderate PUFA intake, 1 year intervention	10 pounds	Total cholesterol 12.1% decline Triglycerides 17.3% decline ($P = 0.01$)
2.	Evaluation of medical benefit of weight loss including improved lipid levels[34]	1981	$n = 71$ men, severe obesity, 8 weeks treatment with very-low-calorie diet followed by 54 months of follow-up	Baseline weight 110.0 ± 2.8 kg 54 months weight 99.9 ± 2.6 kg ($P = <0.005$)	Cholesterol no significant decline Triglyceride significant decline ($P = <0.05$)
3.	Randomized controlled comparisons of the effect of decreased energy intake or increased exercise on fat weight[35]	1988	$n = 131$, overweight sedentary men Exercise group 47 Diet group 42 Control group 42 1 year intervention	Exercise – 4±3.9 kg Diet – 7.2 ± 3.7 kg Control + 06 ± 3.7 kg	HDL increased significantly with exercise TC/HDL declined with exercise TG declined in diet and exercise group
4.	Evaluation of the effect on dyslipidemia of weight loss after gastric bypass surgery[36]	1990	38 patients with gastric bypass with follow-up of 29 months	Baseline: 303 ± 53 kg Follow-up: 251 ± 41 kg	Total cholesterol and triglyceride decreased significantly HDL increased significantly
5.	Longitudinal epidemiologic study of subset of Framingham Study population to determine the health effects of weight loss[37]	1993	2500 adults	Yearly weight changes were variable in between different groups	Man with significant weight loss had decline in total cholesterol
6.	Effect of diet control and exercise on lipid profile of obese men[38]	2014	40 women with obesity Control = 10 Diet = 10 Exercise = 10 Diet + exercise = 10	Diet exercise had significant effect on weight loss	Normalization of lipid with diet and exercise

HDL, high-density lipoprotein; LDL, low-density lipoprotein; TC, total cholesterol; TG, triglycerides.

diet and very-low-calorie diet interventions. Triglycerides are decreased, total cholesterol and LDL cholesterol are reduced and HDL cholesterol is increased with these interventions (Table 11.6).[32,33.]

CONCLUSION

The typical dyslipidemia observed in obesity includes hepatic overproduction of very-low-density lipoprotein VLDL, decreased circulating TG lipolysis and impaired peripheral free fatty acid (FFA) trapping, increased FFA fluxes from adipocytes to the liver and other tissues and the formation of small dense LDL. Treatment should be aimed at weight loss by increased exercise and improved dietary habits with a reduction in total calorie intake and reduced saturated fat intake. Medical therapy can be initiated if lifestyle changes are insufficient. Bariatric surgery is becoming increasingly popular for individuals with greater BMI. Weight loss generally improves lipids in obese patients with dyslipidemia. Statins are the primary lipid lowering drugs and can be used when weight-loss therapy alone cannot achieve lipid targets.

REFERENCES

1. Mokdad AH, Serdula MK, Dietz WH, et al. The spread of the obesity epidemic in the United States, 1991-1998. JAMA. 1999;282:1519-22.
2. Ogden CL, Lamb MM, Carroll MD et al. Obesity and socioeconomic status in adults: United States 1988–1994 and 2005–2008. NCHS data brief no 50. Hyattsville, MD: National Center for Health Statistics. 2010.
3. Boys HE, Chapman RH,Grandy S for the Shield investgators "group, The relationship of body mass index to diabetes mellitus, hypertension and dyslipidaemia: comparison of data from two national surveys. Int J Clin Pract 2007;61:373-374.
4. Gallagher D, Visser M, Sepulveda D, et al. How useful is body mass index for comparison of body fatness across age, sex, and ethnic groups? Am J Epidemiol. 1996;143:228-39.
5. National Heart Lung and Blood Institute. Clinical guidelines on the identification, evaluation, and treatment of overweight and obesity in adults—The evidence report. Obes Res. 1998;6(suppl 2): 51S-210S.
6. Foster GD, Wadden TA, Vogt RA, et al. What is a reasonable weight toss? Patients' expectations and evaluations of obesity treatment outcomes. J Consult Clin Psychol. 1997;65:79-85.
7. Blackburn GL. Effect of degree of weight loss on health benefits. Obes Res. 1995;3(suppl 2):211s-6s.
8. Thomas PR. Weighing the Options: Criteria for Evaluating Weight-Management Programs. Washington, DC: National Academy Press; 1995.
9. Moheney MJ, Lyddon WJ. Recent developements in cognitive approaches to counselling and psychotherapy, Counselling Psycologist 1988,16(2),190-234.
10. National Heart Lung and Blood Institute. The Practical Guide, Identification, Evaluation, and Treatment of Overweight and Obesity in Adults. Bethesda, MD: National Institutes of Health; 2000.
11. Hill JO, Wyatt HR, Phelan S, et al. The National Weight Control Registry: is it useful in helping deal with our obesity epidemic? J Nutr Educ Behav. 2005;37:206-10.
12. Lichtman SW, Pisarska K, Berman ER, et al. Discrepancy between self-reported and actual caloric intake and exercise in obese subjects. N Engl J Med. 1992;327:1893-8.
13. Meichenbaum D. Cognitive Behavior Modification. New York: Plenum; 1977, pp. 133-136.
14. Yang MU, Van Itallie TB. Reducing primary risk factors by therapeutic weight loss. In: Wadden TA, Van Itallie TB (Eds). Treatment of the Seriously Obese Patient. New York: Guilford Press; 1992. pp. 83-106.

15. Wing RR. Physical activity in the treatment of the adulthood overweight and obesity: current evidence and research issues. Med Sci Sports Exerc. 1999;31:S547-52.
16. Pavlou KN, Krey S, Steffee WP. Exercise as an adjunct to weight loss and maintenance in moderately obese subjects. Am J Clin Nutr. 1989;49:1115-23.
17. Klem ML, Wing RR, McGuire MT, et al. A descriptive study of individuals successful at long-term maintenance of substantial weight loss. Am J Clin Nutr. 1997;66:239-46.
18. Hansen D, Astrup A, Toubro S, et al. Predictors of weight loss and maintenance during 2 years of treatment by sibutramine in obesity. Results from the European multi-centre STORM trial. Sibutramine Trial of Obesity Reduction and Maintenance. Int J Obes Relat Metab Disord. 2001;25:496-501.
19. Connolly H, McGoon M. Obesity drugs and the heart. Curr Probl Cardiol. 1999;24:745-92.
20. Sjöström L, Rissanen A, Andersen T, et al. Randomised placebo-controlled trial of orlistat for weight loss and prevention of weight regain in obese patients. European Multicentre Orlistat Study Group. Lancet. 1998;352:167-72.
21. Davidson MH, Hauptman J, DiGirolamo M, et al. Weight control and risk factor reduction in obese subjects treated for 2 years with orlistat: a randomized controlled trial. JAMA. 1999;281:235-42.
22. Gastrointestinal surgery for severe obesity: National Institutes of Health Consensus Development Conference Statement. Am J Clin Nutr. 1992;55:615S-9S.
23. Sjöström L, Larsson B, Backman L, et al. Swedish Obese Subjects (SOS). Recruitment for an intervention study and a selected description of the obese state. Int J Obes. 1992;16:465-79.
24. Sjöström C, Peltonen M, Wedel H, et al. Differentiated long-term effects of intentional weight loss on diabetes and hyper-tension. Hypertension. 2000;36:20-25.
25. Sjöström L, Narbro K, Sjostrom CD, et al. Effects of bariatric surgery on mortality in Swedish obese subjects. N Engl J Med. 2007;357:741-52.
26. Heshka S, Yang MU, Wang J, et al. Weight loss and change in resting metabolic rate. Am J Clin Nutr. 1990;52:981-6.
27. Ong JM, Simsolo RB, Saghizadeh M, et al. Effects of exercise training and feeding on lipoprotein lipase gene expression in adipose tissue, heart, and skeletal muscle of the rat. Metabolism. 1995;44:1596-1605.
28. Despres JP, Moorjani S, Lupien PJ, et al. Regional distribution of body fat, plasma lipoproteins, and cardiovascular disease. Arteriosclerosis. 1990;10:497-511.
29. Krauss RM. Triglycerides and atherogenic lipoproteins: rationale for lipid management. Am J Med. 1998;105:58S-62S.
30. Dattilo AM. Effects of weight reduction on blood lipids and lipoproteins: a meta-analysis. Am J Clin Nutr. 1992;56:320-28.
31. Pi-Sunyer FX. Short-term medical benefits and adverse effects of weight loss. Ann Intern Med. 1993;119:722-6.
32. Schieffer B, Moore D, Funke E, et al. Reduction of atherogenic risk factors by short-term weight reduction. Evidence of the efficacy of National Cholesterol Education Program guidelines for the obese. Klin Wochenschr. 1991;69:163-7.
33. Hall Y, Stamler J, Cohen DB, et al. Effectiveness of a low saturated fat, low cholesterol, weight-reducing diet for the control of hypertriglyceridemia. Atherosclerosis. 1972;16:389-403.
34. Mancini M, Di Biase G, Contaldo F, et al. Medical complications of severe obesity: importance of treatment by very-low-calorie diets: intermediate and long-term effects. Int J Obes. 1981;5:341-52.
35. Wood PD, Stefanick ML, Dreon DM, et al. Changes in plasma lipids and lipoproteins in overweight men during weight loss through dieting as compared with exercise. N Engl J Med. 1988;319:1173-9.
36. Brolin RE, Kenler HA, Wilson AC, et al. Serum lipids after gastric bypass surgery for morbid obesity. Int J Obes. 1990;14:939-50.
37. Higgins M, D'Agostino RB, Kannel W, et al. Benefits and adverse effects of weight loss: observations from the Framingham Study. Ann Intern Med. 1993;119:758-63.
38. Saad S. Al-Zaharani: effect of diet control and exercise on lipid profile of obese men. Int J Res Med Sci. 2014;2(1):95-9.

CHAPTER 12

Statins in Dyslipidemia

Tapan Ghose

- Introduction
- Classification of statins
- Pharmacology
- Biochemical impact of statin therapy
- Clinical impact of statin therapy
- Contraindications
- Prescribing information of various statins
- Conclusion

INTRODUCTION

Statins are chemicals that inhibit the rate-limiting enzyme 3-hydroxy-3-methylglutaryl-coenzyme A (HMG-CoA) in the cholesterol biosynthesis. In early 1970, Japanese microbiologist Dr. Akira Endo discovered mevastatin formerly called compactin from fungus *Penicillium citrinum*. Pravastatin is the first available statin manufactured by Sankyo, Japan (1979). This was commercially launched in 1989 in Japan. It received Food and Drug Administration approval in 1991. Subsequently, lovastatin (Mevacor) was launched by Merck. Pitavastatin (Livalo) was discovered in Japan by Nissan Chemical Industries in 2005.

The discovery of statin is a landmark in human history. For the first time, it was shown that all manifestation of atherosclerotic vascular disease, starting from subclinical to clinical, can be prevented by an oral agent.[1,2]

CLASSIFICATION OF STATINS

Broadly the statins can be classified into two groups based on their source: Type 1 or naturally derived statins and Type 2 or synthetic. The naturally derived statins are obtained from fungus. Type 1 or naturally derived statins are (a) lovastatin, (b) simvastatin, (c) pravastatin and (d) pitavastatins. Synthetic statins or type 2 statins are (a) fluvastatin, (b) atorvastatin and (c) rosuvastatin. Statins can be classified by their solubility also. Water-soluble or hydrophilic statins are pravastatin, pitavastatin and rosuvastatin. Fat-soluble or hydrophobic statins are simvastatin, lovastatin, fluvastatin and atorvastatin (Table 12.1).[3,4]

Table 12.1: Classification of statins

Classification of statins based on the manufacturing method:

    Type 1 (fermentation derived): simvastatin, lovastatin, pravastatin and pitavastatin

    Type 2 (synthetic): fluvastatin, atorvastatin and rosuvastatin

Classification of statins based on the solubility:

    Water-soluble (hydrophilic): pravastatin, rosuvastatin and pitavastatin

    Fat-soluble (lipophilic): simvastatin, lovastatin, fluvastatin and atorvastatin

Classification of statins based on the development:

    First-generation statins

        Lovastatin (prodrug), simvastatin (prodrug) and pravastatin

    Second-generation statins

        Fluvastatin

    Third-generation statins

        Atorvastatin, cerivastatin (withdrawn from the market), rosuvastatin and pitavastatin

Low-Density Lipoprotein (LDL)-Dependent Mechanism of Action

Statins competitively inhibit the rate-limiting enzyme HMG-CoA reductase in the cholesterol biosynthesis. This results in the blockage of conversion of HMG-CoA to mevalonate that leads to a number of changes in the liver cells. The total cholesterol (TC) synthesis and cholesterol pool are reduced. The sterol regulatory element-binding proteins are upregulated. There is increase in the number of low-density lipoprotein (LDL) receptor synthesis in liver. The LDL receptors bind with apolipoprotein (Apo) B and ApoE and very low density lipoprotein (VLDL) particles. This results in the increased clearance of these particles by hepatocytes. The reduction in mevalonate bio-synthesis also results in reduction in dolichols, ubiquinones and isoprenoids. These have varying effect on the lipogenesis and adverse events of statins (Fig. 12.1).[3,5]

Low-Density Lipoprotein-Independent (Pleiotropic) Mechanism of Action

Some of the observed beneficial effects are independent of LDL lowering. They are termed as pleiotropic effects of statins (Greek: pleion—more, tropos—direction). Statins act on anti-inflammatory agents and stabilize the atherosclerotic plaque. The serum C-reactive protein (CRP) is lowered. Endothelial function improves. This occurs much earlier than LDL reduction. Statins also improve endothelial function in smokers with normal LDL levels. Statins led to the reduction in atheroma volume, lipid pool and this leads to regression of atherosclerosis. Statin therapy leads to increased endothelial nitric oxide level, reduction in smooth muscle cell proliferation, inflammation, vasoconstriction, thrombosis, cell migration and changes in actin cytoskeleton. It causes reduction in endothelin 1 level. Inhibition of Rho/Rho kinase signaling pathways by statins is one of the proposed hypotheses to explain these pleiotropic effects. Decreased protein prenylation in peripheral tissues leads to decrease in release of growth hormone. This also reduces platelet aggregation. This could be another possible mechanism of the pleiotropic benefit (Fig. 12.2).[6-8]

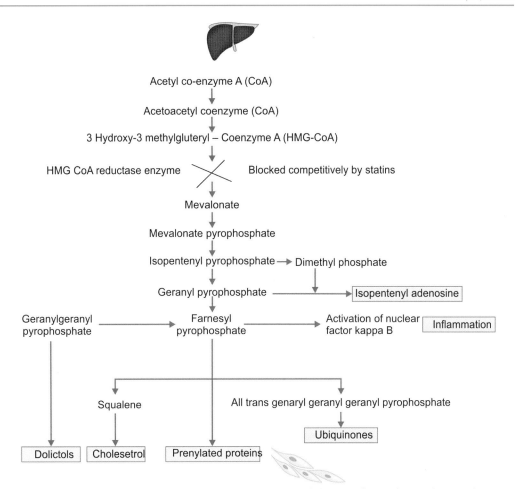

Figure 12.1: Blockade of HMG-CoA reductase results in inhibition of mevalonate biosynthesis that results in upregulation of LDL receptor synthesis, reduction in cholesterol biosynthesis and reduction in formation of prenylated proteins and isoprenoids (isoprenyl adenosyl, dolichols and ubiquinone). LDL, low-density lipoprotein; HMG-CoA, 3-hydroxy-3-methylglutaryl-coenzyme A

PHARMACOLOGY OF STATINS

All statins are absorbed rapidly when orally administered. The peak absorption is by 4 hours. Lovastatin and simvastatin are prodrugs, and they are highly lipid soluble. Fluvastatin and atorvastatin are next lipid-soluble drugs. More lipid-soluble drugs penetrate all membranes easily. Pravastatin and rosuvastatin are more hydrophilic. They are transported across all membranes by organic anion transporting polypeptide. Pravastatin, fluvastatin and rosuvastatin are most bioavailable. Less than 20–25% of the drug reaches circulation. Pitavastatin has the highest bioavailability (51%). Mostly 75–80% of the orally administered drug is eliminated by liver and gastrointestinal tract and minimal amount by the kidneys. Pravastatin and simvastatin have maximum renal elimination (20% and 30%, respectively). In the presence of severely impaired renal function, these statins are to be avoided.

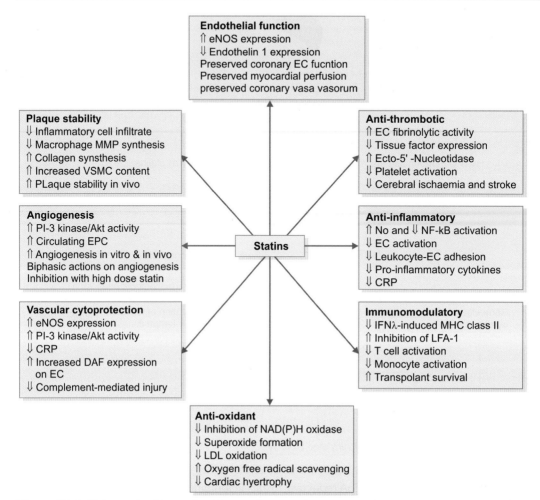

Figure 12.2: Pleiotropic effects of statins on the vasculature

Elimination half-life of older statins like lovastatin, simvastatin, fluvastatin and pravastatin ranges between 1 and 3 hours. Atorvastatin has a half-life of 17 hours, whereas rosuvastatin has a half-life of 19 hours. Pitavastatin has a half-life of 12 hours. Longer half-lives have important therapeutic implication. These three statins can be administered at any time of the day as opposed to bed-time dosing of other statins. This is required because the HMG-CoA enzyme activity is highest at night. The statins are converted to water-soluble salts for elimination. Simvastatin and lovastatin are eliminated by cytochrome p450 3A (CYP3A) enzymes. Atorvastatin also (to a lesser extent) undergoes metabolism by the same pathway. Fluvastatin and rosuvastatin are largely excreted unchanged. Pitavastatin undergoes hepatic glucuronidation and minimal metabolism by CYP2C9 and CYP2C8. Most are excreted in the feces; 10% of the dose is excreted unchanged in the urine. Several clinically important drug interactions need attention. Azole antifungals, macrolide antibiotics, HIV protease inhibitors and grapefruit juice increase the plasma level of statins metabolized by CYP3A pathway, and coadministration of these agents may increase the

Table 12.2: Pharmacology of statins

Oral bioavailability—20–51%

Absorption—absorbed rapidly, peak absorption at 4 hours

Half life—lovastatin, simvastatin, pravastatin, lovastatin and pravastatin—1–3 hours

   Pitavastatin 12 hours, atorvastatin 17 hours, rosuvastatin 19 hours

Metabolism—metabolized by cytochrome p450 pathway

   CYP 2C9—fluvastatin

   CYP 344—atorvastatin, lovastatin and simvastatin.

   Non P450—pravastatin

Excretion—fluvastatin and rosuvastatin are largely excreted unchanged

   75–80% of the rest are excreted by liver and gastrointestinal tract

   <10% excreted by kidneys

chances of rhabdomyolysis. In general, fibrates increase the plasma levels of statins. Gemfibrozil has the highest tendency to increase statin blood concentration by interfering with OATP1B1-mediated transport of statins to hepatocytes and inhibition of CYP2C8. Fenofibrate statin combination avoids these interactions. Statins (with exception of pravastatin) are highly protein-bound molecules. They are likely to replace protein-bound drugs such as warfarin. Rosuvastatin or simvastatin co-administration with warfarin can increase prothrombin time (PT). However, warfarin has no clinically significant interaction with statins (Tables 12.2 and 12.3).[3,9]

BIOCHEMICAL IMPACT OF STATIN THERAPY

Significant reduction in low-density lipoprotein cholesterol (LDL-C) is seen with all the available statins. On mg to mg basis, the LDL-lowering potency is as follows. Rosuvastatin is the most potent statin followed by atorvastatin, pitavastatin, simvastatin and pravastatin. Pravastatin (10–40 mg) lowers LDL by 20–30%, simvastatin (10–80 mg) lowers LDL by 28–46%, atorvastatin (10–80 mg) lowers LDL by 37–51%, rosuvastatin (10–40 mg) lowers LDL by 46–55% and pitavastatin (1–4 mg) lowers LDL by 33.6–47.2%.[10]

Rosuvastatin 10 mg, atorvastatin 20 mg, simvastatin 40 mg and pravastatin 80 mg are comparable in clinical efficiency. National Cholesterol Education Program Adult Treatment Panel III (NCEP ATP III) LDL goals achieved in various treatment groups were rosuvastatin 55%, atorvastatin 43%, simvastatin 31% and pravastatin 11%. However, statin therapy alone may not be able to lower LDL to target levels in some patients.

Plasma triglyceride (TG) levels are decreased by 15–30% by various statins. Their effects follow the same pattern as the effect on LDL-C. Maximum reduction in TG is achieved by atorvastatin and rosuvastatin. Atherogenic dyslipidemia is characterized by high VLDL remnant particles, small dense LDL, low high-density lipoprotein cholesterol (HDL-C) and increase in particle number. Statins are highly efficacious in lowering the number and composition of these particles. Statins reduce LDL, VLDL, ApoCIII, cholesterol and TGs. They also reduce small dense LDL by 44%.

Table 12.3: Statin interactions: Maximum recommended statin doses (mg) and cautions[9-15]

	Simvastatin	Lovastatin	Pravastatin	Atorvastatin	Rosuvastatin	Fluvastatin	Pitavastatin
Itraconazole	0[h]	0[h]	—	20 mg[a]	—	—	—
Ketoconazole	0[h]	0[h]	—	b	—	—	—
Posaconazole	0[h]	0[h]	—	b	—	—	—
Fluconazole	—	—	—	b	—	20 mg BD	—
Erythromycin	0[h]	0[h]	—	b	—	—	1 mg
Clarithromycin	0[h]	0[h]	40 mg	20 mg[a]	—	—	—
Telithromycin	0[h]	0[h]	—	—	—	—	—
HIV protease inhibitors	0[h]	0[h]	—	0–40 mg[c]	10 mg[c,d]	—	—
Telaprevir	0[h]	0[h]	—	Avoid	—	—	—
Boceprevir	0[h]	0[h]	—	—	—	—	—
Nefazodone	0[h]	0[h]	—	—	—	—	—
Gemfibrozil	0[h]	Avoid	Avoid	b,d	Avoid or 10 mg	d	d
Other fibrates	d	20 mg	d	b,d	d	d	d
>1 g niacin/day	b,d	20 mg	b	b	d	b	b
Cyclosporine	0[h]	Avoid	20 mg	Avoid	5 mg	20 mg BD	0[h]
Danazol	0[h]	20 mg	—	d	—	—	—
Amiodarone	10 mg	40 mg	—	—	—	—	—
Dronedarone	10 mg	—	—	—	—	—	—
Verapamil	10 mg	20 mg	—	—	—	—	—
Diltiazem	10 mg	20 mg	—	—	—	—	—
Amlodipine	20 mg	—	—	—	—	—	—

	Simvastatin	Lovastatin	Pravastatin	Atorvastatin	Rosuvastatin	Fluvastatin	Pitavastatin
Ranolazine	20 mg	–	–	–	–	–	–
Digoxin	–	–	–	e	–	–	–
Warfarin	f	f	–	–	d	f	f
Rifampicin	–	–	–	g	–	–	2
Phenytoin	–i	–i	–	–	–	d	–i
Colchicine	d	–	d	–	–	–	–

[a] Caution should be used at doses above this dose (lowest dose necessary should be used).
[b] Consider statin dose reduction when coadministering this drug.
[c] Refer to the section "Statin Dosage".
[d] Coadminister with caution.
[e] Coadministration of atorvastatin and digoxin can increase digoxin level by 20%, these patients should be monitored appropriately.
[f] Monitor INR when statin started.
[g] Administration of atorvastatin with inducers of CYP 450 3A4 (e.g., rifampicin and efavirenz) can lead to variable reduction in plasma concentration of atorvastatin. Thus, atorvastatin should be administered simultaneously with drugs that are 3A4 inducers since delaying the statin administration can result in reduced statin plasma concentration.
[h] Not to be used in this particular combination.
[i] No specific USFDA recommendation.
HIV, human immunodeficiency virus; CYP, cytochrome P450; INR, International Normalized Ratio; BD, twice a day.

The NCEP ATP III non-HDL goal achieved by various statins is as follows: atorvastatin 38%), simvastatin 32%), lovastatin 32%), fluvastatin 26% and pravastatin 26%.

Most statins increase the HDL-C by 5–7%. This is done by upregulating the transport protein ATP-binding cassette transporter A1. Rosuvastatin raises HDL by 8–10%. This also reduces the transfer of cholesteryl ester from HDL to VLDL and LDL via inhibition of cholesteryl ester transfer protein. Pitavastatin increases the HDL concentration to a maximum (24.6%) in patients with low HDL. Reduction in TC, reduction in TG and increase in HDL make this an ideal statin in atherogenic dyslipidemia.[11,12]

CLINICAL IMPACT OF STATIN THERAPY

Statins have shown to reduce cardiovascular (CV) and total mortality in various trials like Scandinavian Simvastatin Survival Study (4S), Long-Term Intervention with Pravastatin in Ischemic Disease (LIPID) and Heart Protection Study (HPS). They reduce coronary heart disease (CHD) death, nonfatal myocardial infarction (MI) and the first CV event. This has been shown in both primary prevention trials and secondary intervention trials involving >1,20,000 patients. In total, 1% reduction in LDL lowers the first major event by 0.88%. Statins reduce the events in all ages and genders. Various trials conducted with statins can be grouped into (1) primary prevention trials, (2) clinical outcome trials, (3) acute coronary syndrome (ACS) trial, (4) stroke trial, (5) high-dose versus low-dose statin trials, (6) chronic heart failure (CHF) trial, (7) trials in border line high lipid situation, (8) trials in low HDL and LDL, (9) atheroma reduction trials and (10) trials in elderly (Table 12.4).[13,14]

Primary Prevention Trials

These are the trials conducted in individuals without overt CHD. Various trials under this category are (1) West of Scotland Coronary Prevention Study (WOSCOPS),[15] (2) The Air Force/Texas Coronary Atherosclerosis Prevention Study (AFCAPS/TexCAPS),[16] (3) Heart Protection Study (HPS),[17] (4) Collaborative Atorvastatin Diabetes Study (CARDS),[18] (5) Anglo-Scandinavian Cardiac Outcomes: Lipid-Lowering Arm (ASCOT-LLA),[19] (6) Atorvastatin Study for Prevention of CHD End Point in Non-insulin-Dependent Diabetes Mellitus (ASPEN),[20] (7) Management of Elevated Cholesterol in the Primary Prevention Group of Adult Japanese (MEGA)[21] trial and (8) Justification for the Use of Statin in Prevention and Intervention Trial Evaluating Rosuvastatin (JUPITER).[22]

In the WOSCOPS trial, 40 mg pravastatin ($n = 3302$) was compared with placebo ($n = 3293$) in men with elevated lipid (LDL 155 mg/dL; TC 252 mg/dL). Pravastatin lowered plasma cholesterol by 20% and LDL by 26%. There were fewer deaths and nonfatal MI in pravastatin arm, 174 versus 248 [relative risk (RR) 31%; 95% confidence interval (CI), 17–43%; $P \leq 0.001$]. The adverse events were comparable, and there was no increase in non-CV mortality.[15]

The AFCAPS/TexCAPS trial was designed to study the role of lovastatin (20–40 mg) for the prevention of first coronary events in individuals with average cholesterol level without having clinically evident atherosclerotic vascular disease. A total of 5608 men and 997 women with mean cholesterol level 222 ± 21 mg/dL and LDL-C level 150 ± 17 mg/dL were randomized to lovastatin versus placebo. After average follow-up for 5.2 years, lovastatin reduced ACS (183 vs. 116; RR 0.63; 95% CI, 0.50–0.79; $P \leq 0.001$), MI (95 vs. 57; RR 0.60; 95% CI, 0.43–0.83; $P = 0.002$). Safety outcomes were comparable to placebo.[16]

The HPS is the largest study with statin in 20,536 adults (aged 40–80 years) with coronary artery disease (CAD) or other vascular disease or diabetes mellitus (DM). The study addressed the benefit of lowering cholesterol with simvastatin in a high-risk population with average

Table 12.4: Various trials with statins

1. **Primary prevention trials**
   WOSCOPS
   AFCAPS/TAXCAPS
   HPS
   CARDS
   ASCOTT—LLA
   ASPEN
   MEGA
   JUPITER

2. **Clinical outcome trials**
   4S
   LIPID
   TNT
   IDEAL
   SEARCH
   BIP

3. **ACS trials**
   MIRACL
   PROVE IT TIMI
   FLORIDA
   PACT
   A TO Z TRIAL (Z. Phase)
   ARMYDA- ACS

4. **High-dose atorvastatin versus angioplasty**
   AVERT

5. **Borderline high lipids**
   CARE

6. **Congestive heart failure**
   CORONA

7. **Atheroma volume reduction**
   ASTEROID
   REVERSAL
   REGRESS
   SATURN
   MARS
   ORION

8. **Postmarketing study**
   LIVES
   ROSUVEES
   CHIBA

9. **Stroke**
   SPARCL

10. **Statins in dementia**
    ROSPER
    LEADe
    CLASP
    ADCLT

11. **New trials**
    REAL CAD
    J-PREDICT
    DIALYSIS

cholesterol. Primary outcome measures were mortality (overall analysis) and fatal and non-fatal vascular events (prespecified subcategory with subsidiary cancer) and other morbidity analysis. All-cause mortality was reduced by simvastatin (1328, 12.9%) compared with placebo (157, 14.7%; $P = 0.0003$). Coronary death was reduced significantly [simvastatin 587 (5.7%) vs. placebo 707 (6.9%); $P = 0.0005$]. Other vascular deaths and nonvascular deaths were not significantly different. Nonfatal MI, coronary death, stroke and revascularization all were reduced with simvastatin. The benefit was seen even in patients with LDL <116 mg/dL (3.0 mmol/L) on average and TC below 193 mg/dL (5.0mmol/L). There was no impact on cancer incidence or hospitalization for any nonvascular cause. In total, 5 years treatment of 1000 patients having high-risk features would prevent 70–100 events irrespective of the initial cholesterol.[17]

The CARDS addressed the benefit of atorvastatin (10 mg) treatment in patients with DM without having prior vascular events and without having high LDL-C concentration. A total of 2838 patients were randomized to atorvastatin ($n = 1428$) versus placebo ($n = 1410$). Mean duration of follow-up was 3.9 years. At baseline, the mean TC was 207 mg/dL (5.35 mmol/L) in placebo arm versus 207 mg/dL (5.36 mmol/L) in atorvastatin arm. The mean LDL was 117 mg/dL

(3.02 mmol/L) versus 118 (3.04 mmol/L) in these two groups. Total cholesterol and LDL-C were reduced by 26% and 40%, respectively by atorvastatin treatment. The primary end point of major CV events including stroke was reduced by 37% (95% CI, 17–52; P = 0.0001, placebo 127 events vs. 83 events in atorvastatin arm). There was no excess of adverse events.[18]

The ASCOT-LLA was one of the arms of the ASCOT trial where effect of lipid lowering was studied, in which 19,257 patients were randomized to blood pressure lowering (ASCOT BPLA beta-blocker ± diuretic vs. calcium channel blocker ± angiotensin-converting enzyme inhibitor. Of these, 10305 patients were again randomized to either atorvastatin 10 mg or placebo. Atorvastatin administration reduced the primary end point (nonfatal MI and fatal CHD) by 36%. The secondary end points were reduced significantly. All coronary events reduced by 19%, fatal and nonfatal stroke by 27% and all CV events and procedures by 21%.[19]

The ASPEN (n = 2410) trial was designed to study the impact of 10 mg atorvastatin versus placebo in diabetic population with LDL-C below guideline targets. The primary end point was composite of CV death, nonfatal MI, nonfatal stroke, recanalization, coronary artery bypass graft (CABG) surgery, resuscitated cardiac arrest and worsening or unstable angina leading to hospitalization. Over a period of 4 years, the primary end point rates were 13.7% and 15.6% [hazard ratio (HR) 0.90; 95% CI, 0.73–1.12]. The composite end point was not significantly reduced.[20]

In MEGA trial, 7832 men aged 40–70 years and postmenopausal woman with TC 220–270 mg/dL (5.69–6.98 mmol/L) were randomized to pravastatin (10–20 mg/day) versus placebo. The primary end point was composite of CAD events defined as sudden death, fatal and nonfatal MI, angina or CV intervention. The secondary end points were stroke, cerebral infarction or CHD composite of any CV event or mortality. Over a period of 5.3 years, mean TC was reduced by 2.1 versus 11.5% in placebo and active treatment group, respectively. Mean LDL-C was reduced by 3.2% and 18% in placebo and active group, respectively. This translated into lower events in the pravastatin arm (66 vs. 101 events; HR 0.67; 95% CI, 0.49–0.9; P = 0.01). Malignant neoplasm and serious adverse events were not different in these two groups.[21]

The JUPITER trial tested the hypothesis that people with elevated high-sensitivity CRP as well as mildly elevated lipid level (LDL <130 mg) might benefit from therapy with rosuvastatin. In total, 17,802 men and women with LDL <130 mg/dL (3.4 mmol/L) and high-sensitivity CRP levels of 2.0 mg/L or higher were randomized to rosuvastatin 20 mg daily versus placebo. The primary end point was the combination of MI, stroke, arterial revascularization, hospitalization for unstable angina or CV death. The trial was stopped at 1.9 year (mean), maximum 5 year follow up. Treatment with rosuvastatin reduced LDL by 50% and C reactive protein (CRP) by 37%. The primary end points were 0.77 versus 1.36 per 100 person follow-up in rosuvastatin versus placebo arm, respectively (HR 0.56; 95% CI, 0.46–0.69; $P \leq$ 0.0001). Myocardial infarction was less (0.17% vs. 0.37% HR 0.46; 95% CI, 0.30–0.70; P = 0.0002). The rates of stroke were less with rosuvastatin (0.18% vs. 0.34%; HR 0.52; 95% CI, 0.34–0.79; P = 0.002). Similarly, revascularization or unstable angina were less (0.41% vs. 0.77%; HR 0.53; 95% CI, 0.40–0.70; P<0.00001). The combined end points of MI, stroke or CV death were less (P = 0.00001). All-cause mortality was less (1.0 vs. 1.25%; HR 0.80; 95% CI, 0.67–0.97; P = 0.02). Myopathy or cancer incidence was not different. However, rosuvastatin arm had higher incidence of DM.[22]

Clinical Outcome Trials

These are the trials conducted on the patients with established CAD. Secondary prevention of the CV events were the end points. The trials under this category are (1) (4 S trial) Scandinavian

Simvastatin Survival Study (4STRIAL),[23] (2) Longterm Intervention with Pravastatin in Ischemic Disease (LIPID),[23] (3) Treating to New Targets (TNT),[24] (4) A comparison of Intensive statin versus low moderate therapy in stable CAD patients with previous MI (IDEAL trial),[25] (5) Study of Effectiveness of Additional Reduction in Cholesterol and Homocysteine (SEARCH)[26] and (6) Early Intensive versus a Delayed Conservative Simvastatin Strategy in patients with Acute Coronary Syndrome, phase Z of the A to Z trial (A to Z trial).[27]

In the 4S trial, 4444 patients with previous history of angina pectoris or MI with elevated cholesterol (5.5–8mmol/L) were randomized to simvastatin ($n = 2221$) and placebo ($n = 2223$). Simvastatin reduced mean TC by 25%, mean LDL-C by 35% and increased HDL-C by 8% over 5.4 years of median follow-up. This translated with reduction in death with simvastatin 182 (8%) versus 256 (12%) in placebo. There was 30% relative risk reduction in death with simvastatin (RR 0.70; 95% CI, 0.58–0.85; $P = 0.003$). Coronary deaths were 111 in simvastatin group versus 189 in placebo group (RR 0.58; 95% CI, 0.46–0.73). Non cardiovascular causes of death were 46 and 49, respectively. Overall, 4311 (19%) in the simvastatin group and 622 (28%) patients in placebo group had major coronary event (RR 0.66; 95% CI, 0.59–0.75; $P<0.00001$). There was 37% relative risk reduction for myocardial revascularization ($P \leq 0.00001$). The number needed to treat (NNT) was 30. There was no excess of adverse events.[23]

In the LIPID trial, 9014 patients aged between 31 and 75 years, who were admitted for unstable angina or acute MI and had cholesterol level between 155 and 271 mg/dL, were randomized to placebo or pravastatin 40 mg/day. The primary end point was mortality for CHD. Over a mean follow-up of 6.1 years CHD death was 8.3% in placebo arm versus 6.4% in the pravastatin arm (RR 0.76; 95% CI, 0.12–0.35; $P \leq 0.001$). Overall mortality was 14.1% in the placebo group versus 11.0% in pravastatin group (RR 0.78; 95% CI, 0.13–0.31; $P \leq 0.001$). The effects were consistent in all predefined subgroups. There were no clinically significant adverse events with pravastatin.[24]

The TNT trial addressed the efficacy and safety of lowering LDL below 100 mg/dL (2.6 mmol/L) in stable CAD patients. A total of 10,001 patients with clinically stable CAD with LDL level <130 mg/dL (34mmol/L) were randomized to atorvastatin 10 mg versus atorvastatin 80 mg dosage. The primary end point was the occurrence of a major CV event, defined as death from CHD, nonfatal procedure-related MI, resuscitation after cardiac arrest, fatal or nonfatal stroke. Over a mean follow-up of 4.9 years, LDL was lowered to mean 77 mg/dL (2.0mmol/L) with 80 mg and to 101 mg/dL (2.6 mmol/L) with 10 mg atorvastatin. Primary event occurred in 434 (8.7%) patients on 80 mg dose versus 548 (10.9%) patent on 10 mg dose. Absolute reduction in risk was 2.2%. There was relative risk reduction with 22% (HR 0.78; 95 CI, 0.69–0.89; $P < 0.007$). The overall mortality was not significantly different. Persistent liver aminotransferase elevation was seen in 0.2% in 10 mg group and 2.2% in 80 mg group ($P<0.001$).[25]

The IDEAL trial assessed the high-dose atorvastatin (80 mg) versus standard dose simvastatin (20 mg) for secondary prevention of CAD following MI. A total of 8888 patients aged 80 years or below were randomized to atorvastatin ($n = 4439$) versus simvastatin ($n = 4449$). The primary end point was major coronary event defined as coronary death, nonfatal MI or resuscitation from cardiac arrest. Over a median follow-up of 4.8 years, mean LDL was lowered to 104 [standard error (SE) 0.3] mg/dL with simvastatin and to 81 (SE 0.3) mg/dL with atorvastatin. Major coronary events occurred in 463 (10.4%) patients in simvastatin group as compared with atorvastatin 411 (9.3%) group (HR 0.89; 95% CI, 0.78–1.01; $P = 0.07$). Intensive lipid lowering did not reduce the primary end point significantly. However, the composite secondary end point and nonfatal MI were reduced. Transaminase elevation was higher, 43 (1%) versus 5 (0.1%; $P<0.001$) with 80 mg dose of atorvastatin.[26]

In the SEARCH trial, 12,064 patients with past MI were randomized to simvastatin 80 mg versus 20 mg dose regimen. This study also had a homocysteine-lowering arm. Overall, 6031 patients received 80 mg and 6033 patients received 20 mg dose of simvastatin. The 80 mg dosage caused a further reduction in TC (0.6 mmol/L), LDL-C (0.5 mmol/L) and TGs (0.2mmol/L). Major vascular events occurred in 1477 (24.5%) patients on 80 mg/dL versus 1553 (25.7%) on 20 mg/dL (RR 0.94; 95% CI, 0.88–1.01; P = 0.010). Hemorrhagic stroke, vascular or nonvascular deaths were not significantly different. Myopathy occurred in 2 (0.03%) with 20 mg versus 53 (0.9%) with 80 mg dosage.[27]

Trials of Statins in Acute Coronary Syndrome

Each and every patient with ACS, including patients with acute ST elevation MI (STEMI), non-ST elevation MI (non-STEMI) and unstable angina, should receive statin therapy at the earliest for secondary prevention of coronary events. The various trials of statins conducted in the setting of ACS are (1) Myocardial Ischemia Reduction with Acute Cholesterol Lowering Trial (MIRACL),[28] (2) Pravastatin or Atorvastatin Evaluation and Infection Therapy—Thrombolysis in Myocardial Infarction 22 (PROVE-IT TIMI-22) trial,[29] (3) the Fluvastatin on Risk Diminishing After Acute MI (FLORIDA) trial,[30] (4) Aggrastat to Zocor (A to Z) trial,[31] (5) the Pravastatin Acute Coronary Syndrome Treatment (PACT)[32] and (6) the LIPID-CAD (L-CAD) study (Table 12.5).[33]

In the MIRACL study, 3806 patients were randomly assigned to receive 80 mg of atorvastatin or placebo within 24–96 hours of a non-QMI (54% patients) or unstable angina (46% patients). In all, 23% of patients had type 2 DM, 55% patients were hypertensive and 28% of patients were smoking at the time of randomization. The follow-up period was 4 months. The composite end point of death, recurrent MI, cardiac arrest and resuscitation or worsening angina with hospitalization had occurred in 14.8% of patients in the atorvastatin group versus 17.4% of placebo group (RR 0.84; P = 0.048). Individually symptomatic ischemia with objective evidence and emergency hospitalization was the only end point that was significant (6.2% vs. 8.4% for atorvastatin vs. placebo, respectively; P = 0.02). The rate of serious advise events was similar (<1%) in both the groups.[28]

In PROVE-IT TIMI-22 trial, 4162 patients who had been hospitalized for ACS within preceding 10 days were randomized to either pravastatin 40 mg daily or atorvastatin 80 mg daily. The primary end point was a composite of all-cause mortality, myocardial infarction, unstable angina requiring hospitalization, revascularization (performed at least 30 days after randomization) and stroke. Follow-up period was 18–36 months (mean 24 months). In the atorvastatin group, the median LDL was 62 mg/dL (1.60 mmol/L) compared with pravastatin group 95 mg/dL (2.46 mmol/L; $P \leq$ 0.001). Kaplan Meier estimates of the rates of the primary end point at 2 years were 26.3% in the pravastatin group and 22.4% in atorvastatin group. There was 16% relative risk reduction with atorvastatin (95% CI, 5–26%; P = 0.005).[29]

In the FLORIDA trial, 540 patients were randomly assigned to receive either fluvastatin 80 mg/day or placebo for 1 year. There was no significant difference of ischemic events at 6 weeks and 1 year. The mortality rate at 1 year was 2.6% with fluvastatin as compared with 4% in the placebo arm (P = NS). The trial did not have statistical power to detect the mortality difference. However, there was a trend toward a lower mortality with fluvastatin (P = 0.08).[30]

Phase Z of the A to Z trial was designed to address the timing and intensity of statin therapy following ACS. Patients with ACS were randomized to 40 mg of simvastatin for 1 month, followed

Table 12.5: Early statin trial in acute coronary syndrome

Sl. No.	Trial	Drugs	Initiation	Duration
1	MIRACL	Atorvastatin vs. placebo	96 h	4 months
2	PROVE-IT TIMI-22	Pravastatin vs. atorvastatin and gatifloxacin vs. placebo	1–10 days	24 months
3	FLORIDA	Fluvastatin vs. placebo		
4	A TO Z	Tirofiban/simvastatin	1–10 days	12 months
5	PACT	Pravastatin vs. placebo	<24 h	1 month
6	L-CAD			
7	PRINCESS	Cervastatin/placebo	96 h	3 months

MIRACL, Myocardial Ischemia Reduction with Acute Cholesterol Lowering; PROVE-IT TIMI-22, Pravastatin or Atorvastatin Evaluation and Infection Therapy–Thrombolysis in Myocardial Infarction 22; FLORIDA, Fluvastatin on Risk Diminishing after Acute; PACT, Pravastatin ACS Treatment; A to Z TRIAL (Z phase), Aggrastat to Zocor; L-CAD, Lipid-Coronary Artery Disease.

by 80 mg/day thereafter (n = 2265) versus placebo for initial 4 months followed by simvastatin 20 mg/day (n = 2232). The primary end point was a composite of CV death, nonfatal MI, readmission for ACS and stroke. Follow-up period was 6 months to maximum 24 months.[30] The primary end point event occurred in 343 (16.7%) patients in placebo plus simvastatin group compared with 309 (14.4%) in the simvastatin only group (HR 0.89; 95% CI, 0.57–1.00; P = 0.05). The beneficial effects were observed after analysis at 4 months onward and persisted till the end of the study. Myopathy [symptoms associated with creatinine kinase (CK)>10 time supper limit of normal (ULN)] occurred in nine patients (0.4%) in simvastatin 80 mg group as compared with one patient in the placebo group (P = 0.02). The trial did not reach the prespecified end points. A favorable trend was observed with intensive statin treatment.[31]

In the PACT trial, 3408 patients for acute MI or stable angina were randomized to 40 mg of pravastatin or placebo. The duration of the treatment was at least 30 days. Post hoc analysis revealed 211/1698 (12.4%) events in placebo arm as compared with 199/1710 (11.6%) in the pravastatin arm. The absolute risk reduction was 0.8% (95% CI, 1.4–3) and the relative risk reduction was 6.4% (95% CI, 13.2–27.6).[32]

In the L-CAD study, 70 patients received pravastatin within 6 days of acute MI or percutaneous coronary intervention (PCI) for ACS. Total 56 patients received lipid-lowering therapy after hospital discharge at the discretion of the family physician and severed as the comparator arm. At 6 months, the lumen diameter was larger than baseline in active group as measured by quantitative coronary angiography where it decreased in the control group. At 2 years, the combined end point (death, MI, stroke, new-onset peripheral vascular disease; coronary intervention) was 23% in the pravastatin group compared with 52% in the control group [odds ratio (OR) 0.28; P = 0.005]. This study had limitations of being an open labeled and single-center study.[33]

In the ARMYDA-ACS trial, high-dose atorvastatin 80 mg initiated 12 hours before angiography and subsequently 40 mg administered, 2 hours before the angioplasty was used. ST elevation MI and high-risk non-STEMI patients requiring emergency PCI were excluded. Duration of 30 days major adverse, cardiac events (MACE) was 5% in statin arm compared with 17% in placebo arm ($P = 0.01$). Post procedure MI was significantly less in atorvastatin arm (5vs.15%; $P = 0.04$).[34]

The ARMYDA trial used 40 mg of atorvastatin initiated 7 days before scheduled PCI in stable CAD patients. Post PCI, troponin I rise was less in statin group (atorvastatin 20% vs. placebo 48%; $P = 0.0004$); 30 days MACE was lower in statin-treated group (5vs. 18%; $P = 0.025$).[35]

Various trial results are available for review regarding the relative benefit of intensive lipid-lowering therapy with different statins (PROVE-IT TIMI-22—pravastatin 40 mg vs. atorvastatin 80 mg; TNT—atorvastatin 10 vs. 80 mg; A to Z—simvastatin 20 mg vs. simvastatin 80 mg; IDEAL—simvastatin 20 mg vs. atorvastatin 80 mg). Intensive lipid-lowering therapy lowers the events and mortality. Mean level of LDL achieved was as low as 62 mg/dL in major international trials and 71 mg/dL in Indian patients. This low level was shown to be safe and also effective.[36,37]

Post-Marketing Studies

The LIVALO Effectiveness and Safety (LIVES) study 20,000 patients with hypercholesterolemia who were treated with pitavastatin for up to 2 years. In this study, the LDL-C target rate recommended by the Japanese Atherosclerosis Society (JAS) was achieved by 88.2% of low-risk patients (<160 mg/dL), 82.7% of intermediate-risk patients (<140 mg/dL), 66.5% of high-risk patients (<120 mg/dL) and 50.3% of secondary prevention patients (<100 mg/dL). In patients with low HDL-C, a significant reduction in TC (−21.0%), LDL-C (−31.3%) and TG (−6.1%) was seen at 104 weeks.[38]

The ROSUVEES ($n = 219$) was a multicenter study of 5, 10 and 20 mg dosage of rosuvastatin in a routine clinical practical setting in patients with LDL >130 mg/dL from India. The primary objective was to establish safety and efficacy of these dosages of rosuvastatin in the general practice setting. The secondary objective was to access the proportion of patients reaching ATP III guidelines in these three groups. There was reduction in LDL in all the three dosage groups over 8 weeks period. 5 mg reduced LDL from 150 mg mean at base line to 110 mg at 8 weeks (26.71%) P ≤ 0.001; 10 mg reduced LDL from 169 mg mean at base line to 108 mg at 8 weeks (35.89%) P ≤ 0.001 ; 53.5% individuals reached ATP III LDL goal and 82.19% reached non-HDL goal. The adverse events were not clinically significant.[39]

In the 12-week open-label trial (Collaborative Study on Hypercholesterolemia Drug Intervention and Their Benefits for Atherosclerosis Prevention), both pitavastatin 2 mg/day and atorvastatin 10 mg/day significantly reduced serum LDL-C by 42.6% and 44.1%, respectively, and serum TG by 17.3% and 10.7%, respectively. An increase in the serum HDL-C was observed (3.2%; $P < 0.033$ vs. baseline), but not after 12 weeks of atorvastatin treatment (1.7%; $P < 0.221$ vs. baseline).[40]

In a multicenter (PIAT) study in patients with hypercholesterolemia and impaired glucose tolerance effect, pitavastatin 2 mg/day was compared with atorvastatin 10 mg/day. The results showed that the percentage change in HDL-C was greater in the pitavastatin than the atorvastatin group (8.2% vs. 2.9%; $P = 0.031$).[41]

A randomized, double-blind, 12-week study to compare pitavastatin and simvastatin reported that the administration of pitavastatin 2 mg/day reduced LDL-C by 39.0% ($n = 307$), which was significantly greater than that achieved with simvastatin 20 mg/day (35.0%, $n = 107$).Pitavastatin 4 mg/day reduced LDL-C by 44.0% ($n = 319$), which was comparable to that of simvastatin 40 mg/day (42.8%, $n = 110$).[42]

In the Japanese dose–response trial, the LDL-C-lowering effect of pitavastatin after 12 weeks was 34% (n = 81) at a dose of 1 mg, 42% (n = 75) at a dose of 2 mg and 47% (n = 76) at a dose of 4 mg.[43]

One report showed that 6 months administration of pitavastatin at 2 mg/day significantly reduced LDL-C, from 155 to 88 mg/dL, in 45 patients with diabetes.[44]

Statins in Stroke

The Stroke Prevention by Aggressive Reduction in Cholesterol Levels trial was a major trial of high-dose atorvastatin in stroke patients.[45] In patients with strokes or transient ischemic attack (TIA) without CHD, atorvastatin 80 mg/day has shown to reduce strokes and TIA by 16% and CHD events were reduced by 35% (P = 0.003). Hemorrhagic stroke was little higher. However, a meta-analysis of more with 90,000 CHD patients participating in 14 trials showed that 39% reduction in LDL-C results in 27% reduction in CHD events and 22% reduction in ischemic strokes with no difference in hemorrhagic strokes incidence. Consequently, all patients of stroke should receive high-dose statin when the risk of hemorrhagic transformation is ruled out.

High-Dose Statins Versus Angioplasty in Stable Coronary Artery Disease

In the AVERT trial, atorvastatin 80 mg (n = 164) was compared with revascularization by PCI (n = 177) in stable ischemic disease. The LDL at entry was at least 115 mg/dL (3.0mmol/L). The follow-up period was 18 months. All patients had normal left ventricular function. Patients had either no angina or mild-to-moderate angina; 23 patients (13%) in the atorvastatin group had an ischemic event compared with 37 (21%) with PCI arm. The mean LDL was 77 mg/dL (2.0mmol/L) versus 119 mg/dL (3.0 mmol/L), respectively. There was 36% event reduction in the high-dose atorvastatin group (P = 0.048), which was not statistically significant after adjustment for interim analysis. The atorvastatin group had a significantly long time to the first ischemic event (P = 0.03).[46]

Statin in Chronic Heart Failure

In the CORONA study, 5011 patients of >60 years age having symptomatic CHF with reduced ejection fraction <35% (class III, IV) and <40% (class II) of ischemic etiology were randomized to rosuvastatin 10 mg or placebo. The primary outcome was combination of CV mortality, nonfatal MI and nonfatal stroke (time to first event). The first secondary end point was all-cause mortality. During a mean follow-up of 32.8 months, the primary outcome occurred in 692 patients in the rosuvastatin arm and 732 patients in the placebo arm (HR 0.92; 95% CI, 0.83–1.02; P = 0.12). Death occurred in 728 and 759 patients in these two groups, respectively (HR 0.95; 95% CI, 0.86–1.05; P = 0.31). There was no deference in death or coronary outcome in between the two groups. There was less rehospitalization for CV cause in the rosuvastatin group (2193 vs. 2,564; P ≤ 0.001). Adverse events were comparable. The trial concluded that rosuvastatin had no impact on mortality in systole heart failure.[47]

Statin in Patients with Borderline High Lipid

The CARE study was designed to address the utility of lipid-lowering therapy with average level of cholesterol. In all, 4159 patients with MI who had TC below 240 mg/dL (mean 269 mg/dL) and

LDL-C level 115–174 mg/dL (mean 139 mg/dL) were randomly assigned to pravastatin 40 mg/day or placebo. The primary outcome was fatal coronary event or a nonfatal MI. The primary end point was reached in 10.2% in the pravastatin group compared with13.2% in the placebo group. There was 3% absolute reduction and 24% relative risk reduction (95% CI, 9 to 3.6%; $P = 0.008$) in the primary end point. Pravastatin reduced the need for CABG surgery by 26% ($P = 0.005$), angioplasty by 23% ($P = 0.01$) and stroke by 30%, $P = 0.03$). There was no difference in overall mortality or death for non-CV causes. Patients with higher pretreatment cholesterol level were benefited the most.[48]

Atheroma Volume Reduction Studies with Statins (Regression Trials)

Intensive lipid-lowering therapy has been shown to halt the progression of the atherosclerosis and cause regression of atheroma volume that results in the disease burden. These trials can be grouped together as regression statin trials. They are (1) Monitor Atherosclerosis Regression Study (MARS),[49] (2) the Reversal of Atherosclerosis with Aggressive Lipid Lowering (REVERSAL),[50] (3) A Study to Evaluate the Effect of Rosuvastatin or Intravascular Ultrasound Derived Coronary Atheroma Burden (ASTEROID),[51] (4) the Regression Growth Evaluation Statin Study (REGRESS),[52] (5)Study of Coronary Atheroma by Intravascular in Ultrasound: Effect of Rosuvastatin versus Atorvastatin (SATURN),[53] (6) Outcome of Rosuvastatin on Carotid Artery Atheroma or Magnetic Resonance Imaging Observation (ORION) study[54] and (7) the Japan Assessment of Pitavastatin and Atorvastatin in Acute Coronary Syndrome (JAPAN-ACS) study.[55]

The MARS trial randomized patients with TC 190–295 mg/dL (4.92–7.64 mmol/L) to either placebo ($n = 124$) or lovastatin 80 mg/day. All patients either had past MI or angiographic CAD. The follow-up period was 2 years. Lovastatin lowered TC by 32%, LDL-C by 38% and ApoB by 26% and increased HDL-C by 8.5% ($P \leq 0.001$).Average percent diameter stenosis increased by 2.2% in placebo group and 1.6% in lovastatin group ($P \geq 0.20$). For lesions of 50% or greater, average percent diameter stenosis increased by 0.9% in placebo group and decreased by 4.1% in lovastatin group ($P = 0.005$).[49]

The REVERSAL study was designed to compare the effect of intensive lipid lowering to moderate lipid lowering on atheroma burden and progression of atherosclerosis. Overall 654 patients were randomized to either 40 mg of pravastatin or 80 mg of atorvastatin. A total of 502 patients had evaluable intravascular ultrasound (IVUS) examination at baseline and at 18-month follow-up. Low-density lipoprotein cholesterol (mean 150.2 mg/dL, 3.89 mmol/L) in both treatment group was reduced to 110 mg/dL (2.85 mmol/L) in atorvastatin arm ($P \leq 0.001$). C-reactive protein also decreased. The primary efficiency end point (percentage change in atheroma volume) showed a lower progression with intensive statin treatment ($P = 0.02$). For the primary end point, progression of coronary atherosclerosis occurred in the pravastatin group (2.7%; 95% CI, 0.2–4.7; $P = 0.001$) compared with baseline. Progression did not occur in the atorvastatin group (–0.4% CI,–2.4 to –1.5; $P = 0.98$) compared with baseline.[50]

The ASTEROID study was designed to determine whether 24 months treatment with 40 mg rosuvastatin would result in regression of atherosclerosis. Patients had to have a clinical indication for coronary angiography and coronary lesion of >20% in a major artery. Total 50 patients had baseline IVUS examination. Any lipid level was permitted. Patients received 40 mg rosuvastatin for 2 years. There was no control group for ethical reasons. At the end of 2 years, 349 patients had repeat IVUS examination. Total cholesterol declined from

204 mg/dL at baseline to 133.8 mg/dL at the end of 2 years (−33.8%; $P \leq 0.001$), LDL-C declined from 130.4 to 60.8 mg/dL (−53.2%; $P \leq 0.001$), HDL-C increased from 43.1 to 43.1 +14.7% ($P \leq 0.001$) and TGs declined from 152.2 to 121.2 mg/dL (−14.5%; $P \leq 0.001$). Percent atheroma volume (PAV) and atheroma volume in most diseased segments (mm^3) were significantly reduced ($P \leq 0.001$). When percentage atheroma volume (PAV) was analysed, 63% of patients showed regression and 36.4% showed progression; when the most diseased subsegment was analyzed, 78.1% and 21.9% showed regression and progression, respectively. Alanine-aminotransferase elevation >3 × upper limit of normal (ULN) was seen in 1.8% and CK >5 × ULN in 0.2%.[51]

The REGRESS trial was designed to assess the effect of 2 years treatment with pravastatin on the progression or regression on the angiographically documented CAD. In all, 221 patients underwent angioplasty, out of which 201 cases were considered successful. A total of 178 (89%) patients underwent repeat angiographic study. Patients in the pravastatin arm ($n = 109$) and placebo arm ($n = 112$) were similar at baseline. Percent diameter before angioplasty was 78±14% in pravastatin arm and 80±14% in the placebo group ($P \leq 0.001$). Clinical restenosis was significantly lower in pravastatin group (7%) compared with placebo group (29%; $P \leq 0.001$). Risk reduction in all events was 58%. The study concluded that intensive lipid lowering reduces restenosis at 2 years.[52]

The SATURN trial was designed to assess the effect of intensive lipid treatment on the disease progression with two available statins. Overall 1039 patients with CAD had IVUS examination at baseline and serially thereafter after 104 weeks of treatment of either atorvastatin 80 mg or rosuvastatin 40 mg daily. The rosuvastatin group had lower LDL-C compared with atorvastatin group at the end of therapy: 62.6 versus 70.2 mg/dL (1.62 vs.1.82 mmol/L; $P \leq 0.001$). High-density lipoprotein cholesterol was higher in rosuvastatin group 50.4 versus 48.6 mg/dL (1.30 vs. 1.26 mmol/L; $P = 0.1$). The primary efficiency end point, PAV, decreased by 0.99% (95% CI, −1.19 to −0.63) with atorvastatin and by 1.22% (95% CI, −1.52 to −0.09) with rosuvastatin ($P = 0.17$). The secondary efficiency end point, normalized total atheroma volume (TAV), was more favorable with rosuvastatin ($P = 0.01$). Both agents induced regression of atherosclerosis. Side effect profiles were comparable.[53]

The ORION trial assessed the effect of rosuvastatin on carotid plaque volume and composition. Only 43 patients with LDL-C >100 to <250 mg/dL and 16–79% carotid stenosis by duplex ultrasound were randomized to receive either low (5 mg) or high (40/80 mg) dose of rosuvastatin for 24 months. Total 33 patients had serial magnetic resonance imaging scan results available for analysis. There was no change in carotid plaque volume in either group. In all the patients with lipid-rich necrotic core (LRNC) at baseline, percentage LRNC decreased by 41.4% ($P = 0.005$).[54]

The JAPAN-ACS study evaluated the effects of pitavastatin and atorvastatin on plaque volume in patients with ACS. Patients received either 4 mg/day of pitavastatin or 20 mg/day of atorvastatin.[3] The mean percentage changes in LDL-C were −36.2 ± 19.5% and −35.8 ± 22.9% in the pitavastatin and atorvastatin groups, respectively. The mean percentage changes in plaque volume measured by IVUS were −16.9 ±13.9% and −18.1 ± 14.2% ($P = 0.5$) in the pitavastatin and atorvastatin groups, respectively. The study demonstrated the noninferiority of pitavastatin when compared with atorvastatin on the plaque volume change.[55]

Statin Rebound or Statin Withdrawal

Cell culture studies and animal experiments showed that statin discontinuation triggers a cascade of changes that results in rebound deterioration of vascular function. There is overshoot activation of heterotrimeric G-protein Rho and Rac. This causes increased production of free oxygen radicals and suppression of endothelium derived relaxing factor (EDRF) bioavailability. Discrimination leads to proinflammatory, prothrombotic state with empirical endothelial function. Retrospective analysis of PRISM database revealed that stopping statins during the first days of admission was associated with worse outcomes in ACS. In a prospective, randomized controlled trial (RCT) in patients with ischemic stroke, stopping statins for 3days was associated with a 4.7-fold increase in the risk of death or dependency, greater neurological deterioration and a larger infarct size. Discontinuing statins during the postoperative period following major vascular surgery was associated with a higher incidence of myocardial ischemia, nonfatal MI and CV death. Under conditions of severe acute vascular stress, removal of statins is contraindicated.[56-58]

Statins in Elderly

The Pravastatin in Elderly Individual at Risk of Vascular Disease (PROSPER)[45] trial assessed the effect of pravastatin 40 mg daily in 5804 men and women aged 70–82 years. Patients received pravastatin 40 mg/day ($n = 2891$) or placebo ($n = 2913$) for 3.2 years. The primary end point was composite of coronary death, nonfatal MI and fatal and nonfatal stroke. Pravastatin reduced LDL-C by 34% and reduced the primary end point to 408 events versus 473 in placebo arm (HR 0.85;95% CI, 0.74–0.97; $P = 0.014$).Coronary death and nonfatal MI were also reduced ($P = 0.006$). Stroke was unaffected.[59]

Elimination half-life of statins is longer in the elderly by a factor of 36%.[60]

In a recent meta-analysis of eight trials ($n = 24,674$) in the age group of >65years, statin therapy reduced the risk of MI by 39.4% ($P = 0.003$), and stroke by 23.8% ($P = 0.006$) in patients without established CVD. Total mortality and cancer incidence were not significantly different. Statin therapy should be considered in the elderly as the benefit is shown in this population also.[61]

Statins in Diverse Clinical Condition

A child above 2 years of age should be screened for dyslipidemia if there is family history of dyslipidemia or premature CAD. The American Heart Association recommends statin therapy after 10 years in boys and after menopause in girls. All major statins can be used in the pediatric age group also. Children with LDC-C >190 mg/dL or >160 mg with family history premature CAD and two or more risk factors need to be treated.LDL goal is <130 mg/dL.[62]

In the presence of reduced glomerular filtration rate (GFR) (<15mL/min), atorvastatin should be used if statin therapy is decided. Fluvastatin is the next alternative. Aggressive lipid lowering in dialysis-dependent patients is not recommended because of lack of proven benefit. In the patient population having stage III (GFR <60mL/min/1.73m^2 BSA) and above chronic kidney disease (CKD), rosuvastatin was shown to be superior to probucol.[63]

Patients with nonalcoholic steatohepatitis and nonalcoholic fatty liver disease are benefited by statin therapy. Patients should be monitored for jaundice, hepatomegaly, malaise, indirect bilirubinemia and elevated PT once statins are initiated. Usually the transaminase level declines over a period. Hepatitis B and C patients are equally benefited by statin therapy from cardiovascular disease (CVD).[64]

Statin therapy benefits patients with peripheral arterial disease (PAD). It improved pain-free walking time and time to onset of claudication in PAD (TREADMILL trial).[65]

Statin in Dementia

Alzheimer's disease occurs because of S S amyloid protein plaque deposition in brain. Amyloid protein generation is cholesterol dependent. Broadly, dementia can be categorized into two groups: vascular dementia and nonvascular dementia. Initial observational studies showed beneficial effects on nonvascular dementia. Subsequently, a number of RCTs were performed with various statins with variable results. In the PROSPER trial ($n = 6000$) conducted in people aged 70–80 years, pravastatin 40 mg/day did not improve the cognitive function over a 3 year follow up period.[47]

In Lipitor's Effect on Alzheimer's Dementia (LEADe) study, 80 mg/day of atorvastatin was used over a 72-week period to delay the cognitive decline in patients with mild-to-moderate dementia. This trial was a negative trial.[66]

In the CLASP study, 20–40 mg/day of simvastatin was used for 18 months in mild-to-moderate dementia. This study was also a negative trial.[67]

The Alzheimer's Disease Cholesterol-Lowering Treatment (ADCLT) trial demonstrated that atorvastatin at a dose of 80 mg/day for 1 year showed a positive effect on cognitive performance after 6 months of therapy when compared with placebo.[68]

A meta-analysis performed on the all RCTs of statin in dementia was published. The analysis concluded that there was not enough evidence to prescribe statin for the treatment of dementia.[69]

Two new studies allayed concerns about cognitive dysfunction being a possible adverse effect of statins.

In the first study, investigations examined whether statin use was associated with new diagnoses of dementia in a random sample of 1 million people covered by Taiwan's National Health Insurance. Total 57,669 individuals older than 65 years had no history of dementia in 1997 and 1998. Of these, 15,200 were on statins. Propensity scoring was used to match these patients with controls not using statins. Patients receiving statins were divided into tertiles according to the dose. There were 5516 new diagnoses of dementia (excluding vascular dementia) during the 4.5 years of follow-up. Results showed an inverse relationship between statin use and dementia, with the risk of dementia decreasing with increasing statin dose. This trend remained in different age, sex, and CV risk subgroups. Higher doses of high-potency statins had the strongest protective effects. All the statins except lovastatin were associated with a decreased risk of new-onset dementia when taken at higher daily doses.[70]

A study from National Taiwan University Hospital included 5221 patients with atrial fibrillation, which is known to be a predisposing factor for dementia. Of these, 1652 were taking statins. During a 6-year follow-up, 2.1% of the patients taking statins developed dementia compared with 3.5% of the nonstatin group (OR 0.565; $P = 0.002$). Other factors that were associated with a reduced risk of dementia included male sex and lower CHADS2 score. History of MI, PAD, CAD, CKD and VHD was not associated with new-onset dementia.[71]

New Statin Trials

Randomized Evaluation of Aggressive or Moderate Lipid Lowering Therapy with Pitavastatin in Coronary Artery Disease (REAL-CAD) evaluated CVD prevention by standard cholesterol lowering (pitavastatin 1 mg/day) or aggressive cholesterol lowering (pitavastatin 4 mg/day) in 12,600 stable CAD patients.[19] The study will also look at whether more aggressive cholesterol-lowering therapy is beneficial, especially in patients with diabetes.[72]

The Japan Prevention Trial of Diabetes by Pitavastatin in Patients with Impaired Glucose Tolerance is a comparative and randomized trial of 1240 subjects to evaluate the prevention of new-onset diabetes using pitavastatin 1–4 mg/day in patients with impaired glucose tolerance. The study has recently been presented at the EASD 2013.It showed that pitavastatin 1–2 mg/day plus lifestyle management reduced new-onset diabetes incidence by 18% ($P = 0.04$) when compared with lifestyle change alone.[73]

The Differential Intervention Trial by Standard Therapy versus Pitavastatin in Patients with Chronic Hemodialysis (DIALYSIS) is a trial to evaluate the effects of pitavastatin 1–4 mg/day on all-cause mortality and the incidence of MI in 1550 hemodialysis patients.[21] It is expected to provide the first evidence of statin use in Asian patients on hemodialysis.[74]

Adverse Events of Statins

Statins are safe drugs. Myalgia (muscle pain or soreness with no CK elevation), myositis (pain with CK elevation), myopathy (muscle pain or soreness with CK > 10 times ULN), rhabdomyolysis (symptoms plus CK >10 times plus brown urine and myoglobinuria), pancreatitis and elevation of transaminase levels are seen in <1% of the treated population. In a meta-analysis of 35 trials involving 74,102 patients, elevated enzymes were noted in 1.4% is statin group versus 1.1% in control group[75] (Table 12.6).

Another meta-analysis involving 1,80,000 patients from 21 major statin trials of average 3-year duration showed myalgias in 1.5–3%, myopathy 5/1,00,000 and rhabdomyolysis in 1.6/1,00,000.[76]

Rarely immune-mediated necrotizing myopathy may occur with statins. This is characterized by persistence of serum CK elevation despite the discontinuation of statin.[77]

Statin-induced myopathy is increased by (a) increasing age, (b) female gender, (c) renal impairment, (d) liver dysfunction, (e) hypothyroidism, (f) dietary factors like grape fruit juice and (g) polypharmacy (Table 12.3). Liver failure occurs in one in 1 million person-years on statin therapy that is similar to general population not taking statin. Baseline liver function should be obtained before initiation. If the transaminase levels are more than three times the ULN, the statin should be discontinued. Between one and three times of ULN, statin should be continued. Routine mentioning of liver function is not required in asymptomatic patients. Lower dosage and alternate day therapy are other strategies in statin-intolerant patients.[78–81]

Cerivastatin is associated with myopathy (8.4 time risk) and has been withdrawn from the market. Pravastatin has not been reported to have myotoxicity. Simvastatin produced myotoxicity in 0.1%. Myalgia occurs in 3–15% cases. Rs 4,363,657 gene polymorphism is associated with myotoxicity. Reduced level of cholesterol in type 2 muscle fibers and reduced level of ubiquinone also called coenzyme Q 10 (CoQ10) may be other mechanisms.

Rare adverse events of statin are cognitive decline and new-onset DM. Cognitive decline in the form of ill-defined memory loss or impairment of memory is reported rarely by patients on statin therapy. Time of onset is variable ranging from 1 day to years. In general, the patients were 50 years of age or older. The occurrence of cognitive defects was not related to fixed or progressive dementia. Adverse effect was not related to a specific statin, age of the individual, statin dosages or concurrent medications. Usually the memory loss is reversible. Statin therapy should be discontinued if memory loss is reported. Other etiologies should be ruled out. If there is no improvement in neurological status after 3 months following discontinuation, statin may be restarted at a lower dose as indicated in the guidelines. Switch over to a hydrophilic statin is another approach.[82]

Table 12.6: Risk markers of myotoxicity of statins

1. Patient-related factors
   a. Increasing age
   b. Female gender
   c. Renal impairment
   d. Liver dysfunction
   e. Hypothyroidism
   f. Asian ethnicity
   g. Low BMI
   h. Family history of myopathy with any statin
   i. Pre-existing muscle disease
2. Statin-related factors
   a. High dose
   b. Lipophilic agent
   c. High bioavailability
   d. Limited protein binding.
3. Pharmacogenetic factor
   a. Carrier of CYP2C9/ABCG2/SLCO1B1 gene polymorphisms
      i. Carrier of rs4363657.
4. Dietary factors
   a. High intake of grape fruit juice
   b. High intake of pomegranate juice.
5. Polypharmacy
   a. Intake of many drugs that interfere with statin metabolism.

BMI, body mass index, CYP, cytochrome p 450.

Incident DM is another area of concern in patients receiving statin therapy. In a collaborative meta-analysis of 13 randomized trials involving 91,140 patients followed up for 4 years, 4278 patients with newly diagnosed DM (2226 on statin and 2052 on placebo) were reported. There was 9% increased risk of incident DM. There was one additional case of DM per 1000 patients taking statins for 1 year. The risk association was stronger in trials with older participants. Baseline body mass index (BMI) and percentage change in LDL concentration were not important factors. Another meta-analysis showed two additional cases of DM per 1000 patients treated for 4.9 years and 6.5 fever CV events per 1000 patients treated with high-dose statins. Number needed to harm for statins is 498 per year and NNT is 155 per year. So, the risk is very small compared to the enormous benefit. Inhibition of β-cell glucose transporters, delayed ATP production, proinflammatory and oxidative β-cell effects of plasma-derived cholesterol, inhibition of calcium channel-dependent insulin secretion and β-cell apoptosis are the various plausible mechanisms.[83,84]

Since statin treatment is a lifelong event, there is a theoretical concern for presumed cancer risk by the patient and the clinicians. Individual statin trials showed the safety of statin as regard to cancer risk.[15,20] A meta-analysis of 1,75,000 people in 27 statin trials showed that statin does not lead to cancer. Recent evidence suggests that statin usage may have a chemoprotective role from bowel cancer.[85,86]

Another area of concern with statin usage is the development of cataract. Observational statins had conflicting evidence. Some statins suggested a protective effect and some an increased risk. In a recent meta-analysis of 14 studies (2,399,200 persons and 25,618 cataracts), statin usage was associated with 20–50% relative risk reduction while the absolute risk reduction was 1.4% + 0.015 (95% CI, 1.1–1.7%; $P \leq 0.0001$).[87]

Emerging Evidence and Future Research

1. Lipid target-based therapy (target to treat) versus therapy based on the persons' 5-year estimated CAD risk (tailored treatment)[88]
2. Role of statins in sepsis,[89] seizure disorders,[90] prevention of hepatocellular carcinoma in hepatitis B virus infection,[91] prevention of infection in cirrhosis of liver[92,93]
3. Alzheimer's disease[94]
4. Prevention of open-angle glaucoma in hyperlipidemia[95]
5. Prevention of human aging by protecting against telomere shortening[96]
6. Prevention of pancreatitis in hypertriglyceridemia.[97]

Clinical Indications of Statin

1. Statins are indicated with an aim to lower LDL in
   (a) Familial hypercholesterolemia
   (b) Mixed (combined) dyslipidemias.
2. Statins are indicated to lower TGs in
   (a) Mixed dyslipidemias
   (b) Dysbetalipoproteinemia.
3. Statins are also indicated to increase the HDL-C in patients with mixed dyslipidemia.
4. Statins are also indicated to lower mortality in patients with
   (a) MI
   (b) ACS.

CONTRAINDICATIONS OF STATINS

1. Pregnancy
2. Breast feeding
3. Active liver disease, transaminitis
4. History of hypersensitivity with statin.

PRESCRIBING INFORMATION OF VARIOUS STATINS

1. Simvastatin[98]
- Dose range is 5–40 mg/day.
- Starting dose 10–20 mg in the evening meal.
- In high-risk patients, starting dose is 40 mg/day.
- Total 80 mg/day simvastatin should only be used when the patient has been tolerating the statin for >1 year without muscle toxicity.
- Coadministration of simvastatin with gemfibrozil, cyclosporine and danazol is contraindicated.
- Dose should be reduced to 10 mg/day when used along with diltiazem or verapamil.

2. **Lovastatin**[99]
   - Dose range is 10–80 mg/day.
   - Statin dose 10 mg with the evening meal.
   - Dose adjustment based on the parameters at 4–6 weeks.
   - In-patients with epidermal growth factor receptor (EGFR)<30mL/min/1.73m^2 BSA, the dose above 20 mg/day should be used with caution.
   - Gemfibrozil and cyclosporine are contraindicated.
   - Maximum dose is 20 mg when used along with danazol, diltiazem or verapamil and 40 mg when used along with amiodarone.
3. **Fluvastatin**[100]
   - Dose range is 20–80 mg/day.
   - Extended release tabs 40–80 mg/day can be given at any time of the day .
   - Dose should be reduced to 20 mg/day when used along with cyclosporine and fluconazole.
   - Caution should be exercised when using along with niacin, fibric acid derivatives, glibenclamide, phenytoin or oral anticoagulants.
   - Safety of dosing above 40 mg/day has not been established in patients with severe renal impairment.
4. **Paravastatin**[101]
   - Dose range is 40–80 mg/day at anytime of the day.
   - 10 mg/day is the starting dose in renal impairment.
   - Maximum dose is 20 mg when used along with cyclosporine and 40 mg when used with clarithromycin.
   - Dose should be reduced when niacin is used in combination.
   - Gemfibrozil should be avoided.
   - Fibrate and colchicines coadministration with pravastatin should be avoided.
5. **Atorvastatin**[102]
   - Dose range is 10–80 mg/day at anytime of the day.
   - 40 mg/day should be used when >45% reduction in LDL is desired.
   - In ACS, patients' 80 mg/day dose can be initiated irrespective of the LDL level.
   - Should be avoided in patients taking cyclosporine, tipranavir, ritonavir and telaprevir.
   - Lowest dose should be used with lopinavir plus ritonavir.
   - Maximum 20 mg/day should be used when coadministered with clarithromycin, itraconazole or in patients taking combination of saquinavir plus ritonavir, darunavir plus ritonavir, fosamprenavir or fosamprenavir plus ritonavir.
   - Maximum 40 mg/day dose should be used along with nelfinavir.
   - Cyclosporine level requires close monitoring when used along with atorvastatin.
6. **Rosuvastatin**[103]
   - Dose range is 5–40 mg/day at anytime of the day irrespective of the meal
   - Starting dose should be 20 mg when LDL >190 mg/dL.
   - Maximum 10 mg/day should be used with gemfibrozil, or ritonavir plus lopinavir or ritonavir plus atazanavir.
   - Maximum 5 mg/day should be used along with cyclosporine.
   - Niacin, fibrate, oral anticoagulant coadministration requires close monitoring.
   - In stage IV CKD (EGFR 15–29mL/min/1.73 m^2 BSA), dose range is 5–10 mg/day.
   - Dose should be reduced in unexplained proteinuria and/or hematuria.

7. Pitavastatin (also called the 7th statin)[104]
- Dose range is 1–4 mg at anytime of the day irrespective of the meals.
- In CKD stage III (EGFR 30–59mL/min/1.73 m² BSA), stage IV, stage V (EGFR<15mL/min/1.73 m² BSA) or on hemodialysis, the dose range is 1–2 mg/day.
- Cyclosporine coadministration is contraindicated.
- Maximum 1 mg dose should be used with erythromycin.
- Maximum 2 mg dose should be used along with rifampicin.
- Should be used with caution along with fibrates and niacin, and the dose should be reduced.

CONCLUSION

Statins are chemicals that block the formation of cholesterol biosynthesis by competitively blocking the enzymes (HMG-CoA reductase) in the liver. Several statins are commercially available. They have shown reduction in total mortality, CV mortality, revascularization and rehospitalization in various primary and secondary intervention trials when they were used in addition to diet and exercise irrespective of LDL level. The benefit has been shown in all spectra of CVD starting from subclinical to clinical atherosclerotic vascular disease. Occasional myalgia and rare liver dysfunctions are the two major limitations. Very rarely rhabdomyolysis may occur. Statins are cost-effective and an excellent tool to arrest the progression or induced regression of atherosclerosis. There is emerging evidence of application of the benefit of the statins in various nonconventional clinical disorders.

REFERENCES

1. Endo A. A gift from nature: the birth of the statins. Nat Med. 2008;14(10):1050-2.
2. Endo A. The discovery and development of HMG-CoA reductase inhibitors. J Lipid Res. 1992;33(11):1569-82. PMID1464741.
3. Stancu C, Sima A. Statins: mechanism of action and effects. J Cell Mol Med. 2001;5(4):378-87.
4. Stein EA. New statins and new doses of old statins. Curr AtherosclerRep. 2001;3:14-8.
5. Stancu C, Sima A. Statins: mechanism of action and effects. J Cell Mol Med. 2001;5(4):378-87.
6. Ikeda U, Shimada K. Pleiotropic effects of statins on the vascular tissue. Curr Drug Targets Cardiovasc Haematol Disord. 2001;1(1):51-8.
7. Marzilli M. Pleiotropic effects of statins: evidence for benefits beyond LDL-cholesterol lowering. Am J Cardiovasc Drugs. 2010;10Suppl 1:3-9.
8. Mason JC. Statins and their role in vascular protection. Clin Sci. 2003;105:251-66.
9. Maron DJ, Fazio S, Linton M F. Current perspectives on statins. Circulation. 2000;101(2):207-13.
10. Jones PH, Davidson MH, Stein EA, et al. Comparison of the efficacy and safety of rosuvastatin versus atorvastatin, simvastatin, and pravastatin across doses (STELLAR* Trial). Am J Cardiol. 2003;92(2):152-60.
11. Vaughan CJ, Gotto AM, Basson CT. The evolving role of statins in the management of atherosclerosis. J Am Coll Cardiol. 2000;35(1):1-10.
12. Chapman MJ, Taggart FM. Optimising the pharmacology of statins: characteristics of rosuvastatin. Atheroscler Suppl. 2000;2(4):33-37.
13. Grundy SM, Cleeman JI, Merz CN, et al. Implications of recent clinical trials for the National Cholesterol Education Program Adult Treatment Panel III Guidelines. J Am Coll Cardiol. 2004;44(3):720-32.
14. Bellosta S, Paoletti R, Corsini A. Atherosclerosis: evolving vascular biology and clinical implications safety of statins focus on clinical pharmacokinetics and drug interactions. Circulation. 2004;109(23-suppl):III-50-7.

15. Shepherd J, Cobbe SM, Ford I, et al. Prevention of coronary heart disease with pravastatin in men with hypercholesterolemia. West of Scotland Coronary Prevention Study Group. N Engl J Med. 1995;333:1301-8.
16. Downs JR, Clearfield M, Weis S, et al. Primary prevention of acute coronary events with lovastatin in men and women with average cholesterol levels: results of AFCAPS/TexCAPS. Air Force/Texas Coronary Atherosclerosis Prevention Study. JAMA. 1998;279(20):1615-22.
17. Heart Protection Study Collaborative Group. MRC/BHF Heart Protection Study of cholesterol lowering with simvastatin in 20,536 high-risk individuals: a randomised placebo controlled trial. Lancet. 2002;360(9326):7-22.
18. Colhoun HM, Betteridge DJ, Durrington PN, et al. Primary prevention of cardiovascular disease with atorvastatin in type 2 diabetes in the Collaborative Atorvastatin Diabetes Study (CARDS). Lancet. 2004;364:685-96.
19. Sever PS, Dahlof B, Poulter NR, et al. ASCOT investigators. Prevention of coronary and stroke events with atorvastatin in hypertensive patients who have average or lower-than-average cholesterol concentrations, in the Anglo-Scandinavian Cardiac Outcomes Trial--Lipid Lowering Arm (ASCOT-LLA): a multicentre randomised controlled trial. Lancet. 2003;361(9364):1149-58.
20. Knopp RH, D'Emden M, Smilde JG, et al. Efficacy and safety of atorvastatin the prevention of cardiovascular end points in subjects with type 2 diabetes: the Atorvastatin Study for Prevention of Coronary Heart Disease Endpoints in Non-Insulin-Dependent Diabetes Mellitus (ASPEN). Diabetes Care. 2006;29:1478-85.
21. Nakamura H, Arakawa K, Itakura H, et al. Primary prevention of cardiovascular disease with pravastatin in Japan (MEGA Study): a prospective randomised controlled trial. Lancet. 2006;368:1155-63.
22. Ridker PM, Danielson E, Fonseca FA, et al. Rosuvastatin to prevent vascular events in men and women with elevated C-reactive protein. N Engl J Med. 2008;359:2195-2207.
23. Randomised trial of cholesterol lowering in 4444 patients with coronary heart disease: the Scandinavian Simvastatin Survival Study (4S). Lancet. 1994;344(8934):1383-9.
24. Prevention of cardiovascular events and death with Pravastatin in patients with coronary artery disease and a broad range of initial cholesterol levels. The Long-Term Intervention with Pravastatin in Ischaemic Disease (LIPID) study group. N Engl J Med. 1998;339:1349-57.
25. LaRosa JC, Grundy SM, Waters DD, et al. Intensive lipid lowering with atorvastatin in patients with stable coronary disease. N Engl J Med. 2005;352:1425-35.
26. Pedersen TR, Faergeman O, Kastelein JJ, et al. High dose atorvastatin vs usual dose simvastatin for secondary prevention after myocardial infarction: the IDEAL study: a randomized controlled trial. JAMA. 2005;294:2437-45.
27. Study of The Effectiveness of Additional Reductions in Cholesterol and Homocysteine Search Collaborative Group, Armitage J, Bowman L, et al. Intensive lowering of LDL cholesterol with 80 mg versus 20 mg simvastatin daily in 12,064 survivors of myocardial infarction: a double-blind randomised trial. Lancet. 2010;376(9753):1658-69.
28. Schwartz GG1, Olsson AG, Ezekowitz MD, et al. Effects of atorvastatin on early recurrent ischemic events in acute coronary syndromes: the MIRACL study: a randomized controlled trial. JAMA. 2001;285(13):1711-8.
29. Christopher P. Cannon, M.D., Eugene Braunwald, M.D., Carolyn H. McCabe, et al. Intensive versus Moderate Lipid Lowering with Statins after Acute Coronary Syndromes for the Pravastatin or Atorvastatin Evaluation and Infection Therapy–Thrombolysis in Myocardial Infarction 22 Investigators. N Engl J Med. 2004;350:1495-1504; April 8, 2004 DOI: 10.1056/NEJMoa040583
30. Liem A, van Boven AJ, Withagen AP, et al. Fluvastatin in acute myocardial infarction: effects on early and late ischaemia events: the FLORIDA trial [abstract]. Circulation. 2000;102:2672-d.
31. de Lemos JA, Blazing MA, Wiviott SD, et al. Early intensive vs a delayed conservative simvastatin strategy in patients with acute coronary syndromes: phase Z of the A to Z trial. JAMA. 2004;292(11):1307-16.

32. Thompson PL, Meredith I, Amerena J, et al. Effect of pravastatin compared with placebo initiated within 24 hours of onset of acute myocardial infarction or unstable angina: the Pravastatin in Acute Coronary Treatment (PACT) trial. Am Heart J. 2004;148:e2.

33. Arntz HR, Agrawal R, Wunderlich W, et al: Beneficial effects of pravastatin (+/- cholestyramine/niacin) initiated immediately after a coronary event (the randomized Lipid-Coronary Artery Disease [L-CAD] Study). Am J Cardiol. 2000;86:1293-8.

34. Patti G, Pasceri V, Colonna G, et al. Atorvastatin pretreatment improves outcomes in patients with acute coronary syndromes undergoing early percutaneous coronary intervention results of the ARMYDA-ACS randomized trial. Am Coll Cardiol. 2007;49(12):1272-8.

35. Pasceri V, Patti G, Nusca A, et al. Randomized trial of atorvastatin for reduction of myocardial damage during coronary intervention: results from the ARMYDA study. Circulation. 2004;110:674-8.

36. Ghose T, Kaur G, Kachru R, et al. Experience with atorvastatin in Indian patients with dyslipidaemia. Indian Heart J. 2000;52:732.

37. Kaul U, Varma J, Kahali D, et al. Post-marketing Study of clinical experience of atorvastatin 80 mg vs 40 mg in Indian patients with acute coronary syndrome- a randomized, multi-centre study (CURE-ACS). J Assoc Physicians India. 2013;61(2):97-101.

38. Teramoto T. Pitavastatin: clinical effects from the LIVES Study. Atheroscler Suppl. 2011;12(3):285-8. doi:10.1016/S1567-5688(11)70888-1.

39. ROSUVEES EF/2011/07/002577 CTRI Website URL-http://ctri.nic.in (Results presented at the EAS annual meeting)

40. Yokote K, Bujo H, Hanaoka H, et al. Multicenter collaborative randomized parallel group comparative study of pitavastatin and atorvastatin in Japanese hypercholesterolemic patients: collaborative study on hypercholesterolemia drug intervention and their benefits for atherosclerosis prevention (CHIBA study). Atherosclerosis. 2008;201(2):345-52. doi:10.1016/j.atherosclerosis.2008.02.008. Epub 2008 Feb 16.

41. Sasaki J, Ikeda Y, Kuribayashi T, et al. A 52-week, randomized, open-label, parallel-group comparison of the tolerability and effects of pitavastatin and atorvastatin on high-density lipoprotein cholesterol levels and glucose metabolism in Japanese patients with elevated levels of LDL-C and glucose intolerance. Clin Ther. 2008;30:1089-101.

42. Ose L, Budinski D, Hounslow N, et al. Comparison of pitavastatin with simvastatin in primary hypercholesterolaemia or combined dyslipidaemia. Curr Med Res Opin. 2009;25(11):2755-64.

43. Saito Y, Teramoto T, Yamada N, et al. Clinical efficacy of NK-104 (Pitavastatin), a new synthetic HMG-CoA reductase inhibitor, in the dose finding, double blind, three-group comparative study. J Clin Ther Med. 2001;17(6):829-55.

44. Nomura S, Shouzu A, Omoto S, et al. Correlation between adiponectin and reduction of cell adhesion molecules after pitavastatin treatment in hyperlipidemic patients with type 2 diabetes mellitus. Thromb Res. 2008;122(1):39-45.

45. Amarenco P, Bogousslavsky J, Callahan A, et al. Design and baseline characteristics of the Stroke Prevention by Aggressive Reduction in Cholesterol Levels Study (SPARCL). Cerebrovasc Dis. 2003;16(4):389-95.

46. Pitt B, Waters D, Brown WV, et al. Aggressive lipid-lowering therapy compared with angioplasty in stable coronary artery disease. Atorvastatin versus Revascularization Treatment Investigators. N Engl J Med. 1999;341:70-76

47. Kjekshus J, Apetrei E, Barrios V, et al. Rosuvastatin in older patients with systolic heart failure. N Engl J Med. 2007;357:2248-61

48. Sacks FM, Pfeffer MA, Moye LA, et al. The effect of pravastatin on coronary events after myocardial infarction in patients with average cholesterol levels. N Engl J Med. 1996;335:1001-9.

49. BlankenhornDH1, AzenSP, KramschDM, et al. Coronary angiographic changes with lovastatin therapy: the Monitored Atherosclerosis Regression Study (MARS). Ann Intern Med. 1993;119(10):969-76.

50. Nissen S, Tuzcu E, Schoenhagen P, et al. Effect of intensive compared with moderate lipid-lowering therapy on progression of coronary atherosclerosis: a randomized controlled trial (REVERSAL). JAMA. 2004;291:1071-80.

51. Nissen SE, Nicholls SJ, Sipahi I, et al. Effect of very high-intensity statin therapy on regression of coronary atherosclerosis The ASTEROID Trial. JAMA. 2006;295(13):1556-65.

52. JukemaJW1, Bruschke AV, van Boven AJ, et al. Effects of lipid lowering by pravastatin on progression and regression of coronary artery disease in symptomatic men with normal to moderately elevated serum cholesterol levels: the Regression Growth Evaluation Statin Study (REGRESS). Circulation. 1995;91(10):2528-40.

53. Nicholls SJ, Ballantyne CM, Barter PJ, et al. Effect of two intensive statin regimens on progression of coronary disease. N Engl J Med. 2011;365:2078-87. doi:10.1056/NEJMoa1110874.

54. Underhill HR, Yuan C, Zhao XQ, et al. Effect of rosuvastatin therapy on carotid plaque morphology and composition in moderately hypercholesterolemic patients: a high-resolution magnetic resonance imaging trial. Am Heart J. 2008;155(3):584.e1-8.

55. Hiro T, Kimura T, Morimoto T, et al. Effect of intensive statin therapy on regression of coronary atherosclerosis in patients with acute coronary syndrome: a multicenter randomized trial evaluated by volumetric intravascular ultrasound using pitavastatin versus atorvastatin (JAPAN-ACS [Japan assessment of pitavastatin and atorvastatin in acute coronary syndrome] study). J Am Coll Cardiol. 2009;54:293-302.

56. Pineda A, Cubeddu LX. Statin rebound or withdrawal syndrome: does it exist? Curr Atheroscler Rep. 2011;13(1):23-30. doi:10.1007/s11883-010-0148-x.

57. Cubeddu LX, Seamon MJ. Statin withdrawal: clinical implications and molecular mechanisms. Pharmacotherapy. 2006;26(9):1288-96.

58. Poldermans D. Statins and noncardiac surgery: current evidence and practical considerations. Cleve Clin J Med. 2009;76Suppl 4:S79-83. doi:10.3949/ccjm.76.s4.13.

59. Shepherd J,Blauw GJ, Murphy MB, et al. Pravastatin in elderly individuals at risk of vascular disease (PROSPER): a randomised controlled trial. Lancet. 2002;360(9346):1623-30.

60. Gibson DM, Bron NJ, Richens A, et al. Effect of age and gender on pharmacokinetics of atorvastatin in humans. J Clin Pharmacol. 1996;36(3):242-6.

61. Waters DD. Meta-analysis of statin trials, clear benefit for primary prevention in the elderly. J Am Coll Cardiol. 2013;62(22):2100-1. doi:10.1016/J.Jacc.2013.67.068.

62. McCrindle BW, Urbina EM, Dennison BA, et al. Drug therapy of high-risk lipid abnormalities in children and adolescents: a scientific statement from the American Heart Association Atherosclerosis, Hypertension, and Obesity in Youth Committee, Council of Cardiovascular Disease in the Young, with the Council on Cardiovascular Nursing. Circulation. 2007;115:1948-67.

63. Yasuda G, et al. Effects of rosuvastatin versus probucol on lipid abnormalities in patients with chronic kidney disease in stage III and above. Abstract No. 244, European Atherosclerosis Congress June 2-5,2013.

64. Riley P, Sudarshi D, Johal M, et al. Weight loss, dietary advice and statin therapy in non-alcoholic fatty liver disease: a retrospective study. Int J Clin Pract. 208;62(3):347-81.

65. Mohler ER 3rd, Hiatt WR, Creager MA. Cholesterol reduction with atorvastatin improves walking distance in patients with peripheral arterial disease. Circulation. 2003;108:1481-6.

66. Feldman HH, Doody RS, Kivipelto M, et al. Randomized controlled trial of atorvastatin in mild to moderate Alzheimer disease: LEADe. Neurology. 2010;74(12):956-64. doi:10.1212/WNL.0b013e3181d6476a.

67. Sano M, Bell KL, Galasko D, et al. A randomized, double-blind, placebo-controlled trial of simvastatin to treat Alzheimer disease. Neurology. 2011;77(6):556-63.

68. Sparks DL, Connor DJ, Sabbagh MN, et al. Circulating cholesterol levels, apolipoprotein E genotype and dementia severity influence the benefit of atorvastatin treatment in Alzheimer's disease: results of the Alzheimer's Disease Cholesterol-Lowering Treatment (ADCLT) trial. Acta Neurol Scand Suppl. 2006;185:3-7.

69. Kasani A, Phillips CO, Foody JM, et al. Risks associated with statin therapy—a systematic review of randomized clinical trials. Circulation. 2006;114:2788-97.
70. T T lin Data presented at the European Society Congress 2013.
71. T T lin Data presented at the European Society Congress 2013.
72. ClinicalTrials.gov Bethesda (MD): National Library of Medicine (US). NCT 01042730-See more at: http://www.modernmedicine.com/node/122896#sthash.0n0ZOMGl.dpuf.
73. EASD European Association for Study of Diabetes annual meeting 2013.
74. Kawai Y, Sato-Ishida R, Motoyama A, et al. Place of pitavastatin in the statin armamentarium: promising evidence for a role in diabetes mellitus. Drug Des Devel Ther. 2011;5:283-97. http://www.modernmedicine.com/node/122896#sthash.0n0ZOMGl.dpuf.
75. Cholesterol treatment trialists (CTT) collaboration, Baigent C, Blackwell L, et al. Efficacy and safety of more intensive lowering of LDL cholesterol: a meta-analysis of data from 170 000 participants in 26 randomised trials. Lancet. 2010;376(9753):1670-81.
76. Kashani A, Phillips CO, Foody JM, et al. Risks associate with statin therapy. A systematic review of randomized clinical trials. J Cardial. 2006;114(25):2788-97.
77. Grable-Esposito P, Katzoerq HD, Grenberg SA, et al. Immune mediated necrotizing myopathy associated with statins. Muscle Nerve. 2010;41(2):185-90.
78. McKenny JM, Davidson MH, Jacobson TA, et al. Final conclusions and recommendations of the National Lipid Association Statin Safety Assessment Task Force. AM J Cardiol. 2006;97(8A):89C-94C.
79. Athyros VG, Tziomalos K, Gossios TD, et al. Safety and efficacy of long-term statin treatment for cardiovascular events in patients with coronary heart disease and abnormal liver tests in the Greek Atorvastatin and Coronary Heart Disease Evaluation (GREACE) Study: a post-hoc analysis. Lancet. 2010;376:1916-22.
80. Bader T. Liver tests are irrelevant when prescribing statins. Lancet. 2010;376:1882-3.
81. Sikka P, Saxsena KK, Kapoor S. Statin hepatotoxicity: is it a real concern? Heart Views. 2011;12(3):104-6.
82. Rojas-Fernandez CH, Cameron JC. Is statin-associated cognitive impairment clinically relevant? A narrative review and clinical recommendations. Ann Pharmacother. 2012;46(4):549-57.
83. Sattar N, Taskinen M-R. Statins are diabetogenic—myth or reality? Atheroscler Suppl. 2102;13:1-10.
84. Sattar N, Preiss D, Murray HM, et al. Statins and risk of incident diabetes: a collaborative meta-analysis of randomised statin trials. Lancet. 2010;375(9716):735-42.
85. Dale KM, Coleman CI, Henyan NN, et al. Statins and cancer risk a meta-analysis. JAMA. 2006;295(1):74-80.
86. Mansouri D, McMillan DC, Roxburgh CS, et al. The impact of aspirin, statins and ACE-inhibitors on the presentation of colorectal neoplasia in a colorectal cancer screening programme. Br J Cancer. 2013;109(1):249-56.
87. Kostis JB, ESC Congress, 2013.
88. Hayward RA, Krumholz HM. Three Reasons to Abandon Low-Density Lipoprotein Targets An Open Letter to the Adult Treatment Panel IV of the National Institutes of Health. Circ Cardiovasc Qual Outcomes. 2012;5:2-5.
89. Gluck EH. Prehospital statin therapy and all-cause mortality in ICU patients. Chest. 2010;138:287A.
90. Media Release | Oct. 25, 2010 Anti-cholesterol drugs could help stave off seizures: UBC-Vancouver Coastal Health research.
91. Tsan YT, Lee CH, Wang JD, et al. Statins and the risk of hepatocellular carcinoma in patients with hepatitis B virus infection. Chen J of ClinOncol.2012;30(6):623-30.
92. Singh S, Singh PP, Singh AG, et al. Statins are associated with a reduced risk of hepatocellular cancer: a systematic review and meta-analysis. Gastroenterology. 2012;144(2):323-32. doi:10.1053/j.gastro.2012.10.005.
93. Motzkus-Feagans C, Pakyz AL, Ratliff SM, et al. Statin use and infections in Veterans with cirrhosis. Aliment Pharmacol Ther. 2013;38(6):611-8.

94. Sparks DL. Statins in the treatment of Alzheimer disease. Nat Rev Neurol. 2011;7:662-3.
95. The relationship between statin use and open-angle glaucoma, Ophthalmology 2012;119:2074–2081 © 2012 by the American Academy of Ophthalmology.
96. Virginia Boccardi, Michelangela Barbieri, Maria Rosaria Rizzo, Raffaele Marfella, Antonietta Esposito, Luigi Marano, and Giuseppe Paolisso. A new pleiotropic effect of statins in elderly: modulation of telomerase activity. FASEB J. September 2013;27:3879-3885, doi:10.1096/fj.13-232066; http://www.fasebj.org/content/27/9/3879.
97. Preiss D, Tikkanen MJ, Welsh P, et al. Lipid-modifying therapies and risk of pancreatitis: a meta-analysis. JAMA. 2012;308(8):804-11.
98. Simvastatin (Zocor) prescribing information. Whitehouse Station, NJ: Merck Co.; 2012.
99. Lovastatin (Mevacor) prescribing information. Whitehouse Station, NJ: Merck Co.; 2012.
100. Fluvastatin (Lescol) prescribing information. East Hanover, NJ: Novartis Pharmaceuticals; 2011.
101. Pravastatin (Pravachol) prescribing information. Princeton, NJ: Bristol Myers Squibb Co.; 2012.
102. Atorvastatin (Lipitor) prescribing information. New York, NY: Pfizer; 2012.
103. Rosuvastatin (Crestor) prescribing information. Wilmington, DE: Astra Zeneca Pharmaceuticals; 2012.
104. Pitavastatin (Livalo) prescribing information. Montgomery, AL: Kowa Pharmaceuticals America Inc.; 2011.

CHAPTER 13

Bile Acid Sequestrants

Anjali Arora

- Introduction
- History of development in BAS
- Physiology of bile acids
- Trials with BAS for atherosclerosis regression
- BAS and hypercholesterolemia
- Plasma lipoproteins and BAS
- Contraindication
- Individual drugs
- Clinical outcome studies of BAS
- Other medical uses of BAS
- Conclusion

INTRODUCTION

Bile acid sequestrants (BAS) are also called bile acid resins or gels. The liver uses cholesterol to produce bile acids, which aid in the digestive process. Bile acid sequestrants bind to bile acids in the intestine. They disrupt the enterohepatic circulation by combining with bile constituents and preventing their reabsorption from the gut. The liver then produces more bile to replace the bile that has been lost. As the body requires cholesterol to make bile, the liver uses the cholesterol in the blood, reducing the amount of low-density lipoprotein cholesterol (LDL-C) circulating in the blood. Bile acid sequestrants are often termed as hypolipidemic agents. They also may be used for purposes other than lowering cholesterol.

HISTORY OF DEVELOPMENT IN BAS

Cholestyramine, the first BAS, was developed at Merck in the late 1950s (MK-135). In 1959, Bergen et al. reported that cholestyramine reduced serum total cholesterol in humans by an average of 20%.

Colestipol was introduced at the beginning of the 1970s. Colestipol has a lower binding capacity for bile salts, and the highest dose of colestipol recommended is 30 g daily.

Colesevelam has an enhanced binding capacity and affinity for bile salts. Its advantages are its lack of drug interactions and low rates of gastrointestinal (GI) side effects.

Colestimide is a BAS shown to be effective as combination therapy for familial hyper-cholesterolemia (FH). Colestimide clinical trials have focused on lowering phosphate in patients undergoing kidney dialysis and also on combined lipid and glucose amelioration in diabetes.

PHYSIOLOGY OF BILE ACIDS

Mechanism of Action

Bile acids are produced by the liver from cholesterol. They exist mostly as glycine or taurine conjugates. The bile acids help in the breakdown of dietary fats and other nutrients through the formation of mixed micelles in the intestinal lumen. This helps in fat-soluble intestinal absorption of nutrients. Bile acids undergo limited absorption until they reach the ileum. The sodium bile acid transporter (ASBT, *SLC10A2*) is expressed in the terminal ileum and is responsible for the uptake of bile acids. In all, 95% of intestinal bile acids are reabsorbed in the small intestine, and <5% are excreted in the feces. Because of binding of the bile acids, the intestinal absorption decreases fecal excretion of the bile acids that can go up threefold (normally 1000 mg). A transport protein, sodium taurocholate cotransporting polypeptide (NTCP), helps the uptake of bile acids by the liver cells. Approximately, 1000 mg of cholesterol

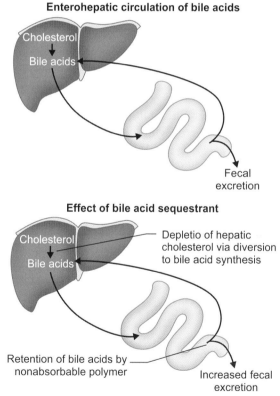

Figure. **13.**1: Entire hepatic circulation of bile acids and effect of intervention. (A) Bile acids are generated in the liver from cholesterol. More than 95% of bile acids are absorbed in ileum return to the liver. (B) Binding of bile acids with resins leads to 3- to 10-fold increase in fecal excretion. Hepatic synthesis in turn increases to a similar degree. As a result, hepatic cholesterol levels falls. This leads to increased expression of hepatic low-density lipoprotein (LDL) receptors. Plasma LDL levels fall as a result of increased uptake by the liver is required per day for bile acid synthesis. Total 800 mg comes from the synthesis and 200 mg comes from diet. An overall 300–500 mg of fecal excretion is the only way of bile acid exertion from human body (Fig. 13.1).

Transcription of Bile Acid Pathway

The key transcriptional regulator of bile acid pathways in the intestine and liver was discovered in 1999 to be the Farnesoid X receptor (FXR). Bile acids are the natural activators of FXR. Farnesoid X receptor forms a heterodimer with its obligate partner 9-*cis* retinoic acid receptor-α (RXR-α), and this heterodimer binds to deoxyribonucleic acid. The hormone-response element to which FXR/RXR-α binds is termed a bile acid response element.

Bile Acid Mechanism: At Molecular Level

Bile acids facilitate the dietary absorption of lipids. They also, act as ligands for the nuclear receptor FXR and the G-protein-coupled receptor TGR5 in the GI tract. Bile acids also exert nonreceptor-mediated effects on cellular responses, such as improvement in the endoplasmic reticulum (ER) stress response.

Farnesoid X receptor is a member of the nuclear receptor superfamily of ligand-activated transcription factors. Liver and intestine have high levels of FXR expression. It is activated by chenodeoxycholic acid. In the liver, as the bile acid pool increases in size, bile acid activation of FXR upregulates expression of the gene encoding the inhibitory nuclear receptor small heterodimer partner. Small heterodimer partner downregulates activation of several transcription factors, including liver X receptor, liver receptor homologue-1 (LRH-1) and hepatocyte nuclear factor-4α (HNF-4α). This in turn suppresses the LRH-1-mediated activation of cytochrome P450 7A1 (CYP7A1). This inhibits the first step in cholesterol catabolism. Bile acid-mediated suppression of HNF-4α also inhibits transcription of CYP7A1, a second pathway of bile acid-mediated repression of its own synthesis involving FXR-mediated induction of fibroblast growth factor-19 (FGF-19; [FGF-15 in mice]) in the intestine.

In addition, bile acids bind and activate TGR5 (also known as GPBAR1, M-BAR and BG37). Bile acid-triggered activation of TGR5 results in internalization of the receptor, activation of extracellular-regulated kinase (the mitogen-activated protein kinase pathway) that stimulates cyclic adenosine monophosphate synthesis.

Bile Acid Sequestrants: Mechanism of Action

Bile acid sequestrants reduce the bile acid pool. Cytochrome P450 7A1 repression mediated by FXR is reduced. Its upregulation stimulates bile acid synthesis. The hepatic level of cholesterol decreases. Reduced hepatic cholesterol triggers the sterol regulatory-binding protein (SRBP). This results in increased LDL receptor expressions. More LDL is cleared from the blood pool. Along with this, there is a rise in very low-density lipoprotein (VLDL) particles and serum triglyceride transiently.

In addition, BAS also increase high-density lipoprotein cholesterol (HDL-C) levels.

The scavenger receptor class B type I is responsible for the hepatic uptake of HDL-C. Additionally, downregulation of apolipoprotein A-I induced by bile acids is blocked by sequestrants. Apolipoprotein A-I level is plasma rise.

TRIALS WITH BAS FOR ATHEROSCLEROSIS REGRESSION

In the Lipid Research Clinics Coronary Primary Prevention trial (LRC-CPPT), 3806 men aged 35–59 years with elevated total cholesterol and without evidence of coronary heart disease were randomized to therapy. The dose response seen in the LRC-CPPT for cholestyramine was over the dose range of 4–24 g/day. A 6.6–28.3% decrease in LDL-C was observed. The National Heart, Lung, and Blood Institute type II Coronary Intervention included patients with type II hyperlipoproteinemia with coronary artery disease (CAD). Patients were randomized to diet plus 6 g cholestyramine 4 times daily versus diet plus matching placebo. Diet alone decreased LDL-C by 6% in both arms. There was additional 5% and 26% reduction of LDL in placebo arm and cholestyramine arm, respectively. After 5 years of treatment, angiographic CAD progressed in 49% in placebo group and 32% in treatment group ($P \leq 0.05$).

In the St. Thomas Atherosclerosis Regression study (STARS), 90 men with angina or past myocardial infarction were randomized to usual care (U) versus dietary interesting (D) versus diet plus cholestyramine (DC). The angiographic progression was reduced significantly by diet and diet plus drug (U 46% vs. D 14% vs. DC 12%).

The Cholesterol Lowering Atherosclerosis Study (CLAS) aimed at demonstrating the angiographic regression of atherosclerosis with combination of colestipol (30 g/day) and niacin (4.3 g/day). Both at 2 years (CLAS I) and 4 years (CLAS 2) there was regression of atherosclerosis. This study also showed new lesions were less in native coronaries (14 vs. 40%) and bypass grafts (16 vs.8%).

Familial atherosclerosis treatment study (FATS) randomized patients to lovastatin (40 mg/day) plus colestipol (30 g/day) versus niacin (4 g/day) plus colestipol (30 g/day) versus placebo. This was first study to demonstrate angiographic regression and also less progression with intensive lipid lowering.

BAS AND HYPERCHOLESTEROLEMIA

Bile acid sequestrants lower the bile and pool and more cholesterol is utilized for bile acid synthesis. Low hepatic cholesterol is sensed by ER protein (ERP). Endoplasmic reticulum protein escorts SRBPs to Golgi complex. After cleavage SRBPs induce increased expressions of 3-hydroxy-3-methylglutaryl-coenzyme A (HMG-CoA) reductive enzymes and LDL receptor in the hepatic nucleus. As a result plasma LDL falls.

PLASMA LIPOPROTEINS AND BAS

Bile acid sequestrants bind bile acids in the intestine and promote their excretion rather than reabsorption in the ileum. To maintain the bile acid pool size, the liver utilizes cholesterol for bile acid synthesis. The decreased hepatic intracellular cholesterol content results in upregulation of the LDL receptor and increased LDL clearance from the plasma. Cholestyramine and colestipol are insoluble resins that must be suspended in liquids. Colesevelam is available as tablets but generally requires up to six to seven tablets per day for effective LDL-C lowering. Bile acid sequestrants are not systemically absorbed. They are safe and are cholesterol-lowering drugs of choice in children and in women of childbearing age (lactating, pregnant or could become pregnant). They are effective in combination with statins as well as in combination with ezetimibe. Bile acid sequestrants are particularly useful with one or both of the above drugs in difficult-to-treat patients or those patients with statin intolerance.

After 2–4 weeks of treatment with BAS, the lipid parameter changes. High-density lipoprotein cholesterol rises by 0–5%. Low-density lipoprotein cholesterol declines by 5–30%. Colesevelam has a greeted bile acid binding capacity and dose in lower.

Increase in cholesterol synthesis through BAS is seen by acting upon HMG-CoA reductase. The use of an HMG-CoA reductase inhibitor, or statin, ameliorates this effect. A substantial LDL-C reduction occurs when BAS are combined with statins. It can lower LDL-C levels by up to 60%.

The decrease in LDL-C through different dose of BAS or statin ranges from 24% to 60% depending upon the dose of BAS and that of the statin.

Bile acid sequestrant reduces LDL by 10–25% additionally when added to statin therapy. In patients who cannot tolerate high-dose statin, a combination of atorvastatin and colesevelam is useful. Combination of colesevelam (3.8 g) plus atorvastatin 10 mg decreased LDL by 48% compared with 53% reduction by 80 mg atorvastatin alone. Cholestyramine and colestipol can interfere with statin absorption. Colesevelam has no such effect on statin absorption.

The combination of statin, BAS and niacin is of great value in patients with heterozygous FH where even greater LDL-C reductions are required. Typical approach to FH would entail the maximum usage of a statin dose, BAS at maximally tolerated dose together with 2 g/day of niacin.

Combining colesevelam and extended-release niacin can produce good effects with lesser side effects. Another possible combination is the addition of ezetimibe to colesevelam, which can lower LDL-C by 32%.

Some patients with high triglycerides and high LDL may require addition of BAS after treatment with fibrates. Clofibrate, bezafibrate, gemfibrozil, or fenofibrate all have been used in combination with BAS.

Adverse Effects Associated with BAS

Adverse effects associated with BAS are mainly GI. Other common adverse effects are as per the following table:

Common adverse events	Other adverse events
Bloating	Nausea and vomiting
Constipation	Diarrhea
Flatulence	Dysphagia, esophageal obstruction
Indigestion and heartburn	Urticaria
Abdominal pain	Elevated transaminase
Increase of plasma triglycerides	Swelling of hands or feet
Aggravation of hemorrhoids	Fatigue, weakness
	Steatorrhea

CONTRAINDICATION

Bile acid sequestrants are contraindicated in individuals having the following conditions:

- High triglycerides
- Familial dysbetalipoproteinemia
- Severe constipation

Recommendations for Minimizing Constipation and Bloating Associated with BAS

Increase fluid intake, increase fiber intake and add stool softeners, such as docusate sodium. For the nonselective BAS (cholestyramine or colestipol), a slow increase in dose has been recommended. Colesevelam or colestipol tablets have been preferred by patients over cholestyramine or colestipol granules. Tablets placed in the mouth should be entirely wet before swallowing to avoid the discomfort of a tablet sticking in the back of the throat. When >18–20% LDL-C lowering is required, granular formulations of BAS are better accepted. Mixing the granules with psyllium powder and ample liquid may help counter constipation and hard stools. There is further LDL lowering from psyllium. With either tablets or granules, it is helpful to advise swallowing without gulping, to minimize air swallowing, which is a major source of intestinal gas.

BAS: Effect on Absorption of Drugs and Vitamins

Bile acid sequestrants bind to a wide range of drugs in GI lumen and retard their absorption. Consequently, the plasma level of various drugs like thiazide, furosemide, penicillin, tetracycline and gemfibrozil is lower when coadministered with BAS. Low level of folic acid lumen detected in children is treated with BAS. Folic acid needs to be supplemented in children treated with cholestyramine. Other vitamins are not significantly altered. As a general rule, all oral drugs are administered either before or 4 hours after BAS administration.

INDIVIDUAL BAS DRUGS

The following are BAS drug names: cholestyramine (brand name: Questran), colestipol (brand name: Colestid), colesevelam (brand name: Welchol).

Indications and Usage

Cholestyramine (Questran)

The powder is indicated as an adjunctive therapy to diet for the reduction of elevated serum cholesterol in patients with primary hypercholesterolemia. It may be useful to lower LDL-C in patients who also have mild hypertriglyceridemia, but is not indicated to the patients of primary hypertriglyceridemia.

Prior to initiation of drug therapy, treatment should begin and continue with therapeutic lifestyle changes. Weight normalization prior to drug therapy is important.

Cholestyramine (oral suspension) helps provide relief of pruritus associated with biliary obstruction.

Serum cholesterol and triglyceride levels should be determined periodically based on National Cholesterol Education Program (NCEP) guidelines. Cholesterol reduction occurs 1 month after therapy. The dose may be increased if there is no substantial reduction or other lipid-lowering agent can be added at that time.

Contraindication

Prior to initiating therapy, secondary causes of hypercholesterolemia should be excluded (e.g., poorly controlled diabetes mellitus, hypothyroidism, nephrotic syndrome, dysproteinemias, obstructive liver disease, other drug therapy and alcoholism).

Dosage

Dosage is expressed in terms of the anhydrous resin:

Children: 240 mg/kg/day in three divided doses.

Adults: 4 g 1–2 times/day to a maximum of 24 g 1–2 times/day, divided in six dosages maximum.

Administration

The powder should be mixed in water or other fluid. Suspension should be consumed immediately after putting in oral cavity. Keeping the mixture for prolonged period in the mouth cavity may cause teeth discoloration or enamel decay.

Colestipol (Colestid)

Adult Dosage: Maintenance dose 2–16 g/day given once daily or in divided doses.

Colestipol tablets must be swallowed as a whole, using plenty of water. Tablet should not be chewed or crushed.

Drug	Major indications	Starting dose	Maximal dose	Mechanism	Common side effects
BAS	Elevated LDL-C			Increased BAS and increased LDL receptors	
Cholestyramine		4 g daily	32 g daily		Bloating
Colestipol		5 g daily	40 g daily		Constipation
Colesevelam		3750 mg daily	4375 mg daily		Elevated triglycerides

Colesevelam (Welchol)

Colesevelam is administered adjunct to diet and exercise to reduce elevated LDL-C. It is advised in adults with primary hyperlipidemia (Fredrickson type IIa). It is given as monotherapy or in combination with a statin.

Colesevelam is indicated as monotherapy or in combination with a statin to reduce LDL-C level with heterozygous FH. When diet plus exercises fails to reduce:

a. Low-density lipoprotein cholesterol below 190 mg/dL or
b. Low-density lipoprotein cholesterol below 160 mg/dL in presence of premature cardiovascular disease or ≥ 2 risk factors of CAD in young (10–17 years of age).

Limitations of Colesevelam

Colesevelam is a contraindicated drug in the treatment of type 1 diabetes or in diabetic ketoacidosis. It has not been studied in Fredrickson type I, III, IV and V dyslipidemias. It has not been studied in children younger than 10 years of age or in premenarchal girls. It has not been studied in type 2 diabetes as monotherapy or in combination with a dipeptidyl peptidase-4 inhibitor on thiazolidinediones.

Adult dosage: Oral monotherapy: 3 tablets twice daily with meals or 6 tablets once daily with a meal; maximum dose: 7 tablets/day.

In combination therapy with an HMG-CoA reductase inhibitor: 4–6 tablets daily; maximum dose: 6 tablets/day, available 625 mg tablet.

Safety of BAS

Bile acid sequestrants are considered safe LDL-lowering agents as systemic exposure to the drugs administered is basically nil. The patients with statin-induced myopathy tolerate colesevelam very well. This should be used in patients with hypercholesterolemia when statin produces toxicity or cannot be tolerated because of myalgia, fatigue and GI side effects.

OTHER CLINICAL OUTCOME STUDIES OF BAS

Individuals with prediabetes are at an increased risk of developing type 2 diabetes (by 5- to 15-fold) and are also at increased cardiovascular risk. Prediabetes is defined by the American Diabetes Association (ADA) and the American Association of Clinical Endocrinologists (AACE), as impaired fasting glucose (IFG) (100–125 mg/dL) and/or impaired glucose tolerance (2-hour poststimulation [with 75 g glucose] 140–199 mg/dL). Prediabetes or IFG antedates clinical diabetes by 5–20 years. At this stage, there is progressive beta cell failure. There is increase in insulin resistance and high level of endogenous glucose production.Colesevelam has been in IFG with hyperlipidemia (colesevelam has been shown to reduce LDL-C (15.6%; $P = 0.001$) and FPG levels (2.0 mg/dL; $P = 0.02$). Evidence suggests that in patients with hypercholesterolemia and IFG, BAS may be a good treatment option.

OTHER MEDICAL USES OF BAS

- In patients with chronic liver disease, e.g., cirrhosis, BAS may be used for preventing pruritus (due to bile acids deposition in the skin).

- Diarrhea may be caused by excess bile salts entering the colon rather than being absorbed at the ileum. Bile acid sequestrants, cholestyramine and colestipol on an empirical basis can be used for the treatment of diarrhea in various clinical settings.
- Cholestyramine is used in the treatment of *Clostridium difficile* infections helping absorb toxins A and B.
- Ileal resection and LDL lowering: Both steatorrhea and diarrhea are features of a rare recessive disorder in which apical sodium-dependent bile acid transporter (ASBT) is nonfunctional. The disorder is treated with BAS.
- Bile acid malabsorption often occurs after surgery to the ileum, in Crohn's disease, with a number of other GI causes, or is commonly a primary, idiopathic condition. The 23-seleno-25-homo-tauro-cholic acid test can be used for diagnosis.
- Bile acid sequestrants are the recommended therapy for diarrhea occurring in bile acid malabsorption. Cholestyramine, colestipol and colesevelam have all been used. Doses may not need to be as high as those previously used for hyperlipidemia. Although the diarrhea may improve, many patients find them hard to tolerate.
- Biliary diarrhea is a side effect of cholecystectomy. Bile acid sequestrants may reduce the frequency of diarrhea in these patients.
- Since BAS sequestrants are not absorbed from the gut, they are regarded as safe in pregnant women. Vitamin supplementation is required when BASs are used in pregnancy and lactating mother.

CONCLUSION

Bile acid sequestrants cause alterations in the bile acid pool with resultant effects on lipid and glucose metabolism. Bile acid sequestrants represent a novel treatment option for patients with type 2 diabetes, unique in their ability to modulate multiple cardiovascular risk factors. To further manage hyperglycemia and hypercholesterolemia. Bile acid sequestrants can be added to existing antidiabetes and lipid-lowering therapies of patients with type 2 diabetes.

Studies suggest that alterations of the enterohepatic circulation may regulate glucose homeostasis by modulating FXR- and TGR5-mediated pathways. Further studies, examining the role of FXR- and TGR5-mediated signaling pathways on lipid and glucose metabolism in animal and human models of T2DM and obesity, are needed to elucidate how these signals are integrated to mediate the lipid- and glucose-lowering effects of BAS.

SUGGESTED READING

1. Bergen SS, Van Itallie TB, Tennent DM, et al. Effect of an anion exchange resin on serum cholesterol in man. Proc Soc Exp Biol Med. 1959;102:676-9.
2. Effects of cholestyramine a bile acid sequestering exchange resin. Nutr Rev. 1961;19:292-3.
3. Kawashiri MA, Higashikata T, Nohara A, et al. Efficacy of colestimide coadministered with atorvastatin in Japanese patients with heterozygous familial hypercholesterolemia (FH). Circ J. 2005;69:515-20.
4. Love MW, Dawson PA. New insights into bile acid transport. Curr Opin Lipidol. 1998;9:225-9.
5. Claudel T, Staels B, Kuipers F, et al. The Farnesoid X receptor: a molecular link between bile acid and lipid and glucose metabolism. Arterioscler Thromb Vasc Biol. 2005;25:2020-30.
6. Grundy SM. Cholesterol metabolism in man. West J Med. 1978;128:13-25.
7. Grundy SM. Treatment of hypercholesterolemia by interference with bile acid metabolism. Arch Intern Med. 1972;130:638-48.

8. Edwards PA, Kast HR, Anisfeld AM, et al. BAREing it all: the adoption of LXR and FXR and their roles in lipid homeostasis. J Lipid Res. 2002;43:2-12.
9. Yabe D, Brown MS, Goldstein JL, et al. Insig-2, a second endoplasmic reticulum protein that binds SCAP and blocks export of sterol regulatory element-binding proteins. Proc Natl Acad Sci USA. 2002;99:12753-8.
10. Shepherd J, Packard CJ, Bicker S, et al. Effect of cholestyramine on low-density lipoproteins. N Engl J Med. 1980;303:943-4.
11. Telford DE, Edwards JY, Lipson SM, et al. Inhibition of both the apical sodium-dependent bile acid transporter and HMG-CoA reductase markedly enhances the clearance of LDL apoB. J Lipid Res. 2003;44:943-52.
12. Buchwald H, Varco RL, Matts JP, et al. Effect of partial ileal bypass surgery on mortality and morbidity from coronary heart disease in patients with hypercholesterolemia. N Engl J Med. 1990;323:946-55.
13. Hofmann AF. The continuing importance of bile acids in liver and intestinal disease. Arch Intern Med. 1999;159:2647-58.
14. Oelkers P, Kirby LC, Heubi JE, et al. Primary bile acid malabsorption caused by mutations in the ileal sodium-dependent bile acid transporter gene (SLC10A2). J Clin Invest. 1997;99:1880-87.
15. Staels B, Kuipers F. Bile acid sequestrants and the treatment of type 2 diabetes mellitus. Drugs. 2007;67:1383-92.
16. Garg A, Grundy SM. Cholestyramine therapy for dyslipidemia in non-insulin-dependent diabetes mellitus. A short-term, double-blind, crossover trial. Ann Intern Med. 1994;121:416-22.
17. Zieve FJ, Kalin MF, Schwartz SL, et al. Results of the glucose-lowering effect of WelChol study (GLOWS): a randomized, double-blind, placebo-controlled pilot study evaluating the effect of colesevelam hydrochloride on glycemic control in subjects with type 2 diabetes. Clin Ther. 2007;29:74-83.
18. Commerford SR, Vargas L, Dorfman SE, et al. Dissection of the insulin-sensitizing effect of liver X receptor ligands. Mol Endocrinol. 2007;21:3002-12.
19. Adridge MA, Ito MK. Colesevelam hydrochloride: a novel bile acid-binding resin. Ann Pharmacother. 2001;35:898-907.
20. Hunninghake DB, Probstfield JL, Crow LO, et al. Effect of colestipol and clofibrate on plasma lipid and lipoproteins in type IIa hyperlipoproteinemia. Metabolism. 1981;30:605-9.
21. Insull W, Toth P, Mullican W, et al. Effectiveness of colesevelam hydrochloride in decreasing LDL cholesterol in patients with primary hypercholesterolemia: a 24-week randomized controlled trial. Mayo Clin Proc. 2001;76:971-82.
22. Research Clinics Program Lipid: The Lipid Research Clinics Coronary Primary Prevention Trial results. II. The relationship of reduction in incidence of coronary heart disease to cholesterol lowering. JAMA. 1984;251:365-74.
23. Insull W, Davidson MH, Demke DM, et al. The effects of colestipol tablets compared with colestipol granules on plasma cholesterol and other lipids in moderately hypercholesterolemic patients. Atherosclerosis. 1995;112:223-35.
24. Davidson MH, Toth P, Weiss S, et al. Low-dose combination therapy with colesevelam hydrochloride and lovastatin effectively decreases low-density lipoprotein cholesterol in patients with primary hypercholesterolemia. Clin Cardiol. 2001;24:467-74.
25. Hunninghake D, Insull W, Toth P, et al. Coadministration of colesevelam hydrochloride with atorvastatin lowers LDL cholesterol additively. Atherosclerosis. 2001;158:407-16.
26. Davidson MH, Dicklin MR, Maki KC, et al. Colesevelam hydrochloride: a non-absorbed, polymeric cholesterol-lowering agent. Exp Opin Invest Drugs. 2000;9:2663-71.
27. Malloy MJ, Kane JP, Kunitake ST, et al. Complementarity of colestipol, niacin, and lovastatin in treatment of severe familial hypercholesterolemia. Ann Intern Med. 1987;107:616-23.
28. Brown G, Albers JJ, Fisher LD, et al. Regression of coronary artery disease as a result of intensive lipid-lowering therapy in men with high levels of apolipoprotein B. N Engl J Med. 1990;323:1289-98.

29. Bays H, Rhyne J, Abby S, et al. Lipid-lowering effects of colesevelam HCl in combination with ezetimibe. Curr Med Res Opin. 2006;22:2191-2200.
30. McKenny J, Jones M, Abby S, et al. Safety and efficacy of colesevelam hydrochloride in combination with fenofibrate for the treatment of mixed hyperlipidemia. Curr Med Res Opin. 2005;21:1403-12.
31. Watts GF, Lewis B, Brunt JN, et al. Effects on coronary artery disease of lipid-lowering diet, or diet plus cholestyramine, in the St. Thomas' Atherosclerosis Regression Study (STARS). Lancet. 1992;339:563-9.
32. Kane JP, Malloy MJ, Ports TA, et al. Regression of coronary atherosclerosis during treatment of familial hypercholesterolemia with combined drug regimens. JAMA. 1990;264:3007-12.
33. National Institutes of Health. Adult Treatment Panel III: Third Report of the National Cholesterol Education Program (NCEP) Expert Panel on Detection, Evaluation, and Treatment of High Blood Cholesterol in Adults. Circulation. 2002;106:3143.
34. Crouse JR. Hypertriglyceridemia: a contraindication to the use of bile acid binding resins. Am J Med. 1987;83:243-8.
35. Hoogwerf BJ, Hibbard DM, Hunninghake DB, et al. Effects of long-term cholestyramine administration on vitamin D and parathormone levels in middle-aged men with hypercholesterolemia. J Lab Clin Med. 1992;119:407-11.
36. Bays HE, Goldberg RB, Truitt KE, et al. Colesevelam hydrochloride therapy in patients with type 2 diabetes mellitus treated with metformin: glucose and lipid effects. Arch Intern Med. 2008;168:1975-83.
37. Goldberg RB, Fonseca VA, Truitt KE, et al. Efficacy and safety of colesevelam in patients with type 2 diabetes mellitus and inadequate glycemic control receiving insulin-based therapy. Arch Intern Med. 2008;168:1531-40.
38. Rigby SP, Handelsman Y, Lai YL, et al. Effects of colesevelam, rosiglitazone, or sitagliptin on glycemic control and lipid profile in patients with type 2 diabetes mellitus inadequately controlled by metformin monotherapy. Endocr Pract. 2010;16:53-63.
39. Insull Jr W. Clinical utility of bile acid sequestrants in the treatment of dyslipidemia: a scientific review. South Med J. 2006;99:257-73.
40. Lambert G, Amar MJ, Guo G, et al. The Farnesoid X-receptor is an essential regulator of cholesterol homeostasis. J Biol Chem. 2003;278:2563-70.
41. Claudel T, Sturm E, Duez H, et al. Bile acid-activated nuclear receptor FXR suppresses apolipoprotein A-I transcription via a negative FXR response element. J Clin Invest. 2002;109:961-71.
42. Ma K, Saha PK, Chan L, et al. Farnesoid X receptor is essential for normal glucose homeostasis. J Clin Invest. 2006;116:1102-9.
43. Beysen C, Murphy E, Deines K, et al. Colesevelam HCl reduces fasting plasma glucose concentrations by improving plasma glucose clearance in subjects with type 2 diabetes. Presented at the 69th Annual Meeting and Scientific Sessions of the American Diabetes Association. New Orleans, LA; June 5–9, 2009.
44. Shang Q, Saumoy M, Holst JJ, et al. Colesevelam improves insulin resistance in a diet-induced obesity (F-DIO) rat model by increasing the release of GLP-1. Am J Physiol Gastrointest Liver Physiol. 2010;298:G419-24.
45. Schwartz SL, Lai YL, Xu J, et al. The effect of colesevelam hydrochloride on insulin sensitivity and secretion in patients with type 2 diabetes: a pilot study. Metab Syndr Relat Disord. 2010;8:179-88.
46. Ballantyne CM. editor. Clinical lipidology: a companion to Braunwald's heart disease. 1st ed. 2009. pp. 281-7.
47. Guyton JR, Goldberg AC. Clinical lipidology: a companion to Braunwald's heart disease. Saunders, an imprint of Elsevier Inc.; p. 281-7.
48. Staels B, Handelsman Y, Fonseca V. Bile acid sequestrants for lipid and glucose control. Curr Diab Rep. 2010;10(1):707.

Niacin in the Lipid Disorders

Bharat Bhusan Kukreti and Tapan Ghose

- Introduction
- Pharmacology
- Clinical studies
- Conclusion

INTRODUCTION

Niacin (nicotinic acid) is the most potent drug commercially available for increasing high-density lipoprotein cholesterol (HDL-C) levels and has been shown to reduce cardiovascular events in pre-statin era.

Nicotinic acid increases HDL-C plasma levels by inducing hepatic production of apoA-I and by inhibiting HDL particle uptake and catabolism in the liver. Nicotinic acid also has broad lipid-modulating actions and has been for many years the principal available therapy besides fibrates for raising HDL-C. Following nicotinic acid therapy, HDL-C increases in a dose-dependent manner up to 25%, and typically reduces both low-density lipoprotein cholesterol (LDL-C) and triglycerides (TGs) by 15–18% and 20–40% respectively. Nicotinic acid is also the only currently available drug that decreases lipoprotein(a) levels by as much as 30%.

High-density lipoprotein is considered to be atheroprotective by virtue of its role in reverse cholesterol transport. In this role, it functions as a transporter of cholesterol from cells to liver and intestines for excretion, thus, reducing cholesterol level at cellular level.

High-density lipoprotein cholesterol and HDL are not synonymous, and there is a clear distinction between them. High-density lipoprotein particle enables lipids-like cholesterol to be transported back to liver, whereas HDL-C represents combination of HDL particle with cholesterol ester inside. Low HDL-C is an independent risk factor for coronary heart disease (CHD). It is inversely associated with CHD risk. In an observational study, it was found to have a 2–3% decrease in the risk of CHD for every 1 mg/dL increase in HDL. Another trial, treating to new targets (TNT), demonstrated a lower risk of CHD in groups with higher HDL. The antiatherogenic effect of HDL-C is related to reverse cholesterol transport and antioxidative and anti-inflammatory properties.

PHARMACOLOGY

Nicotinic acid is absorbed rapidly after oral administration. Peak-plasma level is reached within 30–60 minutes. The plasma half-life is around 1 hour. This is partially metabolized by liver, and the rest are excreted by the kidneys. When it is administrated at low dose, nicotinic acid is converted to *N*-methyl-nicotinamide. This is further converted to *N*-methyl-2-pyridone-5 carboxamide and *N*-methyl-4-pyridone 5-carboxamide. This is then excreted though the kidneys. When it is administered at therapeutic dosage (1–3 g), there is conjugation with glycine, and it is excreted as nicotiuric acid through the urine.

CLINICAL STUDIES

The Coronary Drug Project assessed the effect of four lipid-modifying medications on men with history of previous myocardial infarction (MI) from 1966 to 1975. Estrogen and dextrothyroxine arms of the study were prematurely terminated because of higher mortality. Niacin and clofibrate arms were continued till completion. There was 10% reduction in serum cholesterol with niacin and 6% reduction with clofibrate. Both of these drugs did not affect the cardiovascular mortality significantly. However, there was significant reduction of combined cardiovascular death and MI with both of these agents. Combined end point was reduced by 15% in the niacin arm and by 9% in the clofibrate arm. When compared with placebo, niacin reduced mortality by 11% after 9 years of follow-up.[1]

In the Stockholm Ischaemic Heart Disease Secondary Prevention Study, survivors of MI were randomized to control ($n = 276$) or treatment group ($n = 279$). Open level clofibrate and nicotinic acid were given to treatment group. There was 13 and 19% reduction in cholesterol and TGs in the treatment arm. There was 26% reduction in mortality ($P < 0.05$). Cardiovascular mortality was reduced by 36% ($P < 0.01$). The mortality reductions were more pronounced in the group with higher TGs at baseline.[2]

The safety and efficacy of a combination of extended-release niacin and simvastatin in patients with dyslipidemia (SEACOAST): was randomized controlled trial in patients with elevated non-HDL-C who were already on simvastatin therapy. After the run in phase, 600 patients were randomized to either 20 mg (low-dose) or 40 mg (high-dose) simvastatin. Patients in low-dose group (SEACOAST I) were randomized to extended-release (ER) niacin-simvastatin (1 g/20 mg) combination versus 2g/20 mg combination versus 20 mg simvastatin alone.

Patients in high-dose group (SEACOAST II) were randomized to ER niacin-simvastatin combination (2 g/20 mg) versus 1 g/40 mg versus 80 mg simvastatin alone.

The primary end point in both these two trials was medium percent change in non-HDL-C at 24 weeks.

In SEACOAST I, non-HDL-C was reduced by 23, 14 and 7% with 2 g/20 mg, 1 g/20 mg and simvastatin 20 mg dose alone respectively. High-density lipoprotein cholesterol was also significantly increased by combination therapy. Total 6% of patients discontinued combination therapy compared to 0.8% with simvastatin alone.

In SEACOAST II, non-HDL-C was reduced by 17%, 11%, and 10% with 2 g/40 mg, 1 g/40 mg and simvastatin 80 mg dose respectively.[3]

The OCEAN trial was a randomized, multicenter study that addressed the safety and efficacy of a fixed dose combination of niacin and simvastatin in patients with elevated non-HDL. Long-term safety was the primary end point, and secondary endpoints were the serum levels of non-HDL-C, intermediate-density lipoprotein cholesterol, and TG. In this trial, the subgroup of patients who failed to reach their goals with simvastatin therapy, 82% recipients achieved non-HDL goals, 85% reached HDL goals, 67% reached HDL goals and 64% reached TG target (65% reached all combined goals).[4]

Familial Atherosclerosis Treatment Study was conducted in 146 patients with known CAD. Patients were randomized to either of three arms: (1) niacin-colestipol, (2) lovastatin-colestipol and (3) Conventional therapy. Angiographic change of proximal lesion severity was the primary outcome.

Baseline stenosis average was 34%. After 2.5 years of study intervention, the stenosis increased by 2.1% in the conventional therapy group. Lovastatin–colestipol combination decreased the severity by 0.7% and niacin–colestipol decreased the severity by 0.9% ($P \leq 0.003$). Despite the modest angiographic benefit, the clinical benefit was robust. Myocardial infarction reduction was 19% in the conventional therapy group, 4% in lovastatin–colestipol group and 6% in the niacin–colestipol group.[5]

HDL-Atherosclerosis Treatment Study was a trial to study the effect of niacin, simvastatin and antioxidants on the angiographic progression/regression. Men or women with low HDL with at least one 50% stenosis or three 30% stenoses were randomized to lipid-lowering therapy or placebo versus antioxidant vitamins versus placebo in a 2 × 2 factorial design. Primary end point was angiographic changes and severity of stenosis at 2.5 years. The secondary end points were cardiac death, nonfatal MI, cerebrovascular accident (CVA) or coronary revascularization. Low-density lipoprotein and HDL levels were unchanged in the placebo and antioxidant arms. There was 3.9% stenosis progression in placebo arm, 1.8% in the antioxidant arm, 0.7% with simvastatin plus niacin plus antioxidant ($P = 0.004$) arm and regression (0.4%) with simvastatin niacin alone ($P \leq 0.001$). The clinical end point was 24% with placebo, 3% with simvastatin niacin alone, 21% with antioxidants and 14% with simvastatin-niacin-antioxidant.[6]

The Arterial Biology for the Investigation of the Treatment Effects of Reducing cholesterol (ARBITER) 2 study was a randomized placebo-controlled trial to access the effect of ER niacin added to statin therapy in CHD patients. In total, 167 men and women of more than 30 years of age were included. All patients were on statin (93% on >20 mg/day simvastatin). Niacin-ER formation was titrated up to 1 g/day dose. Primary end point was change in carotid intima media thickness at 1 year. Carotid intima media thickness increased significantly in the placebo group but not in the niacin group in which 38.5% on niacin and 25.40% on placebo-showed stabilization or regression. Clinical cardiovascular events occurred in 9.6% in the placebo arm versus 3.8% in the niacin arm ($P = 0.20$).[7]

AIM-HIGH study addressed the residual risk in the CHD population. Overall, 3414 patients were given simvastatin 40–80 mg/day plus ezetimibe 10 mg/day to maintain LDL 40–80 mg/dL. Patients were then randomized to 1500–2000 mg of ER niacin or placebo. Primary end point was composite of CVA, nonfatal MI, ischemic stroke, hospitalization for acute coronary syndrome (ACS) and revascularization. The trial was stopped at 3 years of lack of benefit. After 2 years, niacin increased HDL from 35 to 42 mg/dL, lowered TG level from 164to 122 mg/dL and lowered LDL-C from 74to 62 mg/dL. The primary end point occurred in 282 patients in the niacin arm (16.4%) compared with placebo arm (16.2%). The study concluded that despite biochemical improvement of reducing TG level and increasing HDL level there was no clinical benefit.[8]

Recently published Heart Protection Study 2-Treatment of HDL to Reduce the Incidence of Vascular Events (HPS2-THRIVE) trial examined the effect of raising HDL-C level in reducing cardiovascular risk. This randomized, controlled trial enrolled 25,673 adults, 50–80 years of age, with clinical CVD. The hypothesis tested in the study was "whether extended-release niacin combined with laropiprant, a new agent that helps prevent flushing could reduce major vascular events, as compared with placebo." Background statin-based therapy was intensified before randomization, resulting in a mean LDL-C level of 63 mg/dL (1.63 mmol/L) before study-drug initiation. Niacin–laropiprant increased HDL-C level by 6 mg/dL (0.16 mmol/L), reduced LDL-C level by 10 mg/dL (0.26 mmol/L) and TG by 33 mg/dL (0.37 mmol/L).[9]

However, there was no significant reduction in the primary end point of major vascular events associated with niacin–laropiprant, with a rate ratio of 0.96 (95% confidence interval, 0.90–1.03). Most worrisome findings of HPS2-THRIVE were the side effects of niacin–laropiprant combination. There were significant and excess adverse events related to gastrointestinal, musculoskeletal, infectious and bleeding complications. Dysglycemia was more. Loss of glycemic control among persons with diabetes and new-onset diabetes among persons without diabetes at baseline was reported.

CONCLUSION

In view of recent large-scale and meticulously conducted trials showing unacceptably high incidence of serious side effects in the absence of add-on benefit over statins use of niacin as a CAD risk modulator appears limited. Previously, failure of cholesteryl ester transfer protein inhibitors to modify CAD risk in spite of significantly raising HDL-C has already raised questions on strategy of artificially raising HDL-C with drugs. Recent data on niacin further raise

Table 14.1: Summary of clinical trials with niacin

	Trials	Population and follow-up	Intervention	Outcome
1	The Coronary Drug Project	Men with history of MI	Estrogen versus dextrothyroxine versus clofibrate versus niacin	Estrogen and dextrothyroxine arm stopped because of excess mortality. Combination of cardiovascular death and nonfatal MI was less with niacin (15%) and clofibrate (9%). 11% reduction of mortality at 9 years in niacin arm
2	Stockholm Ischaemic Heart Disease Secondary Prevention trial	9 years	Clofibrate and placebo versus clofibrate and niacin	13% reduction in serum cholesterol and 36% reduction in mortality with niacin and clofibrate combination
3	SEACOAST I	Mixed dyslipidemia	Niacin ER and simvastatin (1000/20 mg, 2000/20 mg) versus simvastatin alone	HDLC increased by 24% TG reduced by 38% Lp(a) reduced by 25% with combination therapy

	Trials	Population and follow-up	Intervention	Outcome
4	SEACOAST II	Mixed dyslipidemia	Niacin ER and simvastatin (2000/40 mg) versus simvastatin 80 mg	17.1 % reduction in non-HDL-C with combination
5	OCEAN trial	Open level multicenter study to evaluate safety and efficacy of inpatient with non-HDL-C	Niacin–simvastatin combination	Addition of niacin resulted in achievement of non-HDL goal in 82% (combined goals achieved in 65%)
6	FATS study	120 men with CAD	Lovastatin and colestipol versus niacin and colestipol versus placebo	Total cholesterol reduced by 33.8% lovastatin plus colestipol group 22.6% in niacin group 3.5 in placebo group. Stenosis increased by 2.1% in the conventional group. Lovastatin-cholestipol combination decreased the severity by 0.7% and Niacin-cholestipin decreased the severity by 0.9% (P ≤ 0.003). Myocardial infarction was reduction was 19% in the conventional group, 4% in Lovastatin plus Cholestipol group and 6% in the Niacin plus cholestipol group.
7	HATS	160 patients with low HDL and LDL (154 mg/dL)	Placebo vs antioxidant vs antioxidant plus niacin plus simvastatin	There was 3.9% stenosis progression in placebo arm, 1.8% in the antioxidant arm, 0.7% with simvastatin plus niacin plus antioxidant (P = 0.004) arm and regression (0.4%) with simvastatin niacin alone (P ≤ 0.001). The clinical end point was 24% with placebo, 3% with simvastatin niacin alone, 21% with antioxidants and 14% with simvastatin-niacin-antioxidant.

	Trials	Population and follow-up	Intervention	Outcome
8	ARBITER	Niacin ER 1000 once daily plus statin versus statin plus placebo in 160 patients with known CAD and low HDL		Carotid intima media thickness increased by 0.0444 in placebo arm and 0.023 in treatment arm
9	AIM-HIGH	ER niacin after achievement of LDL goal with statin, $N = 3414$	Simvastatin 40/80 mg plus ezetimibe 10 mg/day	Stopped after 2 years because of lack of efficacy
10	HPS2-THRIVE	$N = 20,617$ 4 years F/U	Background statin therapy with niacin–laropiprant versus placebo	No reduction in MACE excess adverse events

MI, myocardial infarction; ER, extended release; HDL-C, high-density lipoprotein cholesterol; TG, triglycerides; Lp(a), lipoprotein(a); CAD, coronary artery disease; LDL, low-density lipoprotein; MACE, major adverse cardiac events.

concern over raising HDL-C with niacin when safer drugs like statins are around. At the present moment, only targets would be the patients who are statin intolerant and have low HDL with high TGs even on adequate life style changes (Table 14.1).

REFERENCES

1. Canner PL, Berge KG, Wenger NK, et al. Fifteen year mortality in Coronary Drug Project patients: long term benefit with niacin. J Am Coll Cardiol.1986;8(6):1245-55.
2. Carlson LA, Rosenhamer G. Reduction in mortality in Stockholm Ischaemic Heart Disease Secondary Prevention Study by combined treatment with clofibrate and nicotinic acid. Acta Med Scand. 1988;223(5):404-18.
3. Ballantyne C, Davidson M, McKenney J, et al. The safety and efficacy of a combination of extended-release niacin and simvastatin in patients with dyslipidemia (SEACOAST): a dose-ranging study. Circulation. 2007;116:II15-II16. Abstract 188.
4. Karas RH, Kashyap ML, Knopp RH, et al. Long-term safety and efficacy of a combination of niacin extended release and simvastatin in patients with dyslipidemia: the OCEANS study. Am J Cardiovasc Drugs. 2008;8(2):69-81.
5. Brown BG, Brockenbrough A, Zhao XQ, et al. Very intensive lipid therapy with lovastatin, niacin, and colestipol for prevention of death and myocardial infarction: a 10-year Familial Atherosclerosis Treatment Study (FATS) follow-up. Circulation. 1998;98:3341.
6. Matthan NR, Giovanni A, Schaefer EJ, et al. Impact of simvastatin, niacin, and/or antioxidants on cholesterol metabolism in CAD patients with low HDL. J Lipid Res. 2003;44(4):800-6. doi:10.1194/jlr.M200439-JLR200.
7. Taylor AJ, Sullenberger LE, Lee HJ, et al. Arterial Biology for the Investigation of the Treatment Effects of Reducing Cholesterol (ARBITER) 2 : a double-blind, placebo-controlled study

of extended-release niacin on atherosclerosis progression in secondary prevention patients treated with statins. Circulation. 2004;110:3512-7.

8. The AIM-HIGH Investigators. Niacin in patients with low HDL cholesterol levels receiving intensive statin therapy. N Engl J Med. 2011;365:2255-67.

9. The HPS2-THRIVE Collaborative Group. Effects of extended-release niacin with laropiprant in high-risk patients. N Engl J Med. 2014;371:203-12.doi:10.1056/NEJMoa1300955.

Cholesterol Absorption Inhibitors

Sudhir S. Shetkar and Sandeep Singh

- Introduction
- Intestinal cholesterol absorption
- Agents affecting cholesterol absorption
- Intraluminal cholesterol processing targets
- Intracellular cholesterol processing targets
- Conclusion

INTRODUCTION

Cholesterol homeostasis is the net result of endogenous production, intestinal absorption and its excretion. Various therapeutic options exist for controlling cholesterol levels. These include targeting endogenous synthesis of cholesterol by statins, interrupting its entero-hepatic circulation by bile acid sequestrants, modulating nuclear hormone receptors by fibrates and many others. Introduction of statins has significantly simplified the pharmacologic treatment of high blood cholesterol levels. This group of drug has shifted the focus on endogenous cholesterol synthesis inhibition as prime therapy for hypercholesterolemia rather than targeting cholesterol absorption. However, monotherapy many a times fails to achieve target cholesterol levels; hence, combination of drugs with different mechanism of action becomes important.

Intestines play an important role not only in cholesterol absorption but also in its efflux and maintenance of plasma levels. Recent molecular studies of intestinal cholesterol absorption have enhanced our understanding of this new therapeutic target.[1] This chapter focuses on the intestinal cholesterol absorption and its metabolism, various therapeutic molecules that interfere with cholesterol absorption and the present clinical status of these agents.

INTESTINAL CHOLESTEROL ABSORPTION

The total plasma cholesterol is derived from two sources: endogenous biosynthesis (both in liver and peripheral tissues) and intestinal absorption. Cholesterol intended for intestinal absorption is primarily derived from two sources: biliary (700–1300 mg) and dietary (300–500 mg). A third source from intestinal cell turnover (200–300 mg) constitutes negligible amount of intestinal luminal cholesterol. As majority (three-fourth) of the intestinal cholesterol is derived from biliary excretion of hepatic cholesterol, intestinal absorption plays a significant role in controlling the hepatic cholesterol content and ultimately its blood level. Dietary cholesterol, which constitutes just one-fourth of total intestinal cholesterol, is considered as a minor contributor to circulating cholesterol, except during states of heavy dietary intake.

In humans, approximately 50% of the cholesterol is absorbed and retained. Cholesterol absorption predominantly occurs at the duodenum and proximal jejunum level. This process is quite complex and involves three distinct phases: its solubilization or micelle formation, uptake into enterocytes and finally its intracellular transport and packaging into chylomicrons. Each of these phases can be targeted for a pharmacological intervention with a goal to minimize the potential systemic adverse and off-target effects (Fig. 15.1).

In the initial phase, cholesterol molecules undergo micelle formation in the intestinal lumen with bile salts. This makes these molecules more water soluble so as to easily cross the intestinal brush border membrane into the intestinal epithelial cells. Niemann–Pick C1-like 1 protein (NPC1L1), the key protein located at the intestinal brush border membrane, is required for this transport of cholesterol from intestinal lumen into the enterocytes and forms the rate-limiting step in this process.[1]

Once inside the enterocytes, the free cholesterol is either excreted back into the intestinal lumen (cholesterol excretion) or packaged into chylomicron particles and absorbed. Cholesterol excretion is mediated by ATP-binding cassette (ABC) transporter G5 and G8. Genetic mutations in these transporters lead to increased intestinal absorption of these molecules, resulting in a condition termed as sitosterolemia.

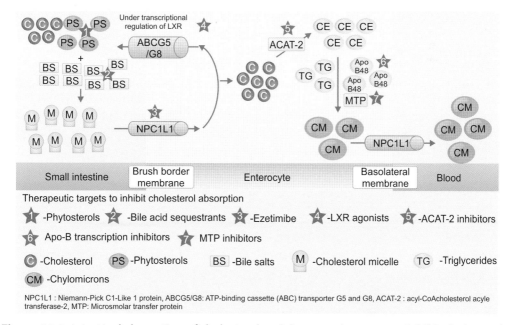

Figure 15.1: Intestinal absorption of cholesterol and therapeutic targets to inhibit cholesterol absorption

The remaining free cholesterol in the enterocytes undergoes esterification through the acyl-coenzyme A: cholesterol acyltransferase (ACAT). Microsomal triglyceride transfer protein (MTP) packages are cholesteryl esters with triglycerides and apolipoprotein B (apoB)-48 into chylomicrons. This process is analogous to the packaging of hepatic cholesterol into very low-density lipoprotein (VLDL) (mediated by ACAT and MTP) and transfer of peripheral tissue cholesterol into low-density lipoprotein (LDL) (mediated by lecithin-cholesterol acyltransferase and cholesteryl ester transfer protein). The chylomicrons are absorbed by lymphatics into the blood, where the action of lipoprotein lipase removes triglycerides and converts chylomicrons into cholesterol-rich chylomicron remnants. These remnants are taken up by the liver through chylomicron remnant receptors, adding cholesterol to the hepatic pool.

Liver is the key regulator of circulating cholesterol by balancing cholesterol syntheses, packaging into lipoproteins, excretion as bile and by down- and upregulating LDL receptors. Concentration of hepatic LDL receptors is under negative feedback control, with high hepatic cholesterol concentration leading to downregulation and low hepatic cholesterol concentration leading to upregulation of LDL receptors. In the event of decreased intestinal cholesterol absorption, there is compensatory increase in hepatic cholesterol synthesis and increased hepatic uptake of cholesterol by upregulation of LDL receptors. The converse holds true in states of increased dietary cholesterol intake.

AGENTS AFFECTING CHOLESTEROL ABSORPTION

Dietary cholesterol consumption affects plasma cholesterol concentrations, especially at high dietary intakes (400–500 mg/day). Thus, restriction of cholesterol and saturated fat in diet is justified as a primary therapeutic intervention for the management of hyperlipidemia. However, as mentioned previously, dietary cholesterol constitutes only 25% of absorbable intestinal cholesterol, thus even significant restrictions in dietary cholesterol intake fail to reduce circulating cholesterol levels appreciably. As majority (75%) of intestinal cholesterol is constituted by biliary excretion, pharmacologic inhibition of cholesterol absorption as a whole, rather than mere dietary restriction, is potentially a more effective way of lowering plasma cholesterol levels. Intestinal cholesterol absorption can be targeted at various steps, resulting in genesis of various therapeutic agents for the management of patients with hypercholesterolemia (Fig. 15.1). Broadly, these can be divided into two groups that affect either intraluminal or intracellular processing of cholesterol (Table 15.1).

Table 15.1: Classification of cholesterol absorption inhibitors

Intraluminal cholesterol modulation	Intracellular cholesterol modulation
Phytosterols	Niemann–Pick C1–like 1 protein inhibitor: ezetimibe
Bile acid sequestrants	Acyl-coenzyme A: cholesterol acyl transferase inhibitors
Direct cholesterol sequestrants	Microsomal transfer protein inhibitors
	ApoB transcription inhibitors
	Liver X Receptor agonists

INTRALUMINAL CHOLESTEROL PROCESSING TARGETS

Phytosterols

Phytosterols in plant food are molecules that are analogous to cholesterol in animals. Vegetable oils have the highest concentration of phytosterols among all plant-derived dietary products. Many phytosterols have been identified, with sitosterol, campesterol and stigmasterol being the predominant sterols in food sources. Even though the dietary intake of phytosterols is equal to that of cholesterol, their bioavailability is quite low, ranging between 0.4% and 3.5% only. Two factors predominantly contribute to low phytosterol levels in plasma: poor absorption and their rapid excretion. Absorption efficiency of plant sterols ranges from 5% to 18%, compared with 30% to 60% for cholesterol. Plant sterols entering the enterocytes are rapidly pumped back into the intestinal lumen by the actions of ABC-G5 and ABC-G8 transporters. Loss of function mutation of these receptors causes the inheritable condition called sitosterolemia. Patients with this condition have high blood and tissue sterol levels, and develop xanthomas and premature atherosclerosis.

Phytosterols successfully reduce plasma cholesterol concentrations. There is considerable debate about the exact mechanism of action of phytosterols. These compounds compete with cholesterol for bile acids during micelle formation and are more efficiently incorporated into micelles as compared with cholesterol. This results in displacement of cholesterol and its precipitation and fecal excretion. Competition between cholesterol and phytosterols for transfer into the brush border membrane also contributes to the inhibitory effect of large amounts of plant sterols on cholesterol absorption. Overall, this leads to decreased hepatic cholesterol delivery resulting in fall in LDL concentration.

Phytosterols are found to be safe, and measured absorption and plasma levels are very small. A recent meta-analysis demonstrated a nonlinear dose–response between LDL-cholesterol (LDL-C) reductions and intake of plant sterols.[2] Daily doses of 2 g produce almost 10% fall in plasma LDL-C levels with minimal improvements to LDL-C lowering at further doses up to 10 g/day.[3] The addition of phytosterols to statin therapy has been shown to be additive, with additional 10% LDL-C lowering above and over statins.[4] Many attempts have been made to modify these compounds to enhance their efficacy. The most studied modified phytosterol is the water-soluble derivative of sitostanol and campestanol, also known as disodium ascorbyl phytostanol phosphate. Though the results were encouraging in preclinical studies, the results of phase II trial hampered its further development.[5]

Bile Acid Sequestrants: Resins

Bile acid sequestrants or resins are positively charged insoluble polymer molecules that bind nonspecifically to negatively charged bile acids in intestinal lumen, thus preventing their absorption and facilitating fecal excretion. This action reduces hepatic delivery of cholesterol by interfering with micelle formation, leading to a fall in hepatic cholesterol pool. To compensate for loss of bile acids and decreased hepatic cholesterol, hepatic bile acid synthesis is increased and LDL receptors are upregulated.

Bile acid sequestrants, such as colesevelam, cholestyramine and colestipol, are safe lipid-lowering drugs. These agents do not have any systemic side effects as these are not absorbed into the circulation, but are frequently associated with undesirable gastrointestinal side effects. The most common side effects are flatulence and constipation, resulting in poor drug compliance and early discontinuation of therapy. By interfering with entero-hepatic circulation, these agents have the propensity to cause malabsorption of fat-soluble vitamins. One more concern of these agents is increase in triglyceride levels, secondary to reflex increase in hepatic production. As such these agents are contraindicated in patients with hypertriglyceridemia.

At their maximal tolerable dose, these agents lower LDL-C by 15–21%, and raise high-density lipoprotein (HDL) cholesterol and triglyceride by 3–9% and 2–16%, respectively.[6] These drugs are used in the treatment of hypercholesterolemia either as monotherapy or in combination with statins, when LDL target levels are not met with statin monotherapy alone. In clinical studies, cholestyramine has shown to reduce LDL levels by 12% and decrease coronary heart disease risk.[7] Colesevelam is a more specific, second-generation bile acid-binding resin that has greater affinity for bile acids and is better tolerated. It lowers LDL-C level up to 16% at a dose of 3.8 g/day, and has additive lipid-lowering effect in combination with statins.[8,9] Lowering of plasma glucose and glycosylated hemoglobin levels is a peculiar property of bile acid-binding resins, which makes them attractive agents in the management of hypercholesterolemia in diabetic patients.[10]

Direct Sequestration of Cholesterol

Bile acid sequestrants like cholestyramine additionally bind and sequester cholesterol directly. Similarly, water-soluble dietary fibers (β-glucan, pectin and psyllium) have the intraluminal cholesterol-binding properties, and these compounds have shown modest reduction in LDL-C.[11] Subsequently, many synthetic fibers (surfomer and Olestra) were developed to improve their efficacy to sequester cholesterol. Despite initial promising results, further development of these agents was stopped due to their lack of efficacy in randomized trial and significant gastrointestinal side effects.[12]

Another, recently developed compound is nanostructured aluminosilicate (NSAS), which is negatively charged in comparison with the positively charged bile acid sequestrants. Surface protons are incorporated to counterbalance these negative charges on NSAS. These protonated NSAS specifically adsorb cholesterol, sequestering it from the aqueous phase of the intestinal milieu as compared with cholestyramine, which nonspecifically binds to bile acids, cholesterol and triacylglycerol.[13] The specificity of cholesterol sequestration, the lack of systemic exposure and the ability to reduce atherosclerotic lesion formation in animal models suggest that protonated NSAS may become a viable adjunct therapy for reducing cholesterol levels.

INTRACELLULAR CHOLESTEROL PROCESSING TARGETS

Ezetimibe

Niemann–Pick C1-like 1 protein is a sterol transporter located at the intestinal brush border membrane, which is responsible for the intestinal uptake of cholesterol and phytosterols. Ezetimibe selectively inhibits NPC1L1 sterol transporter, resulting in potent and selective inhibition of cholesterol and phytosterol absorption. Ezetimibe is effective in reducing LDL-C levels either as monotherapy or in combination with statins. As monotherapy, it reduces LDL-C by 17.2–22.3% compared with placebo, and has an additive effect with statin therapy.[14] Studies suggest that the role of ezetimibe is not just limited to intestinal absorption of cholesterol. Niemann–Pick C1-like

1 protein receptors are also expressed in hepatocytes, and by inhibiting these receptors ezetimibe also regulates hepatic cholesterol uptake and biliary cholesterol concentration. Ezetimibe has been shown to block the uptake of oxidized LDL by human macrophages. Thus, it seems that ezetimibe may reduce plasma cholesterol by inhibiting NPC1L1 function in both the intestine and the liver. Along with reduction in LDL-C levels, ezetimibe either as monotherapy or when added to statins significantly decreases triglycerides, non-HDL cholesterol, high-sensitivity C-reactive protein (hs-CRP), apoB and favorably affects HDL-C levels.[14]

Ezetimibe after oral administration undergoes rapid and extensive glucuronidation in the intestinal wall to yield glucuronides. This glucuronidated ezetimibe is absorbed in portal system and undergoes rapid enterohepatic circulation. Effective enterohepatic circulation exposes the drug repeatedly to the primary site of action (intestine) and is responsible for long duration of action of ezetimibe even after stopping the drug. Unlike bile acid-binding resins, ezetimibe does not interfere in absorption of triglycerides, fatty acids, bile acids or fat-soluble vitamins, and thus results in a highly selective cholesterol absorption inhibition. Inhibition of intestinal absorption of dietary as well as biliary cholesterol leads to decreased hepatic delivery of cholesterol, increased fecal loss of cholesterol and depletion of the hepatic cholesterol pool. However, these same stimuli also lead to a marked compensatory increase in cholesterol synthesis in the liver. This calls for the combination of ezetimibe with statins as a potent and rational cholesterol-lowering strategy. Ezetimibe effectively reduces body concentrations of plant sterols in sitosterolemia, and is an effective treatment of this condition. Ezetimibe administered alone or with statins is generally well tolerated, with safety profiles similar to those of placebo. Adverse reactions may include headache, diarrhea (steatorrhea), myalgia, rhabdomyolysis, deranged liver function tests, hepatitis, pancreatitis and hypersensitivity (rash and angioedema). There were initial concerns of increased risk of incident and fatal cancers in patients receiving ezetimibe; however, these were refuted in a meta-analysis of interim safety data involving patients from the Study of Heart and Renal Protection (SHARP) and study.[15]

Two clinical trials, the Simvastatin and Ezetimibe in Aortic Stenosis (SEAS) and SHARP, showed clinical efficacy of ezetimibe. The SEAS trial compared combination of simvastatin and ezetimibe versus placebo in patients with aortic stenosis. This combination was associated with significant fall in LDL-C levels associated with significant decrease in fatal and nonfatal myocardial infarction.[16] The SHARP trial studied clinical effects of lowering LDL-C with simvastatin plus ezetimibe combination as compared with placebo, in patients with chronic kidney disease. This randomized trial reported that combination of simvastatin 20 mg with ezetimibe 10 mg daily safely reduced major atherosclerotic events by 17%. However, both these trials compared combination of ezetimibe with statins versus placebo, thus the observed clinical benefit could have been driven by statin alone.[17]

The Stop Atherosclerosis in Native Diabetics Study and the Vytorin on Carotid Intima-Media Thickness and Overall Arterial Rigidity study showed addition of ezetimibe over statin to be associated with reduction in carotid intima-media thickness (CIMT), a surrogate marker of progression of atherosclerosis.[18,19] Contrary to these two studies, the Arterial Biology for the Investigation of the Treatment Effects of Reducing Cholesterol 6-HDL and LDL Treatment Strategies trial that studied niacin versus ezetimibe, showed superiority of niacin over ezetimibe in inducing regression of CIMT. Ezetimibe failed to produce any improvement in CIMT.[20] Similar results were seen by the Ezetimibe and Simvastatin in Hypercholesterolemia Enhances Atherosclerosis Regression trial. This study also showed that treatment with ezetimibe plus simvastatin (10 plus 80 mg, respectively) for 2 years did not significantly alter CIMT when compared with simvastatin 80 mg alone.[21]

Studies evaluating impact of ezetimibe on hard clinical cardiovascular outcomes such as mortality are lacking. A recent retrospective cohort study did not found any significant mortality benefit of ezetimibe in combination with statin over statin monotherapy.[22] The recently completed IMPROVE-IT trial (NCT00202878, The Improved Reduction of Outcomes:is a multicenter, randomized, double-blind, active-control trial, testing the addition of ezetimibe to simvastatin therapy on cardiovascular outcomes relative to simvastatin monotherapy in patients with acute coronary syndrome.[23] The primary end points being studied are cardiovascular death, nonfatal myocardial infarction or nonfatal stroke. The trial will continue until a minimum of 5250 subjects have a primary end point event and each subject is followed for at least 2.5 years. Thus, the anticipated completion dates will be adjusted on the basis of actual event occurrence. Results of this study will be pivotal in deciding the impact of ezetimibe on cardiovascular outcomes in patients with coronary artery disease. As of now, due to lack of hard evidence in favor of ezetimibe monotherapy in reducing clinical outcomes, ezetimibe is primarily used as a combination therapy with a statin when statin therapy fails to achieve LDL-C goals.

Acyl-Coenzyme A: Cholesterol Acyltransferase Inhibitors

Free cholesterol that has been moved from the brush border membrane to intracellular must be esterified prior to its assembly into chylomicrons. This esterification process occurs in the endoplasmic reticulum and is catalyzed by ACAT. This process seems to be an important step in enhancing cholesterol absorption. There are two different isoforms of ACAT. Acyl-coenzyme A: cholesterol acyltransferase-1 is expressed ubiquitously (in macrophage, atherosclerotic plaque, liver, intestine etc.), while ACAT-2 is expressed in the liver and intestine only. Lack of ACAT-2 for cholesterol esterification leads to reduced dietary cholesterol absorption and protects against diet-induced hypercholesterolemia. Acyl-coenzyme A: cholesterol acyltransferase-2 knockout mice fed on a high cholesterol diet have a twofold less plasma cholesterol levels as compared with normal wild-type mice.[24]

Avasimibe is the first novel, orally bioavailable ACAT inhibitor. In animal models, avasimibe reduced plasma cholesterol levels, primarily due to decrease in non-HDL cholesterol. Avasimibe significantly reduces plasma total triglyceride and VLDL cholesterol, without any change in total cholesterol, LDL-C or HDL cholesterol. The human studies of avasimibe studying progression of atherosclerosis have shown conflicting results. Few studies showed a synergistic effect of avasimibe and statin combination leading to slowing of atherosclerotic progression, and even regression of plaques as assessed by intravascular ultrasound (IVUS).[25] Another IVUS study evaluating the effect of avasimibe on progression of atherosclerosis surprisingly showed increase in atheroma volume as well as LDL-C with avasimibe monotherapy versus placebo.[26] These conflicting results call for further studies to adequately assess the role of ACAT inhibitors on lipid profile and atherosclerosis progression.

Microsomal Triglyceride Transfer Protein Inhibitors

Microsomal triglyceride transfer protein is involved in assembly and secretion of apoB-containing lipoproteins in the liver and intestine. Abetalipoproteinemia is an autosomal recessive disease caused by mutations in the gene encoding for MTP. This disorder is characterized by the absence of circulating apoB-containing lipoproteins, such as chylomicrons, VLDL and LDL. Microsomal triglyceride transfer protein is a potential therapeutic target for the treatment of both hypercholesterolemia and hyperchylomicronemia. It transfers triglycerides and cholesteryl esters onto apoB-48 and apoB-100 in the assembling chylomicron and VLDL particles, respectively. Absence of functional MTP results in inadequate lipidation of apoB in the endoplasmic reticulum that is then eventually targeted for proteosomal degradation. This degradation of apoB prevents adequate assembly and secretion of chylomicrons (in intestine) and VLDL (in liver) into the circulation. This inhibition leads to a reduction in the synthesis of chylomicrons (in intestines) and VLDL (in liver), resulting in a reduction in plasma LDL-C levels.

Many MTP inhibitors have been studied and have shown to produce a significant fall in apoB-containing lipoprotein levels in animal models. However, development of most of these compounds was halted due to occurrence of significant gastrointestinal adverse events and steatohepatitis. Lomitapide is the only systemic MTP inhibitor that was continued to be developed, tested in clinical trials and is Food and Drug Administration approved for the treatment of homozygous familial hypercholesterolemia. In a phase 2, double-blind, placebo controlled trial, lomitapide at a dose of 10 mg/day as monotherapy significantly reduced LDL-C and apoB by 30% and 24%, respectively. Addition of lomitapide with ezetimibe was additive, with a larger LDL-C reduction (46%).[27] Lomitapide at a dose titrated up to 60 mg/day was studied in a recent multicentric phase 3 study involving 29 patients with homozygous familial hypercholesterolemia. All patients received lomitapide over and above standard therapy. Lomitapide at a median dose of 40 mg/day reduced LDL-C, apoB and triglycerides levels by 50%, 49% and 45%, respectively at 26 week as compared with baseline. This trial confirmed that lomitapide is an effective lipid-lowering agent, and its effects are additive to that of other lipid-lowering drugs.[28]

Gastrointestinal side effects, such as nausea, flatulence and diarrhea, are the most common adverse effects. Gradual escalation of dose can partially control these symptoms. Microsomal triglyceride transfer protein inhibition by virtue of inhibiting chylomicron assembly and secretion leads to intestinal malabsorption of fat-soluble vitamins and essential fatty acids. However, inhibition of MTP by lomitapide at doses used in clinical trials has not shown to cause deficiency of either fat-soluble vitamins or essential fatty acids.[28] Other known side effects of lomitapide include a dose-related increase in hepatic fat content and elevations in transaminase levels.[28] Selective intestinal MTP inhibitors devoid of hepatic MTP inhibition may avoid the hepatic complications of systemic MTP inhibitors. JTT-130 and SLX-4090 are two such molecules that have already entered clinical development.

Apolipoprotein B Transcription Inhibitors

Apolipoprotein B can be directly targeted by inhibiting its production at the transcription level. Apolipoprotein B messenger RNA (m-RNA) can be targeted by oligonucleotides having complementary nucleic acid sequences. One such antisense oligonucleotide, mipomersen, has been studied in a randomized controlled trial of patients with homozygous familial hypercholesterolemia.[29] In this study, mipomersen at a weekly dose of 200 mg given subcutaneously significantly lowered LDL-C as compared with placebo. Injection site reactions were the most common side effects followed by elevated liver enzymes. However, apoB transcription inhibitors are still far from being clinically established as effective hypolipidemic agents.

Liver X Receptor Agonists

ATP-binding cassette transporters are heterodimeric proteins involved in efflux of cholesterol from peripheral cells to nascent HDL particles (by ABCA1 transporter) and from enterocytes to back into the intestinal lumen (by ABC-G5/ABC-G8 transporters). These transporters are under transcriptional regulation of liver X receptor (LXR) receptor, and are attractive targets as lipid-lowering agents. One such LXR activator, T0901317, reduced cholesterol absorption, cholesterol levels and inhibited development of atherosclerosis in murine models.[30] Effects on cholesterol metabolism and clinical utility in humans remain an active area of research.

CONCLUSION

Cholesterol homeostasis is primarily maintained by interplay between its synthesis and absorption. Targeting either of these steps is expected to exert compensatory feedback adjustment. This may be partially responsible for the failure of monotherapy by cholesterol synthesis inhibitors in achieving target cholesterol levels. Combination therapy by adding cholesterol absorption inhibitors is thus complementary to monotherapy with cholesterol synthesis inhibitors. Recent advances have increased our understanding of cholesterol absorption at the molecular level, and have led to the development of whole new armamentarium of lipid-lowering drugs targeting at the level of cholesterol absorption (Table 15.2). Some of these newer molecules such as ezetimibe are already in clinical use and many others are under advance stage of development. However, more data is needed to routinely use these drugs for achieving target lipid goals in patients, especially in patients with high-risk coronary artery disease.

Table 15.2: Cholesterol absorption inhibitors

Drug category	Drug molecule	Mode of action	Dose	Effects	Side effects
Phytosterol	Sitosterol Campesterol Stigmasterol	Compete with cholesterol for micelle formation and absorption at brush border membrane in intestine	2 g/day PO	Decrease in LDL, VLDL and TG	Mild GI side effects: constipation, bloating
Bile acid sequestrants	Colesevelam Cholestyramine Colestipol	Interrupts enterohepatic circulation of bile salts	Colesevelam 2.6–3.8 g/day PO Cholestyramine 4–16 g/day PO Colestipol 5–20 g/day PO	Lowers LDL Raises HDL and TG Lowers blood glucose and HbA1c levels	GI side effects: constipation, bloating Deficiency of fat-soluble vitamins Hypertriglyceridemia

NPC1L1 protein inhibitor	Ezetimibe	Selective inhibition of NPC1L1 protein	10 mg, once a day PO	Lowers LDL, TG, non-HDL cholesterol, apoB and hs-CRP Increases HDL	Headache Steatorrhea Myalgia, rhabdomyolysis Deranged liver function Pancreatitis Hypersensitivity
ACAT inhibitor	Avasimibe	Inhibits ACAT enzyme required in cholesterol esterification	50–750 mg/day PO	Lowers TG, VLDL, non-HDL cholesterol without much effect on LDL or HDL	Increase in liver enzymes
MTP inhibitors	Lomitapide	Inhibits MTP protein leading to inadequate assembly and secretion of chylomicrons and VLDL	10–60 mg/day PO	Lowers LDL, VLDL, TG and apoB	GI intolerance Fatty liver
ApoB transcription inhibitors	Mipomersen	Transcriptional inhibition of apoB synthesis	200 mg SC weekly.	Decreased LDL	Injection site reactions Elevated liver enzymes
Liver X receptor agonists	T0901317	Upregulate transcription of ABC transporters	Decrease cholesterol absorption, cholesterol levels and progression of atherosclerosis in murine models		

LDL, low-density lipoprotein; VLDL, very low-density lipoprotein; TGs, triglycerides; HDL, high-density lipoprotein; GI, gastrointestinal; hs-CRP, high-sensitivity C-reactive protein; ACAT, acyl-coenzyme A: cholesterol acyltransferase; ABC, ATP-binding cassette; PO, per orally; SC, subcutaneous; apoB, apolipoprotein B; NPC1L1, Niemann–Pick C1-like 1 protein; MTP, microsomal triglyceride transfer protein.

REFERENCES

1. Davis HR Jr, Tershakovec AM, Tomassini JE, et al. Intestinal sterol transporters and cholesterol absorption inhibition. Curr Opin Lipidol. 2011;22(6):467-78.
2. Demonty I, Ras RT, van der Knaap HC, et al. Continuous dose-response relationship of the LDL-cholesterol-lowering effect of phytosterol intake. J Nutr. 2009;139(2):271-84.
3. Katan MB, Grundy SM, Jones P, et al. Efficacy and safety of plant stanols and sterols in the management of blood cholesterol levels. Mayo Clin Proc. 2003;78(8):965-78.

4. Blair SN, Capuzzi DM, Gottlieb SO, Nguyen T, et al. Incremental reduction of serum total cholesterol and low-density lipoprotein cholesterol with the addition of plant stanol ester-containing spread to statin therapy. Am J Cardiol. 2000;86(1):46-52.

5. Vissers MN, Trip MD, Pritchard PH, et al. Efficacy and safety of disodium ascorbyl phytostanol phosphates in men with moderate dyslipidemia. Eur J Clin Pharmacol. 2008;64(7):651-61.

6. Ascaso JF. Advances in cholesterol-lowering interventions. Endocrinol Nutr. 2010;57(5):210-9.

7. Lipid Research Clinics Program. The lipid research clinics coronary primary prevention trial results. I. Reduction in incidence of coronary heart disease. JAMA. 1984;251(3),351-64.

8. Knapp HH, Schrott H, Ma P, et al. Efficacy and safety of combination simvastatin and colesevelam in patients with primary hypercholesterolemia. Am J Med. 2001;110(5):352-60.

9. Hunninghake D, Insull W Jr, Toth P, et al. Coadministration of colesevelam hydrochloride with atorvastatin lowers LDL cholesterol additively. Atherosclerosis. 2001;158(2):407-16.

10. Staels B, Kuipers F. Bile acid sequestrants and the treatment of Type 2 diabetes mellitus. Drugs. 2007;67(10):1383-92.

11. Brown L, Rosner B, Willett WW, et al. Cholesterol-lowering effects of dietary fiber: a meta-analysis. Am J Clin Nutr. 1999;69(1):30-42.

12. Mellies MJ, Jandacek RJ, Taulbee JD, et al. A double-blind, placebo-controlled study of sucrose polyester in hypercholesterolemic outpatients. Am J Clin Nutr. 1983;37(3):339-46.

13. Gershkovich P, Sivak O, Contreras-Whitney S, et al. Assessment of cholesterol absorption inhibitors nanostructured aluminosilicate and cholestyramine using in vitro lipolysis model. J Pharm Sci. 2012;101(1):291-300.

14. Bays HE, Neff D, Tomassini JE, et al. Ezetimibe: cholesterol lowering and beyond. Expert Rev Cardiovasc Ther. 2008;6(4):447-70.

15. Peto R, Emberson J, Landray M, et al. Analyses of cancer data from three ezetimibe trials. N Engl J Med. 2008;359(13):1357-66.

16. Rossebø AB, Pedersen TR, Boman K, et al. SEAS Investigators. Intensive lipid lowering with simvastatin and ezetimibe in aortic stenosis. N Engl J Med. 2008;359(13):1343-56.

17. Baigent C, Landray MJ, Reith C, et al. The effects of lowering LDL cholesterol with simvastatin plus ezetimibe in patients with chronic kidney disease (Study of Heart and Renal Protection): a randomised placebo-controlled trial. Lancet. 2011;377(9784):2181-92.

18. Fleg JL, Mete M, Howard BV, et al. Effect of statins alone versus statins plus ezetimibe on carotid atherosclerosis in type 2 diabetes: the SANDS (Stop Atherosclerosis in Native Diabetics Study) trial. J Am Coll Cardiol. 2008;52(25):2198-205.

19. Meaney A, Ceballos G, Asbun J, et al. The VYtorin on Carotid intima media thickness and overall arterial rigidity (VYCTOR) study. J Clin Pharmacol. 2009;49(7):838-47.

20. Villines TC, Stanek EJ, Devine PJ, et al. The ARBITER 6-HALTS Trial (Arterial Biology for the Investigation of the Treatment Effects of Reducing Cholesterol 6-HDL and LDL Treatment Strategies in Atherosclerosis): initial results and the impact of medication adherence, dose, and treatment duration. J Am Coll Cardiol. 2010;55(24):2721-26.

21. Kastelein JJ, Akdim F, Stroes ES, et al.; ENHANCE Investigators. Simvastatin with or without ezetimibe in familial hypercholesterolemia. N Engl J Med. 2008;358(14):1431-43.

22. Patel AY, Pillarisetti J, Marr J, et al. Ezetimibe in combination with a statin does not reduce all-cause mortality. J Clin Med Res. 2013;5(4):275-80.

23. Cannon CP, Giugliano RP, Blazing MA, et al.; IMPROVE-IT Investigators. Rationale and design of IMPROVE-IT (IMProved Reduction of Outcomes: Vytorin Efficacy International Trial): comparison of ezetimibe/simvastatin versus simvastatin monotherapy on cardiovascular outcomes in patients with acute coronary syndromes. Am Heart J. 2008;156(5):826-32.

24. Buhman KK, Accad M, Novak S, et al. Resistance to diet induced hypercholesterolemia and gallstone formation in ACAT2-deficient mice. Nat Med. 2000;6:1341-47.

25. Tardif JC, Gregoire J, Lesperance J, et al. Design features of the Avasimibe and Progression of coronary Lesions assessed by intravascular UltraSound (A-PLUS) clinical trial. Am Heart J. 2002;144:589-96.
26. Tardif JC, Grégoire J, L'Allier PL, et al. Effects of the acyl coenzyme A: cholesterol acyltransferase inhibitor avasimibe on human atherosclerotic lesions. Circulation. 2004;110:3372-77.
27. Samaha FF, McKenney J, Bloedon LT, et al. Inhibition of microsomal triglyceride transfer protein alone or with ezetimibe in patients with moderate hypercholesterolemia. Nat Clin Pract Cardiovasc Med. 2008;5:497-505.
28. Cuchel M, Meagher EA, du Toit Theron H, et al. Efficacy and safety of a microsomal triglyceride transfer protein inhibitor in patients with homozygous familial hypercholesterolaemia: a single-arm, open-label, phase 3 study. Lancet. 2013;381:40-6.
29. Raal FJ, Santos RD, Blom DJ, et al. Mipomersen, an apolipoprotein B synthesis inhibitor, for lowering of LDL cholesterol concentrations in patients with homozygous familial hypercholesterolaemia: a randomised, double-blind, placebo-controlled trial. Lancet. 2010;375(9719):998-1006.
30. Yu L, York J, Von Bergmann K, et al. Stimulation of cholesterol excretion by the liver X receptor agonist requires ATP-binding cassette transporters G5 and G8. J Biol Chem. 2003;278(18):15565-70.

Familial Combined Hyperlipidemia

D J Dutta

- Introduction
- Genetic basis of familial combined hyperlipidemia
- Prevalence of familial combined hyperlipidemia
- Diagnostic criteria of familial combined hyperlipidemia
- Structure and metabolism of lipoproteins in familial combined hyperlipidemia
- Clinical presentation
- Differential diagnosis of familial combined hyperlipidemia
- Principles of management
- Conclusion

INTRODUCTION

Familial combined hyperlipidemia (FCH) is one of the commonest familial lipoprotein disorders.[1] Originally, this condition was described in survivors of young myocardial infarctions. Lipoprotein abnormalities of this disorder fall into the category of type IIb hyperlipidemia (phenotype) as described by Donald Fridrickson et al. in 1967.[2] Familial combined hyperlipidemia was also named as multiple phenotype familial hyperlipidemia, familial mixed hyperlipidemia, familial combined hyperlipoproteinemia and familial combined hypercholesterolemia hypertriglyceridemia.[3]

GENETIC BASIS OF FAMILIAL COMBINED HYPERLIPIDEMIA

Though initially FCH was thought to have a dominant monogenic mode of inheritance, subsequent studies have suggested a complex inheritance pattern.[4] Pakunjnta et al. identified a locus linked to FCH on 1q21:q23 in some Finnish families.[5] This locus was also linked to FCH families of other populations as well as type 2 diabetes. By linkage analysis a newly discovered apolipoprotein A-V (apoA-V) gene with APOAI/AIV cluster was found to be responsible for FCH transmission in a group of 128 European families.[6] Moreover, variable low-density lipoprotein (LDL) particle size in FCH was proposed to be a trait influenced by multiple loci located in 9p, 16q and FIq.[7]

Recently, the gene encoding upstream transcription factor I has appeared to be specifically linked to FCH in the familial study. This factor has been known to regulate several genes controlling glucose and lipid metabolism, and allelic association with triglycerides (TGs), apolipoprotein B (apo B), total cholesterol and LDL particle size has been demonstrated. This finding may explain the monogenic-like transmission of the trait as well as the intra- and interindividual variability in the phenotypic expression.[8]

However, the gene environment interaction could strongly influence the clinical presentation and the different lipid parameters, thereby complicating the detection of FCH.[3]

PREVALENCE OF FAMILIAL COMBINED HYPERLIPIDEMIA

Familial combined hyperlipidemia has been considered as one of the most common genetic hyperlipidemia in the general population with an estimated prevalence of 0.5–2%. Described in 10% of the patients suffering from coronary artery disease, this estimate increases to 11.3%[9] in young survivors of acute myocardial infarctions and 40% when all infarct survivors are considered.[10] However, prevalence estimate depends strongly on the diagnostic criteria applied because of significant phenotypic variation. According to a conservative estimate, over 3.5 million subjects are affected by this disorder in Europe and 2.7 million in the United States. This condition is the cause of approximately 30,000–70,000 infarcts per year in Europe, a good number of those being premature. Geographical distribution of the disease has not been clearly defined since majority studies so far are carried out in Europe and the United States.[9]

DIAGNOSTIC CRITERIA OF FAMILIAL COMBINED HYPERLIPIDEMIA

Combining the old and recent definitions, FCH is now defined as a common metabolic disorder characterized by increase in cholesterol and TG level in at least two members of the same family. Intra and inter individual variability of the lipid phenotype increased the risk of premature coronary artery disease (Table 16.1).[3] Recently, the European Society of Cardiology and European Atherosclerosis Society has laid down the following diagnostic criteria for FCH:[11] *apoB level >120 ng/dL and TG level > 133 mg/dL with a family history of premature cardiovascular disease (CVD).* A number of laboratory abnormalities are commonly found in FCH.[3] They are increase in plasma TG level, increase in cholesterol level, high prevalence of small very low-density lipoprotein (VLDL) and LDL, decrease in high-density lipoprotein(HDL) level (occasionally) and increase in level of apoB level (Table 16.2).

Table 16.1: Diagnostic criteria of familial combined hyperlipidemia

Increase in cholesterol and triglyceride level in at least two members of the same family

Intra- and interindividual variability of the lipid phenotype

Increased risk of premature coronary artery disease

Table 16.2: Lipoprotein abnormality in familial combined hyperlipidemia

Increase in plasma triglyceride level
Increase in cholesterol level
High prevalence of small VLDL and LDL
Decrease in HDL level (occasionally)
Increase in apoB level

VLDL, very low-density lipoprotein; LDL, low-density lipoprotein; HDL, high-density lipoprotein; apoB, apolipoprotein B.

STRUCTURE AND METABOLISM OF LIPOPROTEINS IN FAMILIAL COMBINED HYPERLIPIDEMIA

Very Low-Density Lipoproteins

An increase in the synthesis of VLDL-apoB is usually present. Though the exact reason is not known, the following explanations are put forward by different authors:

1. There is alteration in the incorporation of fatty acids into TGs and/or alteration in the post-prandial metabolism of VLDL with greater conversion to small dense LDL particles[12,13]
2. There are defects in the activities of lipoprotein lipase, lecithin cholesterol acyltransferase and hepatic lipase[3]
3. There is decreased fatty acid oxidation, with fatty acids increasingly being directed to TG synthesis[14]
4. Impaired postprandial plasma component C3 has been observed in FCH that may decrease peripheral postprandial free fatty acid (FFA) uptake, thereby leading to increased hepatic FFA flux and VLDL overproduction.[12]

Low-Density Lipoprotein Cholesterol

There is preponderance of small dense LDL, so-called LDL-B pattern, which is highly athero-genic. This occurs due to overproduction of apoB.[3] In FCH patients with very high LDL level, lipoprotein(a) level also increases.[15]

High-Density Lipoprotein Cholesterol

Reduced level of high-density lipoprotein cholesterol (HDL-C) is a frequent finding in FCH that could be due to TG enrichment of HDL particles and increased activity of hepatic lipase.[3]

CLINICAL PRESENTATION

Familial combined hyperlipidemia has very few physical signs and symptoms. Corneal arcus, xanthelasmas and tendon xanthomas occur less frequently, most common manifestation being the premature CVDs.[1]

DIFFERENTIAL DIAGNOSIS OF FAMILIAL COMBINED HYPERLIPIDEMIA

Familial combined hyperlipidemia shares considerable phenotypic overlap with type 2 diabetes and metabolic syndrome (MS). Common features between FCH and MS are hypertriglyceridemia and/or low HDL-C, frequent association with nonlipid cardiovascular risk factors like hypertension and obesity, and strongly increased cardiovascular risk (Table 16.3).[3]

The main difference between these two conditions is that apoB level is constantly high in FCH. Low-density lipoprotein cholesterol values are normal or low in MS; the phenotypic variability of lipids is more pronounced in FCH than MS; inheritance pattern is more evident in FCH; clinical and laboratory manifestations are much earlier in FCH than MS; markers of low-grade inflammation (high-sensitivity C-reactive protein, adhesion molecules) and/or increased levels of procoagulant factors (fibrinogen, plasminogen activator inhibitor-1) are more associated with MS (Table 16.4).[3]

Differentiation from diabetes may not be relevant clinically since current guideline mandates that diabetic patients should be strongly advised for controlling their risk status in order to minimize CVDs.[1]

Table 16.3: Common clinical features of familial combined hyperlipidemia and metabolic syndrome

Hypertriglyceridemia and/or low HDL-C level
Frequent association with nonlipid cardiovascular risk factors like hypertension and obesity
Strongly increased cardiovascular risk

HDL-C, high-density lipoprotein cholesterol.

Table 16.4: Dissimilarities between familial combined hyperlipidemia and metabolic syndrome

ApoB level is constantly high in FCH. Low-density lipoprotein values are normal or low in MS
Phenotypic variability of lipids is more pronounced in FCH than MS
Inheritance pattern is more evident in FCH
Clinical and laboratory manifestations are much earlier in FCH than MS
Markers of low-grade inflammation (hs-CRP, adhesion molecules) and/or increased levels of procoagulant factors (fibrinogen, PAI-I) are more associated with MS[3]

FCH, familial combined hyperlipidemia; MS, metabolic syndrome; hs-CRP, high-sensitivity C-reactive protein; PAI-I, plasminogen activator inhibitor-1.

Table 16.5: Principles of management

Lifestyle modifications, mainly dietary restriction and physical exercise, are the mainstay of treatment
Proper assessment and meticulous control of associated comorbid conditions to minimize the risk of future vascular events
Drug therapy has been reserved for older children and adolescents particularly nearing 18 years of age considering the increased propensity for early onset of ischemic heart disease. Statins have been found to be quite effective in reducing cholesterol level; however, its effect on reducing triglyceride level is just modest.
Goal of treatment—lipid levels to be brought down to the level as suggested by international guidelines for cardiovascular disease prevention(ATP-III)[3]

ATP-III, Adult Treatment Panel-III.

PRINCIPLE OF MANAGEMENT

The most important risk of FCH is premature coronary artery disease. A recent European guideline has laid out the principle of management of this disorder. Lifestyle modifications, mainly dietary restriction and physical exercise, are the mainstay of treatment. Proper assessment and meticulous control of associated comorbid conditions to minimize the risk of future vascular events. Drug therapy has been reserved for older children and adolescents particularly nearing 18 years of age, considering the increased propensity for early onset of ischemic heart disease. Statins have been found to be quite effective in reducing cholesterol level; however, its effect on reducing TG level is just modest. Goal of treatment is to bring down lipid levels as suggested by international guidelines for CVD prevention (ATP III) (Table 16.5).[11]

Since there is no long-term outcome trial of different drugs on FCH, monitoring should be very stringent in order to identify and modify the serious side effects. Gaddi et al. have suggested periodic performance of carotid ultrasound to assess the effectiveness of different therapies.[3]

CONCLUSION

Familial combined hyperlipidemia is one of the commonly prevalent genetic dyslipidemias and is an important cause of premature coronary artery disease. A high index of suspicion is necessary in order to identify this disorder at the asymptomatic stage and prevent development of overt CVDs. Physicians should be aware about the various phenotypic expressions of this condition since it has a considerable overlap with type 2 diabetes and MS as far as lipid phenotype is concerned.

REFERENCES

1. Genest J, Libby P. Lipoprotein disorders and cardiovascular disease. In: Bonow R O, Mann L D, Zipes P D, Libby P (Eds). Braunwald's Heart Disease—A Textbook of Cardiovascular Medicine, 9th edition. Philadelphia: W B Saunders; 2012. pp. 975-95.

2. Rader DJ, Hobbs HH. Disorders of lipoprotein metabolism. In: Longo DL, Fouci AS, Kasper DL, Hauser SL, Janeson LS, Loscalzo S (Eds). Harrison's Principle of Internal Medicine, 18th edition. Mcgraw Hill Companies, Inc.; 2012. pp. 3145-61.
3. Gaddi A, Cicero AFG, Odoo FO, et al. Practical guidelines for familial combined hyperlipidaemia diagnosis: an up-date. Vasc Health Risk Manag. 2007;3(6):877-84.
4. Austin MA, Brunzell J, Fitch WL, et al. Inheritance of LDL subclass patterns in familial combined hyperlipidaemia. Arteriosclerosis. 1990;10:520-30.
5. PajukantaP, Nuotio I, Terwilliger JD, et al. Linkage of familial combined hyperlipidaemia to chromosome 1q21-q23. Nat Genet. 1998;18:369-73.
6. Eichenbaum-Voline S, Olivier M, Jones EL, et al. Linkage and association between distinct variants of the APOA1/C3/A4/A5 gene cluster and familial combined hyperlipidaemia. Areteriosclero Thromb Vasc Biol. 2004;24:167-74.
7. Badzioch MD,Igo RP Jr, Gagnon F,et al. Low density lipoprotein particle size loci in familial combined hyperlipidaemia: evidence for multiple loci from a genome scan. Arteriosclero Thromb Vasc Biol. 2004;24:1942-50.
8. Pajukanta P, Lilja HE, Sinsheimer JS, et al. Familial combined hyperlipidaemia is associated with upstream transcription factor 1 (USF 1). Nat Gen. 2004;36:371-6.
9. Gaddi A, Galetti C, Pauciullo P, et al. Familial combined hyperlipidaemia: expert panel position on diagnostic criteria for clinical practice. Nutri Metab Cardiovasc Dis. 1999;9:304-11.
10. De Bruin, T.W.A., Castro Cabezas, M., Dallinga-Thie, G.M. et al., Familial combined hyperlipidaemia—do we understand the pathophysiology and genetics? In: Betteridge D.J. (Ed.) Lipids: Current Perspective. Martin Dunitz, London. 1996:101-109.
11. Catapano LA, Reiner Z, et al. for the Task Force for the management of dyslipidaemias of the European Society of Cardiology (ESC) and the European Atherosclerosis Society (EAS). ESC/EAS Guideline for the management of dyslipidaemia. Eur Heart J. 2011;32:1729-818.
12. Meijssen S, Derksen RJ, Bilecen S, et al. In vivo modulation of plasma free fatty acids in patients with familial combined hyperlipidaemiausing lipid lowering medication. J Clin Endocrinol Metab. 2002;87:1576-80.
13. Verseyden C, Meijssen S, Castro C M. Postprandial changes of apoB-100 and apoB-48 in TG rich lipoproteins in familial combined hyperlipidaemia. J Lipid Res. 2002;43:274-80.
14. Evans K, Berdge GC, Wootton SA, et al. Tissue specific stable isotope measurements of postprandial lipid metabolism in familial combined hyperlipidaemia. Atherosclerosis. 2007;197:164-70.
15. Cicero AFG, Martini C, Nativio V, et al. Serum lipoprotein(a) levels in a large sample of subjects affected by familial combined hyperlipidaemia and in general population. J Cardiovasc Risk. 2003;10:149-51.

CHAPTER 17

Dyslipidemia in Children and Adolescents

Rahul Nagpal and Roohi Khan

- Blood lipids and atherogenesis
- Measurement of cholesterol and lipoproteins
- Selected primary lipoprotein disorders
- Hyperlipoproteinemias
- Hypercholesterolemia with hypertriglyceridemia
- Clinical identification of the metabolic syndrome in adults
- Proposed definition of the metabolic syndrome in adolescents
- Hypertriglyceridemias
- Disorders of HDL metabolism
- Disorder associated with low cholesterol
- Disorders of intracellular cholesterol metabolism
- Lipoprotein patterns in children and adolescents
- Secondary dyslipoproteinemia
- Blood cholesterol screening
- Risk assessment and treatment of hyperlipidemia
- Risk assessment for cardiovascular disease or CVD
- Management
- Conclusion

Atherosclerosis begins in early years of life. Detection and control of dyslipidemia in the early years of life are of paramount importance for the prevention of clinical expression of the atherosclerosis vascular disease in adolescent age or later.

The National Cholesterol Education Program (NCEP) provides guidelines for the diagnosis and treatment of dyslipidemia in pediatric age group. The relationship between dietary fat consumption and plasma cholesterol was demonstrated nearly a century ago. In 1977, the Cooperative Lipoprotein Phenotyping Study showed that there is an inverse relationship between high-density lipoprotein (HDL) and coronary heart disease (CHD).

BLOOD LIPIDS AND ATHEROGENESIS

Even if the absolute risk of cardiovascular disease (CVD) during childhood is small, evidence suggests that dyslipidemia is related to fatty streak formation in childhood and to a high incidence of CHD in adulthood.[1,2]

Atherosclerosis starts with subendothelial accumulation of cholesterol-engulfed macrophages (foam cells). Low-density lipoprotein cholesterol (LDL-C) levels submitted to oxidation

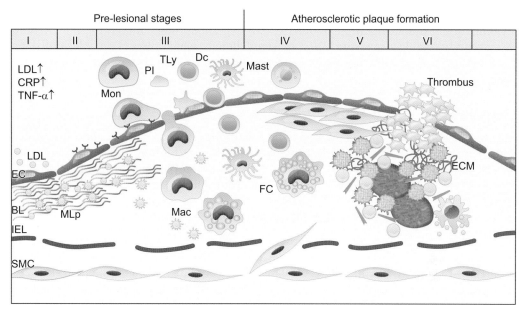

Figure 17.1: Atheroma formation at different stages. Stage I, characterized by modulation of endothelial cell (EC) due to increased concentrations of plasma low-density lipoproteins (LDL), or C-reactive Protein (CRP) and tumor necrosis factor alpha (TNF-α). Stage II, LDL oxidation, glycation, turning into modified lipoproteins (MLp). This is followed by an inflammatory reaction. Stage III, monocytes become activated macrophages (Mac) that express scavenger receptors and turn into foam cells. In stage IV, smooth muscle cells (SMC) migrate from the media into the intima forming the fibrous cap. The fibrolipid plaque comprising defines stage V. Extracellular matrix (ECM), cholesterol crystals (cc) and large calcification cores (Ca) are formed. Thin cap fibroatheroma (TCFA) is a vulnerable plaque. Subsequently damage to the fibrous cap and endothelial cells exposes the matrix leading to activation of the coagulation cascade thrombus formation (stage IV)

(oxLDL) are captured from scavenger cells and, as early as childhood, the oxidative process takes place actively. The antibodies against oxLDL are detectable in children.[3,4] The initial lesions, known as "fatty streaks," are clinically silent but are the precursors of fibrous lesions characterized by the accumulation of lipid-rich debris and smooth muscle cells (Fig. 17.1).

MEASUREMENT OF CHOLESTEROL AND LIPOPROTEINS

Cholesterol levels are reasonably consistent after 2 years of age (with some small increment during adolescence). Cholesterol and LDL levels are not measured before the age of 2 years, and no treatment is recommended for this age group.

1. For the measurement of total cholesterol (TC), the child does not have to be fasting for the test.
2. A lipoprotein analysis is obtained by measuring TC, HDL and triglyceride (TG) levels after an overnight fast of 12 hours. The LDL level is usually estimated by the Friedewald formula:

LDL = total cholesterol – HDL – (triglyceride/5)

This formula is not accurate if the child is not fasting, if the TG level is >400 mg/dL or if chylomicrons or dysbetalipoproteinemia (type III hyperlipoproteinemia) is present. Methods are currently available to measure LDL cholesterol directly, which allow LDL cholesterol determination on TG level >400 mg/dL. Direct LDL cholesterol measurement does not require a fasting specimen.

Normal Levels of Lipids and Lipoproteins

The cross-sectional age and gender-specific distribution of plasma lipids and lipoprotein were reported for American children by NCEP in 1991. Children and adolescents with TC >200 mg/dL, LDL cholesterol >130 mg/dL, HDL cholesterol <40mg/dL or TGs >200 mg/dL need to be evaluated for possible dyslipidemia. (For adults, the desirable level of TGs is <150 mg/dL.)

The following derivatives of lipid profile are useful in the assessment of risks for CVD:

1. TC to HDL-C ratio: The total cholesterol to HDL cholesterol ratio is a useful parameter for assessing the risk of CVD. The usual TC/HDL-C ratio in children is approximately 3 (based on TC of 150 mg/dL and an HDL-C of 50 mg/dL). According to the Framingham study, the ratio for average risk was 5.0 for men and 4.2 for women. The higher the ratio, the higher is the risk of developing CVD. The ratio of 3.4 halves the risk of developing CVD for both men and women.

2. Non-HDL cholesterol: Serum non-HDL cholesterol (TC minus HDL cholesterol) is considered a better screening tool than LDL cholesterol for the assessment of coronary artery disease (CAD) risk in adults because it includes all classes of atherogenic (ApoB-containing) lipoproteins. It includes very low density lipoprotein (VLDL) cholesterol, intermediate-density lipoproteins, LDL, and lipoprotein(a) or Lp(a). An additional advantage of non-HDL-C is that its measurement does not require overnight fasting.

According to the report of the Bogalusa Heart Study, there is no important racial difference, although girls had higher levels than boys. Non-HDL-C was higher than LDL-C by 13.2–17.3mg/dL (with the equation non-HDL cholesterol = 7.56 + 1.05 × LDL cholesterol). Serum non-HDL-C values equivalent to NHCEP's LDL cholesterol cut points of 110, 130, 170, and 200 are 123, 144, 186 and218, respectively.

SELECTED PRIMARY LIPOPROTEIN DISORDERS

Primary lipoprotein disorders may manifest with increased levels of cholesterol or TGs, or both, and/or a decreased level of HDL cholesterol.

1. Primary hypercholesterolemia manifests as familial hypercholesterolemia (FH) and familial combined hyperlipidemia (FCHL), which are the two most common familial lipoprotein disorders with elevated LDL cholesterol levels. One should, however, rule out secondary causes of hypercholesterolemia. Screening of all family members is recommended to determine whether the disorder is familial. Family screening is important not only to detect hypercholesterolemia in other members of the family but also to emphasize the need for all family members to change their eating patterns. Young patients with elevated LDL levels are more likely to have a familial disorder of LDL metabolism.

2. Primary lipoprotein disorders that arise with an increased level of TGs are FCH, familial hypertriglyceridemia (FHTG) and familial dysbetalipoproteinemia (type III hyperlipoproteinemia). Some hypertriglyceridemias are also secondary to other disease state.
3. Familial hypoalphalipoproteinemia (low HDL syndrome).

HYPERLIPOPROTEINEMIAS[5,6]

Hypercholesterolemia (Table 17.1)

Familial Hypercholesterolemia (FH)

Familial hypercholesterolemia is a monogenic autosomal codominant metabolic disease caused by genetic mutations affecting the LDL receptor. The clinical characteristics of the disease are as follows:

1. Strikingly elevated LDL cholesterol
2. Premature CVD and tendon xanthomas.

Of the nearly 800 mutations described, some are mounted with no LDL receptor (receptor negative). Some mutations are associated with poor binding or release of LDL receptor. Five classes of mutations effecting LDL receptor binding have been detected.

The clinical features of hyperlipoproteinemias are summarized in Table 17.2 according to the Fredrickson and Lees phenotype.

Familial Hypercholesterolemia (FH)[8,10]

Familial hypercholesterolemia is a monogenic autosomal codominant metabolic disease caused by genetic mutations of the LDL receptor. Five classes of mutations deffective LDL receptor binding have been identified. The clinical characteristics of the disease are (1) elevated LDL cholesterol, (2) premature CVD and (3) tendon xanthomas. Failure of LDL receptor synthesis is called receptor negative, whereas mutations associated with defective binding or releases from the receptor are called receptor defective mutations. Receptor negative mutations result in more severe phenotypes than receptor defective mutations (Fig. 17.2).

Homozygous FH

These patients inherit two abnormal LDL receptor genes. This causes elevation of plasma cholesterol levels ranging between 500 and 1200 mg/dL. The TG levels are within normal range to mildly elevated, and HDL levels may be slightly low. The frequency in the populations is 1/1,000,000 persons. Receptor negative patients have <2% normal LDL receptor activity, whereas those who are receptor defective may have as much 25% normal activity.

The prognosis is guarded regardless of the specific LDL receptor abnormality. Family history premature vascular disease is present in both parents. The child has tendon xanthomas. Thickening of Achilles tendon or other extensor tendons of hands is present. There can be cutaneous lesion in hands, elbows, knees or buttocks. Corneal arcus is present. Demonstration of defective receptor activity in cultured skin fibroblast is diagnostic. Measurement of receptor activity in the surface of lymphocytes helps in measuring the phenotypic expression (Figs. 17.3 and 17.4).

Table 17.1: Summary of hyperlipoproteinemias

Diseases	Elevated lipid	Clinical picture	Inheritance	Approximate incident
Familial hypercholesterolemia	LDL-cholesterol	Tendon xanthomas, coronary artery disease	AD	1/500
Familial defective ApoB-100	LDL-cholesterol	Tendon xanthomas, coronary artery disease	AD	1/1000
Autosomal recessive hypercholesterolemia	LDL-cholesterol	Tendon xanthomas, coronary artery disease	AR	<1/1,000,000
Sitosterolemia	LDL-cholesterol	Tendon xanthomas, coronary artery disease	AR	<1/1,000,000
Polygenic hypercholesterolemia	LDL-cholesterol	CHD		1 in 300
Familial combined hyperlipidemia (FCHL)	LDL-cholesterol	CHD	AD	1/200
Familial dysbetalipoproteinemia	LDL-cholesterol	Tuberoeruptive xanthomas, peripheral vascular disease	AD	1/10,000
Familial chylomicronemia (Frederickson type I)	TG↑↑	Eruptive xanthomas, hepatosplenomegaly, pancreatitis	AR	1/1,000,000
Familial hypertriglyceridemia (Frederickson type IV)	TG↑	± Coronary artery disease	AD	1/500
Familial hypertriglyceridemia (Frederickson type V)	TG↑↑	Xanthomas ± coronary artery disease	AD	
Familial hepatic lipase deficiency	LDL-cholesterol	Coronary artery disease	AR	<1/1,000,000

AD, autosomal dominant; AR, autosomal recessive; CHD, coronary artery disease; LDL, low-density lipoproteins, TG, triglycerides; VLDL, very low density lipoproteins.

Untreated homozygous patients rarely survive to adulthood. There can be angina on sudden death. Lifestyle change and high-dose statin is recommended in the initial treatment. Low-density lipoprotein apheresis is recommended for many children. Liver transplantation

Table 17.2: Clinical features of different hyperlipiproteinemias

Fredrickson phenotype	Elevated lipids or lipoproteins	Prevalence in childhood	Etiology	Symptoms and signs	Treatment
Type I	Triglyceride (usually >1000 mg/dL) Chylomicrons identified	Rare	LPL deficiency (familial hyperchylomicronemia), ApoC-II deficiency Systemic lupus erythematosus	Childhood onset (70%) Abdominal pain due to pancreatitis Eruptive xanthomas Lack of coronary heart disease during childhood	Very low-fat diet (10%–15% calories), supplemented with medium chain triglycerides
Type IIa	LDL-C (≥130 mg/dL)	Common	FH, FCH, polygenic hypercholesterolemia Hypothyroidism Renal disease, biliary tract disease, diabetes mellitus	Childhood or adulthood onset Xanthomas of eyelids and palms Tendinitis of Achilles tendon Arcus corneae Coronary heart disease(common in homozygotes)	Low cholesterol, high unsaturated fat diet Weight loss if obese Statins, if condition does not respond to diet alone Bile acid sequestrant occasionally
Type IIb	LDL C ≥130 mg/dL and triglycerides (≥125mg/dL)	Uncommon	Similar to type IIa	Late childhood onset. Lack of symptoms and signs often	Low cholesterol, low-fat diet Weight loss if obese Statins, if condition does not respond to diet alone Fibric acid and niacin, occasionally

(Continued)

Table 17.2: Continued

Fredrickson phenotype	Elevated lipids or lipoproteins	Prevalence in childhood	Etiology	Symptoms and signs	Treatment
Type III	Triglycerides and LDL-C (approximately equal values); chylomicron remnant and IDL elevated	Very rare	Dysbetalipoproteinemia ApoE-2 homozygosity (E-2/E-2) plus obesity Diabetes mellitus Renal disease* Hypothyroidism Liver disease	Palmar and tuberosum xanthomas Coronary heart disease (±)	Low-fat, low cholesterol diet Weight control Statins are effective
Type IV	Triglycerides (≥125 mg/dL) VLDL elevated	Relatively uncommon	FCH, FH, familial hypertriglyceridemia, metabolic or endocrine disease† Renal disease Liver disease Ethanol use/abuse Pregnancy Drug use‡	Obesity Eruptive xanthomas Abdominal pain	Low-fat, low cholesterol diet Weight control Statins, if condition does not respond to diet alone Fibric acid and niacin, occasionally
Type V	Triglycerides (>1000 mg/dL); chylomicron and elevated VLDL	Very rare	Usually results from a combination of any two conditions that cause type IV	Obesity Eruptive xanthomas Coronary heart disease (infrequent)	Low fat diet Weight control

Source: Adapted from the following articles: Winter W, Schartz D. Pediatric lipid disorders in clinical practice. eMedicine, last updated January 19, 2005. Trxoler RG, Park MK. Hyperlipidemia in childhood. In: Pediatric Cardiology for Practitioners, 4th edition. St. Louis: Mosby;, 2002. Holmes KW, Kwiterovich PO Jr. Treatment of dyslipidemia in children and adolescents. Curr Cardiol Rep. 2005;7:445–56.

IDL, intermediate-density lipoprotein; LDL-C, low-density lipoprotein cholesterol; VLDL, very low-density lipoprotein.

*Renal disease (e.g., nephrosis).

† Metabolic/endocrine disease (e.g., obesity, diabetes, hypothyroidism, Cushing's disease, acromegaly).

‡ Drug use (e.g., glucocorticoids, growth hormone, androgens, thiazides, β-blockers, estrogen).

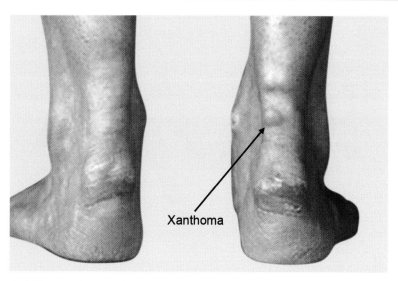

Figure 17.2: Achilles tendon xanthoma

has also been successful in decreasing LDL cholesterol levels. Statin, in combination therapy with ezetimibe, results in decline in LDL levels.

Heterozygous FH

Heterozygous FH is one of the most common single gene mutations associated with acute coronary syndromes and atherosclerotic CHD in adults. Its prevalence is approximately 1/500.

Since heterozygous FH is a codominant condition with nearly full penetrance, 50% of first-degree relatives index case will have the disease, as will 25% of second-degree relatives. An estimated 10 million people have FH worldwide. Symptoms of CHD occur in 45–50 year in men, and a decade later in women.

Measurement of LDL cholesterol does not allow diagnosis of FH heterozygotes, but when values are twice normal for age one should suspect FH. The U.S. MED-PED ("make early diagnosis–prevent early death") Program based in Utah has put forwarded diagnostic criteria. The diagnosis within known FH families is predictable according to LDL levels.

Very high cholesterol levels in children should trigger screening of adult first- and second-degree relatives ("reverse" cholesterol screening). A child of <18 years of age with total plasma cholesterol of 270 mg/dL and/or LDL-C of 200 mg/dL has an 88% probability of having FH. If a first-degree relative has FH, the diagnosis is clinched. If there is a first-degree relative with proven FH, the diagnosis in the child is virtually certain (Table 17.3). Conversely, criteria for diagnosing probable FH in a child whose first-degree relative has known FH require only modest elevation of TC to 220 mg/dL (LDL-C 155 mg/dL). Only modest elevation of LDL (>160 mg/dl) in an individual with a first-degree relative known to have FH points towards a diagnosis of probable FH.

Treatment of children with FH should begin with low-fat diet. National Cholesterol Education Program has formulated guidelines. Child of at least 10 years of age should be given drugs if the LDL-C is >160 mg/day, has a family history of premature heart disease or >190 mg/dL even in the absence of a family history.

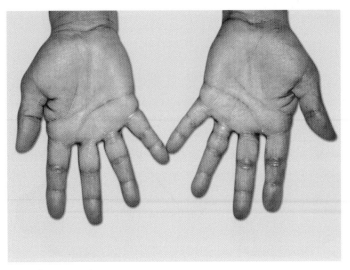

Figure 17.3: Striate palmar xanthomata

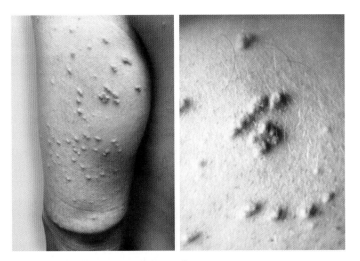

Figure 17.4: Eruptive xanthoma on extensor surface

Bile acid sequestrants are rarely used because of poor patient compliance and modest benefit. Ezetimibe blocks cholesterol adsorption in the gastrointestinal tract and has a low side effects profile: combination of statin and ezetimibe in the treatment of choice.

Familial Defective ApoB–100

This is an autosomal dominant disorder that is similar to heterozygous FH. Low-density lipoprotein cholesterol levels are higher and TGs are normal. Adults often have tendon xanthomas and premature CHD. Familial defective ApoB–100 is caused by mutation in the receptor binding region of ApoB-100, the ligand of the LDL receptor. The estimated

Table 17.3: Percentage of youths under age 18 expected to have FH according to cholesterol levels and closest relative with FH

| Total cholesterol (mg/dL) | LDL Cholesterol (mg/dL) | Percentage with FH at that Level | | | |
| | | Degree of relative | | | General population |
		First	Second	Third	
180	122	7.2	2.4	0.9	0.01
190	130	13.5	5.0	2.2	0.03
200	138	26.4	10.7	4.9	0.07
210	147	48.1	23.6	11.7	0.19
220	155	73.1	47.5	27.9	0.54
230	164	90.0	75.0	56.2	1.8
240	172	97.1	93.7	82.8	6.3
250	181	99.3	97.6	95.3	22.2
260	190	99.9	99.5	99.0	57.6
270	200	100.0	99.9	99.8	88.0
280	210	100.0	100.0	100.0	97.8
290	220	100.0	100.0	100.0	99.6
300	230	100.0	100.0	100.0	99.9
310	210	100.0	100.0	100.0	100.0

Source: From Williams RR, Hunt SC, Schumacher MC, et al. Diagnosing heterozygous familial hypercholest-erolemia using new practical criteria validated by molecular genetics. Am J Cardiol. 1993;72:171-6. FH, familial hypercholesterolemia; LDL, low-density lipoprotein.

frequency is 1/700 people. Familial defective ApoB–100 and FH are clinically similar. Specialized lab tests can differentiate them. However, further testing is not required in clinical practice as the treatment of these two disorders is same.

Autosomal Recessive Hypercholesterolemia

This is present in higher frequency among sardinions. The basic abnormality is the defective receptor-mediated endocytosis of LDL. The cholesterol level is modesty elevated that ranges between homozygous and heterozygous FH. Treatment is with 3-hydroxy-3-methylglutaryl-coenzyme A (HMG-CoA) reductase inhibitors.

Sitosterolemia

This is a rare autosomal recessive disorder. The basic defect is a mutation in the ATP-binding cassette transporter system that is responsible for inhibiting the absorption of plant sterols in the small intestine and also promotes biliary excretion. There is excessive adsorption of plant sterols. Plasma cholesterol is elevated. Tendon xanthomas and premature atherosclerosis are present. The diagnosis is confirmed by elevated plasma sterols. The treatment is with cholesterol absorption inhibitors ezetimibe or bile acid sequestrants. 3-Hydroxy-3-methylglutaryl-coenzyme A reductase inhibitors are not effective.

Polygenic Hypercholesterolemia

Polygenic hypercholesterolemia is a disorder when multiple genes and environment (faulty dietary practice and lack of physical exercise) cluster in different members in the same family. No single gene defect can explain the inheritance. There is modest elevation of total and LDL cholesterol. Triglyceride levels are within normal range. This disorder responds well to physical exercise and dietary changes. Lipid lowering therapy is required only in exceptional cases.

HYPERCHOLESTEROLEMIA WITH HYPERTRIGLYCERIDEMIA

Familial Combined Hyperlipidemia (FCHL)

This is the commonest lipid disorder (occurring 1 in 200) in the general population. Approximately 20% of premature CAD is linked to FCHL. Family history in premature CAD is present. The inheritance is autosomal dominant. There is moderate elevation of plasma LDL cholesterol and TGs; HDL cholesterol is low. Diagnosis is made by the presence of at least two first-degree relatives with dyslipidemia variants as follows: (a) LDL level more than 90th percentile, (b) TG level more than 90th percentile and (C) combined LDL and TG more than 90th percentile.

Individuals' variant may switch from one variant to the other. Tendon xanthomas are absent. Plasma ApoB levels and small dense LDL may be increased. Presence of these phenotypes supports the diagnosis.

Two-third patients with FCHL have clustering of abdominal obesity, atherogenic dyslipidemia, hypertension, insulin resistance, impaired glucose tolerance, vascular inflammation and hypercoagulability. NCEP guideline helps in diagnosis of this metabolic syndrome. South East Asians and Hispanics have this disease with higher frequency.

CLINICAL IDENTIFICATION OF THE METABOLIC SYNDROME IN ADULTS[7]

1. Abdominal obesity: Men, waist circumference ≥40 inches (102 cm); women, waist circumference ≥35 inches (88 cm)
2. Elevated TGs ≥150 mg/dL
3. Reduced HDL cholesterol: Men <40 mg/dL; women <50 mg/dL
4. Hypertension: 130/85 mmHg or greater
5. Elevated fasting glucose: ≥100 mg/dL

The presence of at least three of the preceding abnormalities constitutes metabolic syndrome.

PROPOSED DEFINITION OF THE METABOLIC SYNDROME IN ADOLESCENTS[7,9]

1. Triglycerides ≥110 mg/dL
2. HDL cholesterol ≤40 mg/dL
3. Waist circumference ≥90th percentile or body mass index ≥95th percentile
4. Fasting glucose ≥110 mg/dL
5. Systolic blood pressure ≥90th percentile for age and gender

The presence of at least three of the preceding abnormalities constitutes metabolic syndrome.

The treatment is with dietary changes and physical activity. One hour daily moderate intensity physical activity is recommended. Diet should be low in saturated fat, trans fat and cholesterol. Sugar should be restricted.

Familial Dysbetalipoproteinemia (FDBL, Type III Hyperlipoproteinemia)

Apolipoprotein E (ApoE) gene mutation in association with environmental function like high caloric diet, low physical activity and high alcohol intake causes this disorder. This rare disorder occurs in 1 in 10,000 populations. Plasma cholesterol and TGs are elevated. HDL cholesterol is normal. Apolipoprotein E mediates removal of plasma chylomicrons and VLDL particles from circulation. Three isoforms of ApoE gene have been identified: (a) ApoE2 (b) ApoE3 and (c) ApoE4. Most common mutation in FDBL is ApoE2/E2 (homozygous). Frequency is 1%. However, minority expresses the disease. Diabetes, obesity, hypothyroidism and renal failure precipitates dyslipidemia in the majority. Apolipoprotein E4/E4 allele is associated with Alzheimer's disease. The E4 is the normal allele and present in the majority.

Patients have distinctive xanthomas. Small grape like clusters on the elbows, knees and buttocks are called tuberoeruptive xanthomas. Orange-yellow discoloration of creases (palmar xanthomas) is present. Peripheral vascular disease occurs in fourth or fifth decade. Children presents with milder phenotypic forms along with a precipitating illnesses.

Demonstration of broad beta band of remnant lipoproteins on electrophones is diagnostic. Very low-density lipoprotein is elevated. Very low-density lipoprotein/TG ratio >0.30 is supportive of the diagnosis. *ApoE* genotyping clinches the genetic defect. Negative genetic study does not rule out the diagnosis.

Treatment consists of (a) dietary therapy, (b) physical activity and (c) lipid-lowering therapy. 3-Hydroxy-3-methylglutaryl-coenzyme A reductase inhibitors, nicotinic acid and fibrates have all been used with good clinical result.

HYPERTRIGLYCERIDEMIAS

The generic variant of triglyceridemia includes (1) chylomicronemia (type I), (2) FHTG (type IV) and (3) combined (type I and IV) forms and hepatic lipase (HL) deficiency.

Familial Chylomicronemia (Type I Hyperlipidemia)

This is a single gene defect with autosomal recessive inheritance. The frequency is 1 in 10,00,000. Either there is difference of lipoprotein lipase (LPL) or its cofactor ApoCII. Lipoprotein lipase deficiency causes modest elevation of TG. Plasma becomes turbid on standing. Child may present with acute pancreatitis. Eruptive xanthomas may be present on arms, knees and buttocks. Hepatosplenomegaly may be present. Triglyceride lipolytic activity assessment is diagnostic. Strict fat restriction and supplement of fat-soluble vitamins is the treatment option. Fish oils supplement is beneficial.

Familial Hypertriglyceridemia (FHTG, Type IV Hyperlipidemia)

Familial hypertriglyceridemia is an autosomal dominant disorder characterized by elevated TG (>90th percentile of 250–1000 mg/dL range). Slight mild elevetion of plasma TC and low plasma HDL cholesterol. The frequency is 1 in 500. Familial hypertriglyceridemia usually manifests in adult. However, 20% after individual may present in childhood. Defective breakdown of VLDL particle on overproduction of VLDL is the defect. Differentiated diagnosis includes FCHL and FDBL. Familial hypertriglyceridemia has lower LDL and normal ApoB level. Presence of one first-degree relative with hypertriglyceridemia is diagnostic.

Sometime hypertriglyceridemia may accompany high VLDL particles and chylomicrons (Frederickson type V). Triglyceride levels are often >1000 mg/dL. Lipoprotein lipase or ApoC-II deficiency is not present. Patient has eruptive xanthomas in adulthood. Patient may present with acute pancreatitis. Estrogen and alcohol may precipitate the disease. Secondary cause should be ruled out. Simple sugar, estrogen and alcohol should be avoided, and consumption of carbonated sweetened drinks should be limited. Weight loss and dietary restriction of refined sugar bring down the level of TG drastically. Drug therapy in children is reserved for TG >1000 mg/dL to prevent acute pancreatitis. Fibrate and niacin are recommended in adults. 3-Hydroxy-3-methylglutaryl-coenzyme A reductase inhibitors are the treatment of choice in children.

Hepatic Lipase Deficiency

This is a rare autosomal recessive disorder characterized by HL deficiency associated with elevation of TG and TC. Hepatic lipase is responsible for hydrolysis of TGs, phospholipids in VLDL and IDL. HDL level is higher. Hepatic lipase activity measurement establishes the diagnosis.

DISORDERS OF HDL METABOLISM

Primary Hypoalphalipoproteinemia

It is the common disorder of HDL metabolism. High-density lipoprotein level is less than the 10th percentile for age and gender. The inheritance is autosomal dominant. Low-density lipoprotein cholesterol and TG level are normal. Reduced ApoA1 synthesis and increased HDL catabolism are linked in this condition. The disorder that may be associated with low HDL like metabolic syndrome, lecithin–cholesterol acyltransferase (LCAT) deficiency and Tangier disease must be ruled out.

Familial Hyperalphalipoproteinemia

The members of the family with this disorder have HDL level >80 mg/dL. There is increased longevity and decreased rate of CAD in these families.

Familial ApoA–I Deficiency

Here two types if mutations may occur. Mutations in *apoA-I* gene may result in the absence of HDL cholesterol in plasma. Liver and small intestine are the source of nascent HDL particles. Esterification of free cholesterol by the enzyme LCAT forms mature HDL particles. ApoA-I is required for the completion of the reaction. Mutation results in high cholesterol level in circulation and associated corneal opacities, planar xanthomas and premature atherosclerosis vascular disease.

In some patients, mutations may result in very rapid clearance of the cholesterol. These patients may not have atherosclerosis in spite of low HDL cholesterol levels in the range of 15–30 mg/dL.

Tangier Disease

This phenotype is recognized by enlarged orange-colored tonsils, hepatosplenomegaly low HDL (<5 mg/dL). Peripheral neuropathy may result from cholesterol accumulation in the Schwann cells of the nerve fibers. The inheritance is autosomal dominant. The basic defect is mutation in the gene coding for ABCA1. ABCA1 facilitates the binding of cholesterol to ApoA-I.

Familial Lecithin–Cholesterol Acyltransferase (LCAT) Deficiency

Genetic mutation of LCAT hinders the esterification of cholesterol. Formation of mature HDL particles is prevented. Plasma cholesterol level is very high. Patient develops corneal opacities. High-density lipoprotein level is low (<10 mg/dL). Partial LCAT deficiency patients have corneal opacities and are known as "fish-eye" disease. Complete deficiency is associated with renal failure and hemolytic anemia. Premature atherosclerosis does not occur.

Cholesteryl Ester Transfer Protein (CETP) Deficiency

Cholesteryl ester transfer protein transports TGs from VLDL or LDL and exchange them for cholesteryl esters from HDL particles and vice versa. The gene is located in 16q21 position. Mutations are associated with accelerated atherosclerosis, and 1405V polymorphism of CETP gene is associated with increased longevity.

DISORDER ASSOCIATED WITH LOW CHOLESTEROL

Abetalipoproteinemia

This is caused by mutation in the gene encoding for microsomal TG transfer protein. Inherence is autosomal recessive. The protein is responsible for the transfer of lipids to chylomicrons in small gut and VLDL in liver. There is absence of chylomicrons, VLDL particles, LDL cholesterol and ApoB. Plasma cholesterol level and TG level are low.

Diarrhea results due to fat malabsorption and vitamin E deficiency. There is failure to thrive. Spinocerebellar degeneration presents as ataxia. The tendon reflexes are lost. Spasticity may develop. There is pigmented retinopathy with progressive visual loss leading to blindness. The differential diagnosis includes Friedreich's ataxia. Presence of malabsorption and acanthocytosis in peripheral blood smear examination points towards abetalipoproteinemia. Patients have normal ApoB level and lipids.

Familial Hypobetalipoproteinemia

Clinically this mimics abetalipoproteinemia. The inheritance is autosomal codominant. ApoB = 100 gene mutation is responsible for the disease. Parents have plasma LDL cholesterol and ApoB level <50% of normal. Heterogygotes do not have any clinical disorder.

Inability to secrete ApoB-48 from the small intestine results in a condition resembling abetalipoproteinemia or homozygous hypobetalipoproteinemia. This is sometimes referred to as Anderson disease. There is steatorrhea and fat-soluble vitamin deficiency. The blood level of ApoB-100 is normal.

Smith–Lemli–Opitz Syndrome

This is a rare (1:20,000) autosomal recessive disorder that results from mutation in 7 dehydrocholesterol-Δ^7 reductase gene. The enzyme 7 dehydrocholesterol-Δ^7 reductase level is low. The child develops multiple congenital abnormalities (Table 17.4 and 17.5). The plasma cholesterol is low. All the procurer levels are very high (Fig. 17.5).

There is spontaneous abortion. Death occurs in neonatal period if TC is <20 mg/dL. Multiple variations in phenotypes have been reported. Cholesterol supplement (egg yolk) and statin to block toxic precursors are the treatment of choice.

Table 17.4: Major clinical characteristics of Smith-Lemli-Opitz syndrome: frequent anomalies (>50% of patients)

Craniofacial
Microcephaly
Blepharoptosis
Anteverted nares
Retromicrognathia
Low-set, posteriorly rotated ears
Midline cleft palate
Broad maxillary alveolar ridges
Cataracts (<50%)
Skeletal anomalies
Syndactyly of toes II/III
Postaxial polydactyly (<50%)
Equinovarus deformity (<50%)
Genital anomalies
Hypospadias
Cryptorchidism
Sexual ambiguity (<50%)
Development
Pre- and postnatal growth retardation

Feeding problems

Mental retardation

Behavioral abnormalities

Source: From Haas D, Kelley RI, Hoffmann GF. Inherited disorders of cholesterol biosynthesis. Neuropediatrics. 2001;32:113-22.

Table 17.5: Characteristic malformations of internal organs in severely affected Smith-Lemli-Opitz patients

Central nervous system

Frontal lobe hypoplasia

Enlarged ventricles

Agenesis of corpus callosum

Cerebellar hypoplasia

Holoprosencephaly

Cardiovascular

Atrioventricular canal

Secundum atrial septal defect

Patent ductus arteriosus

Membranous ventricular septal defect

Urinary tract

Renal hypoplasia or aplasia

Renal cortical cysts

Hydronephrosis

Ureteral duplication

Gastrointestinal

Hirschsprung disease

Pyloric stenosis

Refractory dysmotility

Cholestatic and noncholestatic progressive liver disease

Pulmonary

Pulmonary hypoplasia

Abnormal lobation

Endocrine

Adrenal insufficiency

Source: From Haas D, Kelley RI, Hoffmann GF. Inherited disorders of cholesterol biosynthesis. Neuropediatrics. 2001;32:113-22.

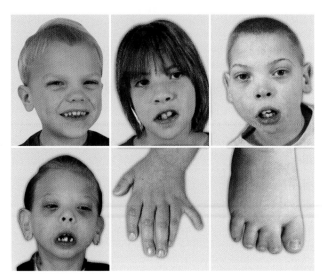

Figure 17.5: Major clinical features of Smith-Lemli-Opitz syndrome

DISORDERS OF INTRACELLULAR CHOLESTEROL METABOLISM

Cerebrotendinous Xanthomatosis

This is an autosomal recessive disorder caused by mutation of gene encoding sterol 27 hydroxylase. This enzyme is responsible for the formation of bile acids in the mitochondria. There is accumulation of bile acid precursors. The adolescent presents with tendon xanthomas, cataracts and neurodegeneration. Treatment is with chenodeoxycholic acid.

Cholesterol Ester Storage Disease and Wolman Disease

This rare autosomal disorder is caused by deficiency of lysosomal acid lipase. Low-density lipoprotein enters the cell by endocytosis. Low-density lipoprotein is delivered to lysosomes. Lysosome lipase hydrolyzed the LDL. Failure of hydrolysis causes increased level of cholesteryl esters. There is steatorrhea, hepatosplenomegaly and failure to thrive. Cholesterol ester storage disease patients may live longer and have detectable level of lipase actively. Wolman disease is the severe form and child dies by 1 year of age.

Niemann–Pick Disease Type C

This is an autosomal recessive disorder. Intracellular cholesterol transport is defective. Cholesterol and sphingomyelin accumulate in central nervous system and reticuloendothelial systems. Death occurs in early years.

LIPOPROTEIN PATTERNS IN CHILDREN AND ADOLESCENTS

The mean plasma level at birth ranges between 50 and 68 mg/dL. The level develops by the end of 1 year. There is very gradual rise until puberty. The level is reduced 160 mg/dL. Total

Table 17.6: Plasma cholesterol and triglyceride levels in childhood and adolescence

	Total triglyceride (mg/dL)					Total cholesterol (mg/dL)					Low-density lipoprotein cholesterol (mg/dL)					High-density lipoprotein cholesterol (mg/dL)*				
	5TH	Mean	75th	90th	95th	5th	Mean	75th	90th	95th	5th	Mean	75th	90th	95th	5th	10th	25TH	MEAN	95TH
Cord	14	34	—	—	84	42	68	—	—	103	17	29	—	—	50	13	—	—	35	60
1–4 yr																				
Male	29	56	68	85	99	114	155	170	190	203	—	—	—	—	—	—	—	—	—	—
Female	34	64	74	95	112	112	156	173	188	200	—	—	—	—	—	—	—	—	—	—
5–9 yr																				
Male	28	52	58	70	85	125	155	168	183	189	63	93	103	117	129	38	42	49	56	74
Female	32	64	74	103	126	131	164	176	190	197	68	100	115	125	140	36	38	47	53	73
10–14 yr																				
Male	33	63	74	94	111	124	160	173	188	202	64	97	109	122	132	37	40	46	55	74
Female	39	72	85	104	120	125	160	171	191	205	68	97	110	126	136	37	40	45	52	70
15–19 yr																				
Male	38	78	88	125	143	118	153	168	183	191	62	94	109	123	130	30	34	39	46	63
Female	36	73	85	112	126	118	159	176	198	207	59	96	111	29	137	35	38	43	52	74

Source: Data for cord blood from Strong W. Atherosclerosis: its pediatric roots. In: Kaplan N, Stamler J (Eds). Prevention of Coronary Heart Disease. Philadelphia: WB Saunders; 1983. Data for the children aged 1–4 years from Tables 6, 7, 20 and 21, and all other data from Tables 24, 25, 32, 33, 36 and 37 in Lipid Research Clinics Population Studies Data Book, Vol. 1, The Prevalence Study. NIH publication No. 80–1527. Washington, DC: National Institutes of Health' 1980.

*Note that different percentiles are listed for HDL cholesterol.

cholesterol decreases during puberty very transiently. In males it is due to decrease in HDL, and in females due to decrease in LDL cholesterol. There is tracking of the cholesterol level in individuals, within families and communities (Table 17.6)

An acceptable TC among children and adolescents is <170 mg/dL; borderline is 170–199 mg/dL and high >200 mg/dL. An acceptable LDL cholesterol is <110 mg/dL, borderline 110–129 mg/dL and high >130 mg/dL. HDL cholesterol should be >40 mg/dL.

SECONDARY DYSLIPOPROTEINEMIA

Secondary dyslipoproteinemias result from other underlying disorders, but they may mimic primary forms of hyperlipidemia and can have similar consequences. They may result in increased predisposition to premature CAD, or when associated with marked hypertriglyceridemia, they may lead to the development of pancreatitis and other features of hyperchylomicronemia. Common causes in children include obesity, oral contraceptive use and isotretinoin (Accutane) use or anabolic steroid therapy. Medications such as diuretics, β-blockers and estrogens; medical conditions including hypothyroidism, renal failure and nephritic syndrome and alcohol usage are less common causes of secondary dyslipoproteinemia. Table 17.7 lists causes of secondary dyslipoproteinemia.

Table 17.7: Secondary causes of hyperlipidemia

Hypercholesterolemia
Hypothyroidism
Nephrotic syndrome
Cholestasis
Anorexia nervosa
Drugs: progesterone, thiazides, Tegretol, cyclosporine
Hypertriglyceridemia
Obesity
Type II diabetes
Alcohol
Renal failure
Sepsis
Stress
Cushing syndrome
Pregnancy
Hepatitis
AIDS, protease inhibitions
Drugs: anabolic steroids, β-blockers, estrogen, thiazides
Reduced HDL

Smoking

Obesity

Type II diabetes

Malnutrition

Drugs: β-blockers, anabolic steroids

HDL, high-density lipoprotein.

Certain medications exacerbate hyperlipidemia, including isotretinoin (Accutane), thiazide diuretics, oral contraceptives, steroids, β-blockers, immunosuppressants and protease inhibitors used in the treatment of HIV.

BLOOD CHOLESTEROL SCREENING

NCEP's Expert Panel on Blood Cholesterol Levels in Children and Adolescents established guidelines for cholesterol measurement that were published in 1991. The panel recommended a *selective* approach to screening based on the following criteria:
- Screen children and adolescents whose parents or grandparents have documented CAD before the age of 55 years.
- Screen the offspring of a parent who has been found to have a blood cholesterol level of >240 mg/dL.
- Screen children and adolescents for whom family history is unobtainable, particularly those with other risk factors.

RISK ASSESSMENT AND TREATMENT OF HYPERLIPIDEMIA

Cholesterol-Lowering Strategies

The NCEP Expert Panel has recommended two complementary approaches to lowering blood cholesterol levels for children and adolescents: a population approach and an individualized approach.

Population Approach

The population approach encourages changes in nutrient intake and eating patterns for the entire population. For children older than 2 years, the following are recommended:

1. Nutritional adequacy should be achieved by eating a wide variety of foods.
2. Adequate calories should be provided for normal growth and development.
3. The following pattern of nutrient intake is recommended:
a. Saturated fatty acids <10% of total calories.
b. Total fat ≤30% of total calories.
c. Dietary cholesterol <300 mg/day.

These recommendations are the same as a step-one diet (Table 17.8 below). Children younger than 2 years may require a higher percentage of calories from fat.

Table 17.8: Nutrient composition of step-one and step-two diets

Nutrient	Step-one diet	Step-two diet
Total fat (% of total calories)	<30%	<30%
Saturated fatty acids	<10%	<7%
Polyunsaturated fatty acids	Up to 10%	Up to 10%
Monounsaturated fatty acids	10–15%	10–15%
Carbohydrates (% of total calories)	50–60%	50–60%
Protein (% of total calories)	10–20%	10–20%
Cholesterol (per day)	<300 mg	<200 mg
Total calories	To achieve and maintain desirable weight	To achieve and maintain desirable weight

Individualized Approach

The individualized approach identifies and treats children and adolescents at risk of having high cholesterol levels.

The NCEP Expert Panel recommends *selective* screening of children and adolescents with family histories of premature CVD or at least one parent with high serum cholesterol levels because there is strong evidence demonstrating a familial aggregation of CHD, high serum cholesterol levels and other risk factors. Patients who meet the following specific criteria should be screened:

1. Children and adolescents whose parents or grandparents, at 55 years of age or younger for men and 65 years of age or younger for women, had coronary atherosclerosis after angiography or underwent balloon angioplasty or coronary artery bypass surgery.
2. Children and adolescents whose parents or grandparents, at 55 years of age or younger for men and 65 years of age or younger for women, had documented myocardial infarction, angina pectoris, peripheral vascular disease, cerebrovascular disease or sudden cardiac death.
3. The offspring of a parent who had high TC levels (≥240 mg/dL).
4. Children and adolescents whose parental or grandparental history is unobtainable, particularly those with other risk factors.

The recommendations for selective screening are somewhat controversial. Several studies published in the pediatric literature have indicated that about 50% of children with high LDL levels will be missed if a positive family history of premature CHD is used as the sole screening criterion. The results of the Bogalusa Heart Study, in particular, show that 60% of white and 80% of African American children with high LDL cholesterol levels (95th percentile) did not have positive family histories of CAD (Denison et al., 1989). Universal screening should theoretically detect all children with high LDL levels, and some authorities recommend general screening of preschool children. Although the NCEP Expert Panel believed that, given the current state of knowledge, universal screening should not be recommended, optional cholesterol testing by the

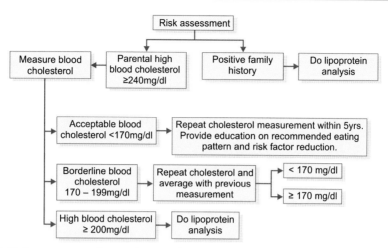

Figure 17.6: Risk assessment for cardiovascular disease or CVD. Source: From Expert Panel on Blood Cholesterol Levels in Children and Adolescents: National Cholesterol Education Program. NIH Publication No. 91-2732, September 1991

practicing physician may be appropriate in children judged to be at higher risk of CHD (such as those who smoke, have high blood pressure, are obese, or have excessive fat intake).

The panel's recommendations are summarized in Fig. 17.6. The screening protocol varies according to the reasons for testing.

RISK ASSESSMENT FOR CARDIOVASCULAR DISEASE OR CVD

1. For young people being tested because they have at least one parent with high blood cholesterol levels, the initial step is measurement of TC.
2. For children who have family histories of premature CVD, a lipoprotein analysis is recommended because a high proportion of these children have some lipoprotein abnormality.

Depending on TC and LDL levels, patients' conditions are categorized as acceptable, borderline or high.

1. For those who had TC levels measured (see Fig. 17.2), the patient's condition is categorized as *acceptable* (<170 mg/dL), *borderline* (170–199 mg/dL) or *high* (≥200 mg/dL).
   a. If TC levels are acceptable (<170 mg/dL), cholesterol measurement is repeated within 5 years.
   b. If TC levels are borderline (170–199 mg/dL), a second measurement is taken.
   c. If the average is borderline or high (>200 mg/dL), a lipoprotein analysis is recommended.
2. For those who had lipoprotein analysis done (Fig. 17.4), regardless of indications, a lipoprotein analysis should be repeated and the average LDL levels determined. The patient's condition is then categorized as *acceptable* (LDL cholesterol <110 mg/dL), *borderline* (110 to 129 mg/dL) or *high*(≥130 mg/dL).
   a. If LDL levels are acceptable (<110 mg/dL), education about the eating pattern recommended for all children and adolescents and about CHD risk factors is provided. Lipoprotein analysis is repeated in 5 years.

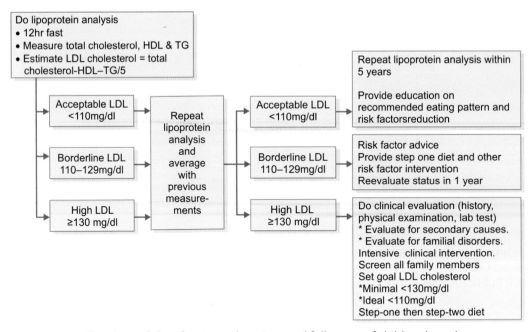

Figure 17.7: Flowchart of classification, education, and follow-up of children based on low-density lipoprotein (LDL) cholesterol levels. TG, triglycerides; CVD, cardiovascular disease; HDL, high-density lipoprotein (10). *Source*: From Williams CL, Hagman LL, Daniels SR, et al, Cardiovascular health in childhood. Circulation. 2002;106:143-60

    b. If LDL levels are in the borderline range (110–129 mg/dL), advice about risk factors is provided, the step-one diet is initiated (Table 17.8) and the patient's status is evaluated in 1 year.

    c. If LDL levels are high (≥130 mg/dL), the patient is evaluated for secondary causes and familial disorders; all family members are screened and the step-one diet is initiated, followed, if necessary, by the step-two diet (see Table 17.8) and, in extreme cases, by drug therapy (see later section) (Fig. 17.7).

MANAGEMENT

Diet Therapy

Diet therapy is prescribed in two steps that progressively reduce the intake of saturated fatty acids and cholesterol. The step-one diet calls for the same nutrient intake recommended in the population approach to lowering cholesterol levels (see Table 17.8): <10% of total calories from saturated fatty acids, no >30% of calories from total fat, <300 mg of cholesterol per day and adequate calories to support growth and development and to reach or maintain a desirable body weight. Involvement of a registered dietitian or other qualified health professional is recommended.

    If the step-one diet fails to achieve the minimal goals of therapy in 3 months, the step-two diet is prescribed (see Table 17.8). This diet further reduces the saturated fatty acid intake to

<7% of calories and the cholesterol intake to <200 mg per day. Adequate amounts of nutrients, vitamins and minerals should be provided. A registered dietitian or other qualified nutrition professional should be consulted.

Drug Therapy (Tables 17.9–17.12)[11,12,13]

The NCEP Expert Panel for Children and Adolescents recommends that consideration be given to pharmacologic treatment of hyperlipidemia if the child is at least 10 years of age and an adequate period of dietary restriction, at least 6 months, has not achieved therapeutic goals. Drug therapy should be considered when:
- LDL cholesterol remains >190 mg/dL.
- LDL cholesterol remains >160 mg/dL and there is a positive family history of premature CVD before 55 years of age or two or more other risk factors for CVD are present after vigorous attempts at lifestyle modification.

The maintenance dosage of the drug is decided by periodic determinations of cholesterol levels.

1. Atorvastatin: Starting dose of 10 mg is increased to 20 mg at 4–6 weeks and further to a dose of 40 mg/day (maximum adult dose is 80 mg/day).
2. Lovastatin: Starting dose 10 mg/day for 6–8 weeks, with a 10-mg increase every 6–8 weeks, to a maximum 40 mg/day.
3. Pravastatin: Starting dose of 10 mg/day is increased to 20 or 40 mg/day.
4. Simvastatin: Starting dose 10 mg, increment of 10 mg every 6–8 weeks to maximum 40 mg/day.

Table 17.9: Drugs used for the treatment of hyperlipidemia

Drug	Mechanism of action	Indication	Starting dose
HMG-CoA reductase inhibitors (statins)	↓ Cholesterol and VLDL synthesis ↑ Hepatic LDL receptors	Elevated LDL	5–80 mg qhs
Bile acid sequestrants:	↑ Bile and excretion	Elevated LDL	
Cholestyramine			4–32 g daily
Colestipol			5–40 g daily
Nicotinic acid	↓ Hepatic VLDL synthesis	Elevated LDL Elevated TG	100–2,000 mg tid
Fibric acid derivatives:	↑ LPL	Elevated TG	600 mg bid
Gemfibrozil	↓ VLDL		
Fish oils	↓ VLDL production	Elevated TG	3–10 g daily
Cholesterol absorption inhibitors:			
Ezetimibe	↓ Intestinal absorption cholesterol	Elevated LDL	10 mg daily

LDL, low-density lipoprotein; LPL, lipoprotein lipase; TG, triglyceride; VLDL, very low density lipoprotein; HMG-CoA, 3-hydroxy-3-methylglutaryl-coenzyme A.

Table 17.10: Summary of lipid lowering drugs

Agent	Mechanism of action	Side effects	Daily dosage range
Bile acid sequestrants: cholestyramine (Questran), colestipol (Colestid), colesevelam (WelChol)	Increases excretion of bile acids in stool; increases LDL receptor activity	Constipation, nausea, bloating, flatulence, transient increase in transaminase and alkaline phosphatase levels, increased triglyceride levels (±), possible prevention of absorption of fat-soluble vitamins	Related to levels of cholesterol, not body weight; for specific dosage, see Table 17.11 below for pediatric dosages
HMG-CoA reductase inhibitors ("statins"): atorvastatin (Lipitor), fluvastatin (Lescol), lovastatin (Mevacor), pravastatin (Pravachol), rosuvastatin (Crestor), simvastatin (Zocor)	Inhibits HMG-CoA reductase, with resulting decrease in cholesterol synthesis; increases LDL receptor activity; and reduces LDL and VLDL secretion by the liver	Mild gastrointestinal symptoms, myositis syndrome, elevated hepatic transaminase levels, increased CPK levels (contraindicated during pregnancy because of potential risk to a developing fetus)	Children: See text for suggested pediatric dosages Adult dose ranges (of statins approved for pediatric use): Atorvastatin: 10–80 mg Lovastatin: 20–80 mg Pravastatin: 10–40 mg Simvastatin: 10–80 mg
Cholesterol absorption inhibitors: ezetimibe (Zetia; Ezetrol)	Selective inhibition of intestinal sterol absorption	Abdominal pain, rhabdomyolysis (±)	Adult: 10 mg/day
Nicotinic acid (niacin, vitamin B3)	Decreases plasma levels of free fatty acid; possibly inhibits cholesterol synthesis; decreases hepatic VLDL synthesis	Cutaneous flushing, pruritus, gastrointestinal upset, liver function abnormalities, increased uric acid levels, increased glucose intolerance	Children: only short term efficacy reported for homozygous FH; not recommended for routine use Adults: 1–3 g
Fibric acid derivatives: Gemfibrozil (Lopid), Clofibrate	Decrease hepatic VLDL synthesis; increase LPL activity	Increased incidence of gallstones and perhaps gastrointestinal cancer, myositis, diarrhea, nausea, rash, altered liver function, increased CPK levels, potentiation of warfarin	Children: not recommended Adults: gemfibrozil, 600–1200 mg; clofibrate, 1–2 g

CPK, creatine phosphokinase; FH, familial hypercholesterolemia; HDL, high-density lipoprotein; HMGCoA,3-hydroxy-3-methylglutaryl coenzyme A; LDL, low-density lipoprotein; LPL, lipoprotein lipase; VLDL, very low-density lipoprotein.
Based on published clinical trials in children and adolescents, the following may be reasonable pediatric dosages of the four statins that are approved for pediatric use (Holmes KW, Kwiterovich PO Jr. Treatment of dyslipidemia in children and adolescents. Curr Cardiol Rep. 2005;7:445–56).

Table 17.11: Suggested initial dosage of a bile acid sequestrant for the treatment of familial hypercholesterolemia in children and adolescents

Daily doses*	TC	LDL
1	<245	<195
2	245–300	195–235
3	301–345	236–280
4	345	

LDL, low-density lipoprotein; TC, total cholesterol.
TC and LDL levels after diet (mg/100 dL).
*One dose is the equivalent of a 9-g packet of cholestyramine (containing 4 g of cholestyramine and 5 g of filler), one bar of cholestyramine, or 5 g of colestipol.

In pediatric trials, starting doses were usually half of the adult lower range dose, depending on the age of the child, increased by 10 mg every 4–8 weeks to the half or full dose of the upper range dosage with periodic measurements of cholesterols.

For High Levels of Triglycerides

Treatment of this condition includes a very low fat diet (10% to 15% of calories) that can be supplemented by medium-chain TGs (see Table 17.7). Portagen, a soybean-based formula enriched in medium chain TGs, is available for infants with LPL deficiency. Lipid-lowering drugs are ineffective in LPL deficiency.

In adult patients, the primary aim of therapy is to reach the LDL goal by the use of statins, intense weight management and increasing physical activity. If TGs are ≥200 mg/dL when the LDL goal is reached, nicotinic acid or fibrate alone, or better in combination with a statin, may be used to reduce the non-HDL cholesterol level to the level of 30 mg/dL plus the LDL goal. A prescription omega-3 fatty acid product (e.g., Omacor) at 4 and 8 g/day reduced TG levels by 30% and 43%, respectively, from baseline values. (Most fish oil capsules have an omega-3 fatty acid content only one third of that in Omacor.) Omega-3 fatty acid plus a statin may be an effective alternative to a fibrate or niacin plus a statin.

For Low Levels of HDL Cholesterol

A low HDL level is defined as <40 mg/dL in men and <50 mg/dL in women. High-density lipoprotein cholesterol is inversely related to fatal myocardial infarction. A rise of 1 mg/dL in HDL cholesterol lowers the risk of fatal myocardial infarction by about 3%. Statins that are effective in lowering LDL cholesterol are not very effective in raising HDL cholesterol.

CONCLUSION

Lipid abnormality occurs early in childhood. Recognition of the clinical syndrome is very important for the future adult. Most of the clinical expression of these abnormalities takes place in adolescent or later years in life. Diet and exercise are the mainstay of therapy. Statins are safe after 10 years of age. Combination of statin, ezetimibe, fibrates has been used with good outcome. Several genetically determined dyslipidemias require further research and newer mode of treatment.

REFERENCES

1. Elsevier, Kleigman, Behrman, Jenson, Stanton, Nelson Textbook of Pediatrics, 18th edition, volume 1, Chapter 86, part X, pp. 580-93.
2. MOSBY, Elsevier, Park MK. Pediatric Cardiology for Practitioners, 5th edition, Chapter 33, Part VII, pp. 635-59.
3. Winter W, Schartz D. Pediatric lipid disorders in clinical practice. eMedicine, last updated January 19, 2005.
4. Trxoler RG, Park MK. Hyperlipidemia in childhood. In: Pediatric Cardiology for Practitioners, 4th edition. St. Louis: Mosby; 2002.
5. Holmes KW, Kwiterovich PO Jr. Treatment of dyslipidemia in children and adolescents. Curr Cardiol Rep. 2005;7:445-56.
6. Williams RR, Hunt SC, Schumacher MC, et al. Diagnosing heterozygous familial hypercholesterolemia using new practical criteria validated by molecular genetics. Am J Cardiol. 1993;72:171-6.
7. Cook S, Weizman M, Auinger P, et al. Prevalence of a metabolic syndrome phenotype in adolescents: findings from the third National Health and Nutrition Examination Survey, 1988-1994. Arch Pediatr Adolsc Med. 2003;157:821-7.
8. Haas D, Kelley RI, Hoffmann GF. Inherited disorders of cholesterol biosynthesis. Neuropediatrics. 2001;32:113-22.
9. Expert Panel on Blood Cholesterol Levels in Children and Adolescents: National Cholesterol Education Program. NIH Publication No. 91-2732, September 1991.
10. Williams CL, Hagman LL, Daniels SR, et al. Cardiovascular health in childhood. Circulation. 2002;106:143-60
11. Knopp RH. Drug treatment of lipid disorders. N Engl J Med. 1999;341:498-512.

Dyslipidemia in Diabetes Mellitus

Suchitra Behl and Misra A

- Introduction
- Definitions and mechanisms
- Dyslipidemia in Asian Indians
- Dyslipidemia and macrovascular complications in diabetes mellitus
- Dyslipidemia and microvascular complications in diabetes mellitus
- Diagnosis and management of dyslipidemia
- Guidelines for initiating therapy
- Other medications and supplements
- Newer medicines
- Summary

Dyslipidemia is common in patients with diabetes and is related to increased risk of coronary heart disease (CHD). There is also evidence associating dyslipidemia with microvascular complications of diabetes. Management of dyslipidemia in patients with diabetes includes lifestyle modification and pharmacotherapy.

INTRODUCTION

Diabetes mellitus has emerged as one of the major health problems worldwide. The International Diabetes Federation (IDF) estimated that 366 million people worldwide had diabetes in 2011 and 80% of the people with diabetes live in low- and middle-income countries. The prevalence of diabetes in India is estimated at 61.3 million as per the fifth Atlas released by the IDF.

Patients with diabetes have high risk of premature atherosclerosis and CHD due to insulin resistance, metabolic abnormalities, dyslipidemia and other pro atherogenic factors.[1-3] The causes of CHD in diabetic population include dyslipidemia (the following alone or in combination; increased concentration of total cholesterol and low-density lipoprotein cholesterol (LDL-C), decreased concentration of high-density lipoprotein cholesterol (HDL-C) and hypertriglyceridemia), hypertension, smoking and obesity.[4-6] Aggressive management of dyslipidemia is indicated in view of the improvement in cardiovascular outcomes with the treatment of dyslipidemia.

DEFINITION AND MECHANISM

Dyslipidemia refers to the derangement of one or many of the lipoproteins; elevation of total cholesterol, LDL-C and/or triglycerides (TG); or low levels of HDL-C, while elevation of lipoproteins alone is labeled as "hyperlipidemia."

Diabetic dyslipidemia refers to the lipid abnormalities observed in diabetic patients. These changes are both quantitative and qualitative. The most common pattern of dyslipidemia seen in patients with type 2 diabetes mellitus (T2DM) is that of elevated TG and low levels of HDL-C. There is an increased preponderance of small dense LDL even when LDL-C values are not very high. Studies have noted that dyslipidemia is present in patients with T2DM in prediabetic phase and at diagnosis.[7,8] This pattern of dyslipidemia with low HDL-C, elevated TG and small dense LDL particles is also referred to as "atherogenic dyslipidemia" and is seen in patients with obesity, metabolic syndrome and T2DM.

Mechanism

Insulin is an anabolic hormone and is responsible for promoting lipid synthesis and inhibiting breakdown of stored lipids. In adipocytes, it promotes increased glucose uptake and activation of enzymes involved in lipid synthesis. Insulin inhibits lipolysis in adipocytes by inhibiting the enzyme hormone-sensitive lipase.[9] Lipoprotein lipase (LPL) hydrolyzes TG in lipoproteins like chylomicrons and very low-density lipoprotein (VLDL). Insulin activates LPL in the adipocytes but inhibits LPL in the muscle.

Dyslipidemia in T2DM is linked with insulin resistance, a condition in which a normal amount of insulin produces a less than normal biologic response.[10] Insulin resistance is associated with increased lipolysis and decreased fatty acid uptake in the striated muscle. There is increased supply of nonesterified fatty acid to the liver leading to increased hepatic TG synthesis. Decreased activity of endothelial insulin-dependent LPL leads to decreased TG clearance from TG-rich lipoproteins.[11] Increased VLDL levels and decreased catabolism of TG-rich lipoproteins result in elevated TG-rich lipoproteins.[12]

The HDL-C in diabetics is TG enriched and there is increased glycosylation of apoproteins in HDL particles that leads to accelerated HDL catabolism, and hence lower HDL levels.[13,14] Triglycerides from VLDL are exchanged for cholesterol ester from LDL particles, and due to increased VLDL levels there is an increased generation of TG-rich LDL particles in diabetic individuals. The TG in the LDL particles are hydrolyzed to form small dense LDL particles that are more atherogenic.[15,16]

Elevated TG and low HDL-C level is the most common pattern of dyslipidemia in T2DM.[2] The median TG level is <200 mg/dL, and 85–95% of patients have TG levels below 400 mg/dL.[5] Elevated TG may be present at diagnosis as well as in prediabetic phase.[8] Elevated TG level is the most predominant dyslipidemia in patients with type 1 diabetes mellitus (T1DM) too. The elevated TG is related to insulin deficiency and levels normalize with improvement in glucose control on initiation of insulin.

DYSLIPIDEMIA IN ASIAN INDIANS

Recent decades have witnessed increasing prevalence of chronic diseases like obesity, T2DM, dyslipidemia and CHD in India. The increased prevalence of obesity and abdominal obesity in

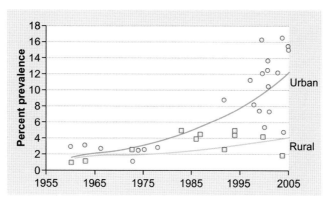

Figure 18.1: Trends in prevalence of diabetes in urban (•) and rural (○) India.
Source: Adapted from Ref. 22.

urban India has been documented,[17] and the prevalence of obesity by body mass index criteria in various cities is reported as 50.1% in New Delhi,[18] 45.9% in Chennai[19] and 55.5% in Jaipur.[20] Diabetes has increased in prevalence in both rural and urban India with exponential increase in urban India (Fig.18.1) related to socioeconomic and dietary changes accompanied by decrease in physical activity. Alongside, there has been an increase in the prevalence of CHD, and a meta-analysis of CHD prevalence found a nine- and twofold increase in the prevalence of CHD in urban and rural India, respectively.[21]

Although total cholesterol levels in Asian Indians are similar to Caucasians,[23] atherogenic dyslipidemia with elevated TG, small dense LDL-C and low levels of HDL-C is more common. A review of studies on dyslipidemia in Asian Indians noted that the overall prevalence of dyslipidemia in India in various studies ranged from 10% to 73%.[24] There was high serum TG in urban Asian Indians (up to 73% in obese and 61% in nonobese) and migrant Asian Indians,

Table 18.1: Prevalence of obesity and cardiometabolic risk factors in New Delhi

Variable	Total	Percentage (%)
Obesity (BMI criteria)*	230	50.1
Impaired fasting glucose	110	24
Diabetes	39	8.5
Hypercholesterolemia	122	26.6
Hypertriglyceridemia	196	42.7
LDL-C ≥ 100 mg/dL	237	51.6
HDL-C < 40 mg/dL (males) and <50 mg/dl (females)	170	37

Source: Adapted from Ref. 18.
*BMI ≥25 kg/m² defined as obesity.
BMI, body mass index; LDL-C, low-density lipoprotein cholesterol; HDL-C, high-density lipoprotein cholesterol.

Table 18.2: Dyslipidemia in Indian diabetic patients*

	Males (422)	Females (366)
Prevalence of dyslipidemia	85.5%	97.8%
Most common dyslipidemia	Combined dyslipidemia (44.9) 1. High LDL and low HDL (19.4) 2. High TG and high LDL (10.2) 3. High TG and low HDL (8.8)	Combined dyslipidemia (47.8) 1. High LDL and low HDL (32.2) 2. High TG and low HDL (9.3) 3. High TG and high LDL (5.2)
Second most common dyslipidemia	Isolated single parameter dyslipidemia (41) 1. High LDL (18.2) 2. Low HDL (10.4) 3. High TG (6.4)	Isolated single parameter dyslipidemia (27.7) 1. Low HDL (13.1) 2. High LDL (12.6) 3. High TG (1.4)
Third most common dyslipidemia	Mixed dyslipidemia (14.1) High TG, high LDL and low HDL	Mixed dyslipidemia (24) High TG, high LDL and low HDL

Source: Adapted from Ref. 27.
Mixed dyslipidemia: all three parameters outside recommended targets; combined dyslipidemia: two parameters outside targets; isolated single parameter dyslipidemia: single parameter not meeting target either HDL or LDL or TG.
*Prevalence in parentheses is given in %.
LDL, low-density lipoprotein; HDL, high-density lipoprotein TG; triglycerides.

and while the average level of serum TG in rural areas was comparatively lower, it was still higher than Caucasians. The results from a recent cross-sectional study in urban New Delhi that noted a high prevalence of hypertriglyceridemia (42.7%)[18] are summarized in Table 18.1. In addition, the average HDL-C in all Asian subgroups is lower than Caucasians and a study that included Singapore Indians noted that 34% of the subjects with low HDL-C levels were Asian Indians.[25] Studies in Indian diabetics have shown elevated levels of small dense LDL that is associated with diabetes and coronary artery disease.[26] Some of the determinants of dyslipidemia in Asian Indians are low physical activity, vegetarian diet that is carbohydrate rich and low in ω-3 polyunsaturated fatty acids, body composition with excess truncal fat and intra-abdominal fat and genetic predisposition.[24]

There are few published studies on the prevalence of dyslipidemia in patients with diabetes in India. Results of a study done by Parikh et al.[27] that looked at pattern of dyslipidemia in 788 diabetic patients are summarized in Table 18.2. Total 97.8 % of the female patients and 85.5 % of the male patients had dyslipidemia. Combined dyslipidemia with high LDL and low HDL was the most common pattern observed in both males and females. Isolated high LDL was the second most common dyslipidemia in males, and isolated low HDL was the second most common dyslipidemia in females.[27]

Another study on patients with T2DM in a metropolitan city in India (Mumbai) that looked for the presence of metabolic syndrome in 5088 diabetic patients found that 57.86% of the patients had elevated fasting TG levels (>150 mg/dL) and 52.28% of the patients had low HDL levels (<40 mg/dL).[28]

DYSLIPIDEMIA AND MACROVASCULAR COMPLICATIONS OF DIABETES MELLITUS

Several studies have established the association of dyslipidemia in diabetic patients with increased cardiovascular mortality and the reduction in cardiovascular mortality and morbidity with statin therapy.[29-35] While the statin used has differed in these studies, reduction in the frequency of coronary events in diabetic patients with established CHD[30,31] and in risk of major cardiovascular events in diabetic patients without CHD[33,35] has been documented. While there is evidence of lowering of cardiovascular risk with lowering of LDL-C levels with statin therapy, there is much less evidence in favor of lowering of cardiovascular disease (CVD) risk with therapy, which primarily targets low HDL-C and elevated TG.[34,36]

However, elevated TG and low HDL-C levels are predictors of CVD independent of LDL-C, and the Prospective Cardiovascular Münster study showed substantial risk of myocardial infarction with low HDL-C and/or high TG levels, particularly if LDL-C is low.[37] The Action to Control Cardiovascular Risk in Diabetes study did not show significant cardiovascular benefits with combination treatment of simvastatin plus fenofibrate, but a subgroup analysis showed benefit with combination therapy for men and possible benefit for patients with both TG $\geq$204 mg/dL and HDL-C $\leq$ 34 mg/dL.[38] A recent meta-analysis including 29 studies showed that after adjustment for risk factors, the odds ratio of CHD was 1.72 (95% confidence interval = 1.56–1.90) when individuals in the highest TG tertile were compared with those in the lowest tertile.[39] The Atherothrombosis Intervention in Metabolic Syndrome with Low HDL/High Triglycerides: Impact on Global Health Outcomes (AIM-HIGH) trial, which included patients with diabetes and assessed benefits of addition of extended release niacin to statin therapy in patients with established cardiovascular disease, found no difference in outcome and a possible increase in ischemic stroke in those on combination therapy.[40] However, the patients in this trial had LDL-C levels that were well controlled with statin therapy, and the role of niacin in patients with high LDL-C levels is still under study. These factors must be considered when prescribing for the treatment of diabetic dyslipidemia and treatment individualized.

DIABETIC DYSLIPIDEMIA AND MICROVASCULAR COMPLICATIONS OF DIABETES MELLITUS

There is evidence associating diabetic dyslipidemia with microvascular complications of diabetes. Retinal hard exudates are twice as common in patients with higher baseline total cholesterol and LDL-C compared with patients with normal levels.[41] Elevated TG levels have been identified as a risk factor for proliferative diabetic retinopathy,[42] and the severity of retinopathy is positively associated with TG and negatively associated with HDL-C levels.[43] Data derived from studies that included diabetic patients on treatment with statins or fibrates for lowering of cardiovascular risk suggests that there are beneficial effects on diabetic retinopathy. In one study, patients with T2DM who were on treatment with fenofibrate were less likely to experience laser treatment for retinopathy, and in patients with preexisting retinopathy, fewer patients had progression of retinopathy.[44] In another study, patients with T2DM on treatment with simvastatin had less worsening in angiographic findings compared with patients who were on placebo.[45]

Both diabetes and renal insufficiency are associated with dyslipidemia. In the United Kingdom Prospective Diabetes Study (UKPDS), elevated TG levels were independently associated with incident microalbuminuria and macroalbuminuria.[46] There are studies that show that hypertriglyceridemia is a predictive factor for the development and progression of renal complications.[47] It has been noted that diabetic (both T2DM and T1DM) patients without nephropathy have higher HDL-C values than those with nephropathy, suggesting a protective role of HDL-C.[48,49] Diabetic dyslipidemia (high TG and low HDL-C) was identified as a predictor of more rapid progression of microalbuminuria in patients with well-controlled blood pressure.[49] A study on multifactorial intervention in patients with T2DM and microalbuminuria for a mean follow-up interval of 7.8 years showed significantly lower risk of nephropathy and retinopathy,[50] and hence patients with or at risk of diabetic nephropathy are advised intensive management, including lipid-lowering medications.

Elevated TG along with higher levels of total and LDL-C has been associated with diabetic neuropathy in T1DM.[51] Low HDL-C and elevated fasting TG have been associated with autonomic neuropathy.[52] Based on these findings, it is suggested to target elevated TG and low HDL-C in addition to glycemic control, control of LDL-C and blood pressure control[53] to reduce the risk of diabetic microvascular complications.

DIAGNOSIS AND MANAGEMENT OF DYSLIPIDEMIA

Dyslipidemia is diagnosed with a fasting lipid profile that is recommended at diagnosis in all adult patients with diabetes. A minimum of 9–12 hours of fasting is recommended in order to minimize the postprandial effect on lipid panel. As per Adult Treatment Panel III (ATP III) classification, optimal LDL-C is <100 mg/dL, desirable TC is < 200 mg/dL and HDL-C <40 mg/dL is defined as low. In diabetic individuals, low-risk lipid values are LDL-C <100 mg/dL, HDL-C >50 mg/dL and TG<150 mg/dL.[34]

Patients with diabetes may have primary dyslipidemia (e.g., familial hypercholesterolemia), but secondary dyslipidemia due to diabetes itself is more common. Lifestyle factors related to lack of exercise and faulty eating habits and other diseases may contribute to dyslipidemia. These secondary causes of dyslipidemia must be ruled out by appropriate investigations (see Table 18.3). After the first measurement of lipid profile, patients with low-risk lipid values (LDL-C <100 mg/dL, HDL-C >50 mg/dL and TG <150 mg/dL) may have fasting lipid profiles checked every 2 years,[34] while patients who are on the treatment for diabetic dyslipidemia may need more frequent monitoring of lipid profiles. Glycemic control is an important consider-

Table 18.3: Secondary causes of dyslipidemia

1	T2DM
2	Cholestatic liver disease
3	Nephrotic syndrome, chronic kidney disease
4	Hypothyroidism
5	Drugs, e.g., thiazides, beta blockers, protease inhibitors, anabolic steroids, estrogen, progesterone, clozapine, olanzapine
6	Obesity

T2DM, type 2 diabetes mellitus.

Table 18.4: Treatment goals and desired levels for diabetic dyslipidemia

Parameter	Treatment goal/desired level
LDL-C	Treatment goal (patients without CVD): <100 mg/dL
	Treatment goal (patients with overt CVD): <70 mg/dL
	Alternative goal: reduction of 30–40% from baseline
HDL-C	Desired level(men): >40mg/dL
	Desired level(women): >50 mg/dL
TG level	Desired level: <150 mg/dL

Source: Adapted from Ref. 34.
LDL-C, low-density lipoprotein cholesterol; HDL-C, high-density lipoprotein cholesterol; TG, triglyceride; CVD, cardiovascular disease.

ation in the management of dyslipidemia as good glycemic control significantly improves TG levels and modestly lowers LDL-C. This is discussed in further detail in the section "Guidelines for Initiating Therapy."

Management

The American Diabetic Association (ADA) has outlined an order of priorities for the treatment of diabetic dyslipidemia and this is summarized in Table 18.4. Lowering of LDL-C is ranked as the first priority in the management of diabetic dyslipidemia due to considerable data showing benefits of statin therapy on primary and secondary prevention of CVD events in diabetic patients.[34] Since there is less evidence in the support of drugs (nicotinic acid and fibrates) targeting elevated TG and low HDL-C in terms of lowering of CVD events, they are ranked further down in the order of priorities despite their high prevalence in diabetic patients.[2] Measurement of non-HDL-C, apolipoprotein B (apoB) or lipoprotein particles is routinely not advised as clinical management is not impacted.[34]

GUIDELINES FOR INITIATING THERAPY

The following suggested management is partly based on the position statement on the management of dyslipidemia issued by ADA and the standard of medical care in diabetes released by the ADA. Drugs used in the management of diabetic dyslipidemia are summarized in Table 18.5.

1. Lifestyle modification should be recommended to all patients. Medical nutrition therapy, increased physical activity and weight loss are essential components of lifestyle modification. Nutritional intervention should be done by a certified nutritionist. Reduction in intake of saturated fat, cholesterol and trans unsaturated fat and increased intake of omega-3 fatty acids, viscous fiber and plant sterols are recommended.[54] Patients should be advised to perform at least 150 min/week of moderate-intensity aerobic physical activity.
2. Low-density lipoprotein cholesterol lowering is the first goal of therapy for the management of diabetic dyslipidemia, and statins are the first drug of choice. Improved glycemic control will only modestly reduce LDL-C, and hence statin therapy may be initiated simultaneously

Table 18.5: Drugs used in the treatment of diabetic dyslipidemia

Type	Mechanism of action	Effect on lipid profile	Some common adverse drug reactions
HMG-CoA reductase inhibitors (statins) Lovastatin Simvastatin Atorvastatin Pravastatin Fluvastatin Rosuvastatin	↓Cholesterol synthesis ↑LDL receptor	↓LDL-C ↓TG	GI upset Muscle aches Hepatitis Myopathy Peripheral neuropathy
Fibrates Gemfibrozil Fenofibrate Bezafibrate Ciprofibrate	↑Fatty acid oxidation→hepatic TG synthesis ↑LPL→↑TG hydrolysis	↓TG ↑HDL-C ↑or ↓LDL-C	GI upset Gall stones Myositis Erectile dysfunction
Bile acid sequestrant Cholestyramine Colestipol	↓Reabsorption of bile acids in intestine→↑synthesis of new bile acids and ↑LDL receptor	↓LDL-C ↑HDL-C ↑TG	Constipation GI upset Rash
Nicotinic acid	↓Hepatic TG synthesis ↓Secretion of apoB100 containing lipoprotein; ↓VLDL→LDL conversion	↓LDL-C ↓VLDL-C ↓Lp(a) ↓HDL-C ↓TG	Flushing Pruritus Hyperpigmentation Orthostatic hypotension Hepatotoxicity
Azetidinone (cholesterol absorption inhibitors) Ezetimibe	↓Absorption of cholesterol from intestinal micelles	↓LDL-C	Upper respiratory infection Diarrhea Myalgia Fatigue

Source: Adapted from Ref. 55.
apoB, apolipoprotein B; LDL, low-density lipoprotein; LDL-C, low-density lipoprotein cholesterol; HDL, high-density lipoprotein; HDL-C, high-density lipoprotein cholesterol; VLDL, very low-density lipoprotein; GI, gastrointestinal; HMG-CoA, 3-hydroxy-3-methylglutaryl-coenzyme A; TG; triglycerides; LPL, lipoprotein lipase.

with the management of hyperglycemia. Statin therapy is added to lifestyle modification for patients with overt CVD and to patients who are above 40 years and have at least one CVD risk factor irrespective of the baseline lipid levels.[34] For other diabetic patients, treatment with statins should be started if LDL-C is >100 mg/dL or there are multiple CVD risk factors.

Low-density lipoprotein cholesterol should be lowered to <100 mg/dL in all diabetic patients and to <70 mg/dL in high-risk diabetic patients with overt CVD.[54] A lowering of

LDL-C of 30–40% from baseline is acceptable for patients in whom these goals cannot be met or for those who have LDL-C minimally >100 mg/dL at baseline. There is not enough evidence to support the use of combination therapy for patients who do not achieve 30% reduction in LDL-C from baseline after maximum tolerated doses of statins.[34] For patients who cannot tolerate statins, bile acid-binding resin or fibrates may be used. In patients with severe hypercholesterolemia, statins may be combined with ezetimibe.

3. Lifestyle modification with weight loss, increased physical activity and smoking cessation is the first step in raising HDL-C. Niacin is the most effective drug for raising HDL-C but high doses can worsen glycemic control significantly and the patient should be followed up carefully. If used, niacin should be used at doses between 750 and 2000 mg/day for raising HDL-C. Alternatively, fibrates may be used.

4. Weight loss, increased physical activity and moderation of alcohol consumption are advised for lowering TG. Improvement in glycemic control improves TG levels and should be achieved before fibrates are advised. For TG between 200 and 400 mg/dL, it is up to the physician to decide on the need for initiation of pharmacotherapy. Pharmacological treatment should be strongly considered for TG >400 mg/dL, and fibric acid derivatives are the first choice of pharmacotherapy. High-dose statins are moderately effective in hypertriglyceridemic (≥300 mg/dL) patients who also have elevated LDL. In patients with severe hypertriglyceridemia (≥1000 mg/dL), severe dietary fat restriction (<10% of calories) in addition to pharmacotherapy is advised. Gemfibrozil use in combination with statins is associated with increased risk of muscle toxicity, and fenofibrate is considered safer as it does not increase the level of statins.

5. Combination therapy (e.g., statin plus fibrate or statin plus niacin) is associated with increased risk of abnormal transaminase levels, myositis and rhabdomyolysis, and patients must be monitored for these adverse drug reactions. The risk of rhabdomyolysis is higher in patients with renal insufficiency and with higher dose of statins.

OTHER MEDICATIONS AND SUPPLEMENTS

Orlistat that is used in the treatment of obesity is a pancreatic lipase inhibitor. It has been shown to reduce the total cholesterol, LDL-C, TG and apoB concentration in obese diabetic patients. Fish oil supplements containing ω-3 polyunsaturated fatty acids have been shown to lower TG levels, and a meta-analysis in diabetic patients did not find any worsening of glycemic control. In addition, dietary soluble fibers, like guar gum and pectin, cause lowering of cholesterol levels.

NEWER MEDICINES

Newer medicines under clinical trial include pitavastatin and nisvastatin. Colesevelam is a bile acid sequestrant that significantly lowers LDL-C in patients with primary hypercholesterol-emia and has been shown to improve glycemic control in adults with T2DM.[56] Inhibitors of squalene synthase, an enzyme involved in cholesterol synthesis, are under investigation as in animal studies they were found to lower LDL-C and TG levels.[57-59] Microsomal triglyceride transfer protein (MTP) inhibitors that block the hepatic secretion of VLDL and the intestinal secretion of chylomicrons[60] and naringenin, a grapefruit flavonoid, which may inhibit hepatic MTP activity,[60] are under study. Inhibitors of ileal apical sodium-dependent bile acid cotransporter, sterol regulatory element-binding protein cleavage-activating protein ligands and many more agents are currently under investigation.[11]

SUMMARY

Diabetic dyslipidemia with elevated TG, low levels of HDL-C and small dense LDL-C is highly prevalent in diabetic patients. Due to the higher risk of cardiovascular disease in diabetic patients and considerable evidence in favor of lowering of CVD risk, statins are the most commonly used medications in diabetic dyslipidemia, and lowering of LDL-C is the first step in the treatment of diabetic dyslipidemia. There is emerging evidence relating elevated TG and low HDL-C levels with macrovascular and microvascular complications of diabetes. Correction of these lipid abnormalities are of immense importance for the prevention of cardio vascular disease. Combination therapy may be needed in certain patients, but the risk of combination therapy should be discussed with the patient and treatment individualized on a case-to-case basis.

REFERENCES

1. Kannel WB, McGee DL. Diabetes and glucose tolerance as risk factors for cardiovascular disease: the Framingham study. Diabetes Care. 1979;2(2):120-6.
2. Haffner SM. Management of dyslipidemia in adults with diabetes. Diabetes Care. 2003;26(Suppl 1): S83-6.
3. DeFronzo RA, Ferrannini E. Insulin resistance. A multifaceted syndrome responsible for NIDDM, obesity, hypertension, dyslipidemia, and atherosclerotic cardiovascular disease. Diabetes Care. 1991;14(3):173-94.
4. Bierman EL. George Lyman Duff Memorial Lecture. Atherogenesis in diabetes. Arterioscler Thromb. 1992;12(6):647-56.
5. Haffner SM. Management of dyslipidemia in adults with diabetes. Diabetes Care. 1998;21(1):160-78.
6. Turner RC, Millns H, Neil HA, et al. Risk factors for coronary artery disease in non-insulin dependent diabetes mellitus: United Kingdom Prospective Diabetes Study (UKPDS: 23). BMJ. 1998;316(7134):823-8.
7. U.K. Prospective Diabetes Study 27. Plasma lipids and lipoproteins at diagnosis of NIDDM by age and sex. Diabetes Care. 1997;20(11):1683-7.
8. Haffner SM, Stern MP, Hazuda HP, et al. Cardiovascular risk factors in confirmed prediabetic individuals. Does the clock for coronary heart disease start ticking before the onset of clinical diabetes? JAMA. 1990;263(21):2893-8.
9. Insulin Resistance: A Multifaceted Syndrome Responsible for NIDDM, Obesity, Hypertension, Dyslipidemia, and Atherosclerotic Cardiovascular Disease. Ralph A DeFronzo, MD and Eleuterio Ferrannini, MD Diabetes Care. March 1991;14(3):173-94.
10. Kahn CR. Insulin resistance, insulin insensitivity, and insulin unresponsiveness: a necessary distinction. Metabolism. 1978;27(12 Suppl 2):1893-902.
11. Chowdhury S, Pandit K. Dyslipidemia in diabetes. In: Tripathy BB, Chandalia HB, Das AK, et al. (Eds). RSSDI Textbook of Diabetes Mellitus, 2nd edition. New Delhi: Jaypee Brothers; 2008. pp. 664-80.
12. Johnstone MT, Nesto R. Diabetes mellitus and heart disease. In: Kahn CR, Weir GC, King GL, et al. (Eds). Joslins's Diabetes Mellitus, 14th edition. Boston (MA): Lippincott Williams & Wilkins; 2005. p. 978.
13. Witztum JL, Fisher M, Pietro T, et al. Nonenzymatic glucosylation of high-density lipoprotein accelerates its catabolism in guinea pigs. Diabetes. 1982;31(11):1029-32.

14. Gowri MS, Van der Westhuyzen DR, Bridges SR, et al. Decreased protection by HDL from poorly controlled type 2 diabetic subjects against LDL oxidation may be due to the abnormal composition of HDL. Arterioscler Thromb Vasc Biol. 1999;19(9):2226-33.

15. Tsai EC, Hirsch IB, Brunzell JD, et al. Reduced plasma peroxyl radical trapping capacity and increased susceptibility of LDL to oxidation in poorly controlled IDDM. Diabetes. 1994;43(8):1010-4.

16. Stewart MW, Laker MF, Dyer RG, et al. Lipoprotein compositional abnormalities and insulin resistance in type II diabetic patients with mild hyperlipidemia. Arterioscler Thromb. 1993;13(7):1046-52.

17. Misra A, Khurana L. Obesity and the metabolic syndrome in developing countries. J Clin Endocrinol Metab. 2008;93(11 Suppl 1):S9-30.

18. Bhardwaj S, Misra A, Misra R, et al. High prevalence of abdominal, intra-abdominal and subcutaneous adiposity and clustering of risk factors among urban Asian Indians in North India. PLoS One. 2011;6(9):e24362.

19. Deepa M, Farooq S, Deepa R, et al. Prevalence and significance of generalized and central body obesity in an urban Asian Indian population in Chennai, India (CURES: 47). Eur J Clin Nutr. 2009;63(2):259-67.

20. Gupta R, Agrawal M. High cardiovascular risks in a North Indian Agarwal community: a case series. Cases J. 2009;2:7870.

21. Gupta R, Gupta VP, Sarna M, et al. Prevalence of coronary heart disease and risk factors in an urban Indian population: Jaipur Heart Watch-2. Indian Heart J. 2002;54(1):59-66.

22. Gupta RM, A. Type 2 diabetes in India: regional disparities. Br J Diabetes Vasc Dis. 2007;7:12-6.

23. Gama R, Elfatih AB, Anderson NR. Ethnic differences in total and HDL cholesterol concentrations: Caucasians compared with predominantly Punjabi Sikh Indo-Asians. Ann Clin Biochem. 2002;39(Pt 6):609-11.

24. Misra A, Luthra K, Vikram NK. Dyslipidemia in Asian Indians: determinants and significance. J Assoc Physicians India. 2004;52:137-42.

25. Tai ES, Emmanuel SC, Chew SK, et al. Isolated low HDL cholesterol: an insulin-resistant state only in the presence of fasting hypertriglyceridemia. Diabetes. 1999;48(5):1088-92.

26. Mohan V, Deepa R, Velmurugan K, et al. Association of small dense LDL with coronary artery disease and diabetes in urban Asian Indians-the Chennai Urban Rural Epidemiology Study (CURES-8). J Assoc Physicians India. 2005;53:95-100.

27. Parikh R.M., Joshi S.R., Menon P.S., Shah N.S. Prevalence and pattern of diabetic dyslipidemia in Indian type 2 diabetic patients. Diabetes Metab Syndr Clin Res Rev. 2010;4:10-12.

28. Surana SP, Shah DB, Gala K, et al. Prevalence of metabolic syndrome in an urban Indian diabetic population using the NCEP ATP III guidelines. J Assoc Physicians India. 2008;56:865-8.

29. National Cholesterol Education Program (NCEP) Expert Panel on Detection, Evaluation, and Treatment of High Blood Cholesterol in Adults (Adult Treatment Panel III), Circulation 2002, 106(25):3143-421.

30. Pyorala K, Pedersen TR, Kjekshus J, et al. Cholesterol lowering with simvastatin improves prognosis of diabetic patients with coronary heart disease. A subgroup analysis of the Scandinavian Simvastatin Survival Study (4S). Diabetes Care. 1997;20(4):614-20.

31. Goldberg RB, Mellies MJ, Sacks FM, et al. Cardiovascular events and their reduction with pravastatin in diabetic and glucose-intolerant myocardial infarction survivors with average cholesterol levels: subgroup analyses in the cholesterol and recurrent events (CARE) trial. The Care Investigators. Circulation. 1998;98(23):2513-9.

32. Shepherd J, Barter P, Carmena R, et al. Effect of lowering LDL cholesterol substantially below currently recommended levels in patients with coronary heart disease and diabetes: the Treating to New Targets (TNT) study. Diabetes Care. 2006;29(6):1220-6.

33. Sever PS, Poulter NR, Dahlof B, et al. Reduction in cardiovascular events with atorvastatin in 2,532 patients with type 2 diabetes: Anglo-Scandinavian Cardiac Outcomes Trial—lipid-lowering arm (ASCOT-LLA). Diabetes Care. 2005;28(5):1151-7.

34. Standards of medical care in diabetes–2013. Diabetes Care. 2013;36(Suppl 1):S11-66.

35. Colhoun HM, Betteridge DJ, Durrington PN, et al. Primary prevention of cardiovascular disease with atorvastatin in type 2 diabetes in the Collaborative Atorvastatin Diabetes Study (CARDS): multicentre randomised placebo-controlled trial. Lancet. 2004;364(9435):685-96.

36. Singh IM, Shishehbor MH, Ansell BJ. High-density lipoprotein as a therapeutic target: a systematic review. JAMA. 2007;298(7):786-98.

37. Assmann G, Cullen P, Schulte H. Non-LDL-related dyslipidaemia and coronary risk: a case-control study. Diab Vasc Dis Res. 2010;7(3):204-12.

38. Ginsberg HN, Elam MB, Lovato LC, et al. Effects of combination lipid therapy in type 2 diabetes mellitus. N Engl J Med. 2010;362(17):1563-74.

39. Sarwar N, Danesh J, Eiriksdottir G, et al. Triglycerides and the risk of coronary heart disease: 10,158 incident cases among 262,525 participants in 29 Western prospective studies. Circulation. 2007;115(4):450-8.

40. Boden WE, Probstfield JL, Anderson T, et al. Niacin in patients with low HDL cholesterol levels receiving intensive statin therapy. N Engl J Med. 2011;365(24):2255-67.

41. Chew EY, Klein ML, Ferris FL, et al. Association of elevated serum lipid levels with retinal hard exudate in diabetic retinopathy. Early Treatment Diabetic Retinopathy Study (ETDRS) Report 22. Arch Ophthalmol. 1996;114(9):1079-84.

42. Davis MD, Fisher MR, Gangnon RE, et al. Risk factors for high-risk proliferative diabetic retinopathy and severe visual loss: Early Treatment Diabetic Retinopathy Study Report #18. Invest Ophthalmol Vis Sci. 1998;39(2):233-52.

43. Lyons TJ, Jenkins AJ, Zheng D, et al. Diabetic retinopathy and serum lipoprotein subclasses in the DCCT/EDIC cohort. Invest Ophthalmol Vis Sci. 2004;45(3):910-8.

44. Keech AC, Mitchell P, Summanen PA, et al. Effect of fenofibrate on the need for laser treatment for diabetic retinopathy (FIELD study): a randomised controlled trial. Lancet. 2007;370(9600):1687-97.

45. Sen K, Misra A, Kumar A, et al. Simvastatin retards progression of retinopathy in diabetic patients with hypercholesterolemia. Diabetes Res Clin Pract. 2002;56(1):1-11.

46. Retnakaran R, Cull CA, Thorne KI, et al. Risk factors for renal dysfunction in type 2 diabetes: U.K. Prospective Diabetes Study 74. Diabetes. 2006;55(6):1832-9.

47. Hadjadj S, Duly-Bouhanick B, Bekherraz A, et al. Serum triglycerides are a predictive factor for the development and the progression of renal and retinal complications in patients with type 1 diabetes. Diabetes Metab. 2004;30(1):43-51.

48. Jenkins AJ, Lyons TJ, Zheng D, et al. Lipoproteins in the DCCT/EDIC cohort: associations with diabetic nephropathy. Kidney Int. 2003;64(3):817-28.

49. Smulders YM, Rakic M, Stehouwer CD, et al. Determinants of progression of microalbuminuria in patients with NIDDM. A prospective study. Diabetes Care. 1997;20(6):999-1005.

50. Gaede P, Vedel P, Larsen N, et al. Multifactorial intervention and cardiovascular disease in patients with type 2 diabetes. N Engl J Med. 2003;348(5):383-93.

51. Tesfaye S, Chaturvedi N, Eaton SE, et al. Vascular risk factors and diabetic neuropathy. N Engl J Med. 2005;352(4):341-50.

52. Kempler P, Tesfaye S, Chaturvedi N, et al. Autonomic neuropathy is associated with increased cardiovascular risk factors: the EURODIAB IDDM Complications Study. Diabet Med. 2002;19(11):900-9.

53. Wanner C, Krane V. Recent advances in the treatment of atherogenic dyslipidemia in type 2 diabetes mellitus. Kidney Blood Press Res. 2011;34(4):209-17.

54. Standards of medical care in diabetes–2012. Diabetes Care. 2012;35(Suppl 1):S11-63.

55. Chowdhury S, Pandit K. Dyslipidemia in diabetes. In: Tripathy BB, Chandalia HB, Das AK, et al. (Eds). RSSDI Textbook of Diabetes Mellitus, 2nd edition. New Delhi: Jaypee Brothers; 2008. p. 672.

56. Fonseca VA, Rosenstock J, Wang AC, et al. Colesevelam HCl improves glycemic control and reduces LDL cholesterol in patients with inadequately controlled type 2 diabetes on sulfonylurea-based therapy. Diabetes Care. 2008;31(8):1479-84.

57. Charlton-Menys V, Durrington PN. Squalene synthase inhibitors: clinical pharmacology and cholesterol-lowering potential. Drugs. 2007;67(1):11-6.

58. Nishimoto T, Amano Y, Tozawa R, et al. Lipid-lowering properties of TAK-475, a squalene synthase inhibitor, in vivo and in vitro. Br J Pharmacol. 2003;139(5):911-8.

59. Seiki S, Frishman WH. Pharmacologic inhibition of squalene synthase and other downstream enzymes of the cholesterol synthesis pathway: a new therapeutic approach to treatment of hypercholesterolemia. Cardiol Rev. 2009;17(2):70-6.

60. Chang G, Ruggeri RB, Harwood HJ, Jr. Microsomal triglyceride transfer protein (MTP) inhibitors: discovery of clinically active inhibitors using high-throughput screening and parallel synthesis paradigms. Curr Opin Drug Discov Devel. 2002;5(4):562-70.

CHAPTER 19

Lipids and Kidney Disease

Upendra Singh and Sanjeev Gulati

- Introduction
- Pathophysiology of dyslipidemia in chronic kidney disease and dialysis-dependent patients
- Evidence of association between lipid disorders and cardiovascular outcome in chronic kidney disease
- Management of lipid disorders in chronic kidney disease
- Therapeutics for dyslipidemia in chronic kidney disease
- Conclusion

INTRODUCTION

Hyperlipidemia is a well-established cardiovascular (CV) risk factor in the general population. However, in patients with chronic kidney disease (CKD), the evidence is not similar. Epidemiologic studies[1-3] and clinical trials[4-12] have raised uncertainties regarding the impact of dyslipidemia on clinical outcomes and, consequently, the optimal lipid profile.

The pathophysiology of dyslipidemia in CKD and hemodialysis patients, and its association with clinical outcome and the effects of therapy will be addressed in this chapter.

PATHOPHYSIOLOGY OF DYSLIPIDEMIA IN CHRONIC KIDNEY DISEASE AND DIALYSIS-DEPENDENT PATIENTS

The nature of dyslipidemia in patients with CKD and dialysis-dependent patients is different from that of the general population. It involves the majority of lipoprotein classes and shows variations depending on the stage of CKD (Table 19.1). There seems to be a gradual shift to a distinct (uremic) lipid profile as kidney function declines.[13,14] Diabetes[15] and nephrotic syndrome[16] further modify this pattern.

Chronic kidney disease is not only associated with quantitative changes, but also qualitative changes like increased level of oxidized low-density lipoprotein (LDL), which makes the LDL more atherogenic.

Hypertriglyceridemia

Plasma triglycerides (TGs) start rising in early stages of CKD (Table 19.2), and the highest concentrations are noted in nephrotic syndrome and in dialysis patients, especially those who are

Table 19.1: Trend of changes in lipids, lipoproteins and apoprotein A-IV in various stages of chronic kidney disease[a]

Parameter	CKD 1–5	Nephrotic syndrome	Hemodialysis	Peritoneal dialysis
Total cholesterol	M	11	72	1
LDL-C	M	11	72	1
HDL-C	2	2	2	2
Non-HDL-C	M	11	72	1
TG	M	11	1	1
Lp(a)	m	11	1	11
ApoA-I	n	m	2	2
ApoA-IV	m	1n	1	1
ApoB	m	11	72	1

[a]These trends are derived from the composite of the literature. Non-HDL-C includes cholesterol in LDL, VLDL, IDL and chylomicron and its remnant. Explanation of symbols: normal (7), increased (1), markedly increased (M) and decreased (2) plasma levels compared with nonuremic individuals; increasing (m) and decreasing (n) plasma levels with decreasing GFR.
LDL-C, low-density lipoprotein cholesterol; HDL-C, high-density lipoprotein cholesterol; Lp(a), lipoprotein(a); Apo, apoprotein; TG, triglyceride.

Table 19.2: Association of dyslipidemia and clinical outcomes in dialysis patients

Study[a]	N	Outcome	High TC
Longitudinal studies			
Iseki et al. (1996)[17]	1,491	Incident stroke	7
Degoulet et al. (1982)[2]	1,453	Cardiovascular and all-cause mortality	2
CHOICE study[18,19]	833	Cardiovascular and all-cause mortality	2 in presence of inflammation/ malnutrition; 1 in absence of inflammation/ malnutrition
CHOICE study[18,19]		Incident fatal or nonfatal atherosclerotic cardiovascular events	
Kronenberg et al. (1999)[3]	440	Incident coronary events	7
Koda et al. (1999)[20]	390	Cardiovascular mortality	
Zimmermann et al. (1999)[21]	280	Cardiovascular and all-cause mortality	7

Study[a]	N	Outcome	High TC
Ohashi et al. (1999)[22]	268	Cardiovascular mortality	7
Shoji et al. (2001)[23]	265	Cardiovascular and all-cause mortality	
Hocher et al. (2003)[24]	245	Cardiovascular and all-cause mortality	7
Schwaiger et al. (2006)[25]	165	Cardiovascular events	7
Cressmann et al. (1992)[26]	129	Incident atherosclerotic cardiovascular events	7
Cross-sectional studies			
Stack et al. (2001)[27]	4,025	History of coronary artery disease	7
Koch et al. (1997)[28]	607	History of MI or more then 50% coronary artery disease	7
Cheung et al. (2000)[29]	936	Presence or history of cardiovascular events	7
Güz et al. (2000)[30]	269	Carotid artery intima media thickness	7
Overall			7

[a]Included are only reports with at least 125 patients in prospective studies and at least 200 patients in cross-sectional studies. Presented are outcome measures that were increased (1), unchanged (7) or decreased (2) associated with the indicated dyslipidemia. LMW, low molecular weight; TC, total cholesterol; MI, myocardial infarction.

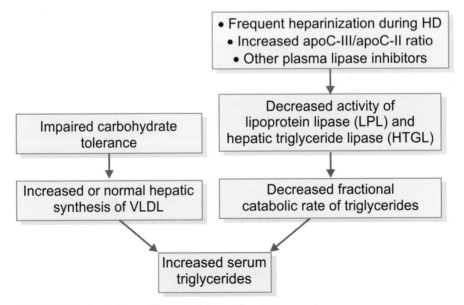

Figure 19.1: Pathophysiology of hypertriglyceridemia in uremia

treated with peritoneal dialysis (PD). Both a high production rate and a low fractional cata-bolic rate[31] (Fig. 19.1) are the causes of hypertriglyceridemia. Increased production of TG-rich lipoproteins is a consequence of impaired carbohydrate tolerance and enhanced hepatic very low-density lipoprotein (VLDL) synthesis.[32] Decreased activity of two endothelium-associated lipase SB-1, lipoprotein lipase and two hepatic TG lipases causes reduced catabolism and as a consequence the hypertriglyceridemia rises further.

High-Density Lipoprotein

Patients with CKD generally have lower plasma high-density lipoprotein cholesterol (HDL-C) concentrations compared with nonuremic counterparts (Table 19.2). The distribution of HDL subfractions is different because of the low apolipoprotein-AI (apoA-1) level and decreased lecithin–cholesterol acyltransferase (LCAT) activity. The esterification of free cholesterol and hence the conversion of HDL_3 to HDL_2 are reduced in uremia. Inflammation might convert HDL from an antioxidant into a pro-oxidant particle.[33,34] All of these contribute to atherogenesis in CKD.

Apolipoprotein A-IV

Apolipoprotein A-IV (apoA-IV) is a glycoprotein that is synthesized primarily in enterocytes of the small intestine. Studies suggest that apoA-IV might protect against atherosclerosis by promoting several steps in the reverse cholesterol transport pathway. This removes cholesterol from periph-eral cells and directs the cholesterol to liver and other organs for biochemical activity.[35,36,37]

Apolipoprotein A-IV has also been identified as a marker of primary CKD, and its plasma levels are already increased when glomerular filtration rate (GFR) is still in normal range (Table 19.2).[20] Furthermore, high plasma apoA-IV concentrations predicted the progression of primary nondiabetic kidney disease. In dialysis patients, apoA-IV levels are twice as high as in the general population.[38,39,40,41]

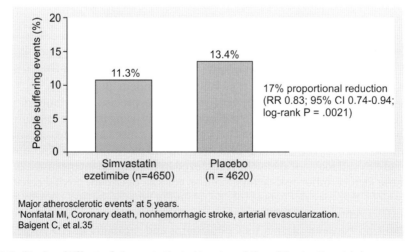

Major atherosclerotic events' at 5 years.
'Nonfatal MI, Coronary death, nonhemorrhagic stroke, arterial revascularization.
Baigent C, et al.35

Figure 19.2: Study of Effect of simvastatin in Heart and Renal Protection trial

Low-Density Lipoprotein

Elevated plasma LDL cholesterol (LDL-C) concentration is seen in nephrotic syndrome but this is not a typical feature of patients with advanced CKD (Table 19.2). Furthermore, qualitative changes in LDL in patients with CKD and dialysis patients are also seen. The proportions of LDL and intermediate-density protein (IDL), which are considered to be highly atherogenic, are high. Oxidized fractions of these trigger the process of atherosclerosis. Decreased hepatic lipase activities in hemodialysis (HD) patients causes impaired conversion IDL to LDL and as a result IDL accumulates in plasma.[42]

A vicious cycle sets in uremic patients. Decreased catabolism of IDL and LDL cause increased plasma dwelling time of these particles. Further modification of the apoB contained in these lipoproteins by oxidation, carbamylation and glycation occurs.[43] Recently, it has been demonstrated that the plasma residence time of LDL and IDL is more than twice as long in individuals on HD compared with nonuremic counterparts (Fig. 19.2). This reduced catabolism, is further modified by the decreased production of LDL, resulting in near-normal plasma levels of LDL.[43]

Lipoprotein(a)

Population-based studies have shown that lipoprotein(a) [Lp(a)] is a genetically determined risk predictor for CVD.[44,45] However, in CKD, plasma Lp(a) levels are also influenced by GFR. Plasma Lp(a) levels begin to increase in stage 1 CKD before GFR starts to decrease.[19] After kidney transplantation, a decrease in plasma Lp(a) can be regularly observed in HD patients with large apo(a) isoforms,[46,47] and in PD patients with all apo(a) isoform groups.[48] In contrast to the general population, the elevation of Lp(a) in CKD is an acquired abnormality. This is mostly influenced by the degree of proteinuria[19,49] and to a lesser extent by the etiology of kidney disorder.[41]

EVIDENCE OF ASSOCIATION BETWEEN LIPID DISORDERS AND CARDIOVASCULAR OUTCOME IN CHRONIC KIDNEY DISEASE

Population-based studies have shown that high plasma concentrations of LDLC, low concentrations of HDL-C, and to some extent high total TG concentrations are associated with increased atherosclerotic CV risk.[50] However, in the dialysis-dependent populations,[2,3,17-30] association between dyslipidemia and CVD is not very strong. The precise contributions of lipids to atherogenicity should probably be evaluated longitudinally using multiple measurements over time, because the plasma lipid patterns change as kidney disease progresses. Moreover, the atherogenic potential of dyslipidemia in CKD may depend more on the apolipoprotein than on lipid abnormalities and may not always be recognized by measurement of plasma lipids alone.[51] On top of these factors, other risk factors, such as volume overload, medial calcification and arrhythmogenicity that may not necessarily be related to atherosclerosis, contribute to clinical expression of CV events.

The relationship between plasma total cholesterol and mortality in HD patients follows a U-shaped distribution pattern.[52,53] Interestingly, the group with total cholesterol between 200 and 250 mg/dL had the lowest risk for death, whereas those with levels > 350 mg/dL had a 1.3-fold relative risk of death and those with levels <100 mg/dL had a 4.2-fold relative risk of death. These observations are compatible with the hypothesis that the inverse association of total cholesterol levels with mortality in dialysis patients is mediated by the cholesterol-lowering effect of malnutrition and/or systemic inflammation.

MANAGEMENT OF LIPID DISORDERS IN CHRONIC KIDNEY DISEASE

In the general population, plasma levels of total, HDL- and LDL-C as well as TGs are the parameters that usually are measured clinically. The total and LDL-C levels are often normal in the CKD and HD populations, but there are increased levels of LDL, IDL and modified (oxidized, glycated or carbamylated) LDL that are presumably more atherogenic. The commonly used biochemical assays do not differentiate among LDL and Lp(a) and its low molecular weight isoform. Clinically used assays for HDL-C also do not capture the alterations in the distribution of cholesterol subclasses.

Based on the recent works, the use of non-HDL-C, calculated as total cholesterol minus HDL-C, was suggested as an alternative.[54] Non-HDL-C includes and does not distinguish among LDL-C and subfractions that are considered to be highly atherogenic, such as Lp(a) and lipoprotein remnant particles. At present, there are insufficient data to establish the role of non-HDL-C for atherosclerosis risk assessment in CKD population.

THERAPEUTICS FOR DYSLIPIDEMIA IN CHRONIC KIDNEY DISEASE

Diet, exercise and statins remain the three prongs approach to the treatment of dyslipidemia in kidney disease patients similar to the approach in general population. However, there are subtle differences.

Statins

As in the general population, statins are very effective in lowering total and LDL-C in CKD patients.[12] The efficacy of statins in reducing CV events, however, may differ depending on the stage of CKD. In several randomized controlled trials of statins, *post hoc* analyses of subgroups with impaired kidney function have been performed. In the Pravastatin Pooling Project,[10] which combined data from three randomized trials, a total of 4991 patients with stage 3 CKD were analyzed. A total of 40 mg/day pravastatin was associated with a 23% reduction in the composite outcome of nonfatal myocardial infarction (MI), coronary mortality and coronary revascularization in stage 3 CKD over 5 years in this analysis. In a prespecified subgroup analysis of 6517 patients with kidney dysfunction in the Anglo-Scandinavian Cardiac Outcomes Trial,[6] 10 mg/day atorvastatin significantly reduced the risk for the primary composite end point of nonfatal MI and cardiac death by 39% over a median of 3.3 years. In both of these studies, individuals with known CVD or high CV risk were recruited; therefore, it is unclear whether these positive results are generalizable to all patients with moderate CKD.

In a retrospective analysis of a registry of 3716 incident dialysis patients, the use of statins at baseline was associated with a significant (36%) reduction in CV and 32% reduction in all-cause mortality.[55] This study, however, was limited by the small number of patients who were on statins (*n* = 362) and possible selection bias. These findings were in general not consistent with the Die Deutsche Diabetes-Dialyse Studie (4D study), a randomized, controlled trial of 1255 HD patients with diabetes.[12] In the 4D study, randomization to 20 mg/day atorvastatin resulted in the reduction in plasma LDL-C levels by 40%, compared with placebo.[12] Despite this difference in cholesterol, there were no statistically significant differences (8% reduction) between the groups in the primary composite end point of cardiac death, stroke or nonfatal MI. In the atorvastatin group, there was also an 18% decrease in cardiac events (205 vs. 246; $P = 0.03$) but a twofold increase in fatal strokes (27 vs. 13; $P = 0.04$).

These results, along with the seemingly paradoxic epidemiologic relationship between plasma cholesterol levels and mortality,[12] have prompted a less aggressive statin therapy in CKD. Proponents of the use of statins in dialysis patients, however, point out that the 4D study was powered only to detect a 27% difference in the primary end point and not a more modest effect size of, for example, even 15%. Despite the twofold increase in fatal stroke in the 4D study, the absolute number of events was small, compared with the number of cardiac events, which seemed to respond favorably to atorvastatin. Moreover, approximately 15% of the patients in the placebo arm received a non-study statin, and 15% of the patients who received atorvastatin required a dosage reduction to 10 mg/day. These drop-ins and dropouts might have resulted in the convergent trend in plasma LDL-C levels between the two treatment arms over time. Nevertheless, the time-averaged difference in plasma LDL-C was approximately 0.9 mmol/L, which was similar in magnitude to that observed in many positive statin trials. Many of the CV events in dialysis patients were due to arrhythmia or nonischemic cardiomyopathy, which might not be related to atherosclerosis and could have diluted the potentially beneficial effects of statins. Finally, even though statins were effective in lowering plasma LDL-C, they have minimal effects on plasma TGs and HDL-C and no effects on Lp(a). Because uremic dyslipidemia is complex and characterized by these three components and not elevated LDL-C alone, lowering of plasma LDL-C levels in uremic patients might not produce substantial clinical benefits. It is reasonable to conclude from the 4D study that, in dialysis patients without overtly high plasma LDL-C levels, the effect of statins on clinical outcome are probably not large enough. However, a modest effect cannot be ruled out.

Evidence for Primary Prevention

The Justification for the Use of Statin in Prevention: an Intervention Trial Evaluating Rosuvastatin (JUPITER) demonstrated the benefits of targeting inflammation in patients at risk for CVD.[56] The JUPITER trial included 17,802 apparently healthy adults who had normal LDL-C levels (<130 mg/dL) but elevated high-sensitivity CRP (hs-CRP) levels (≥2.0 mg/L). Patients were randomly assigned to treatment with rosuvastatin 20 mg/day or placebo. After a median follow-up of 1.9 years, statin therapy reduced the risk of major CV events 44% compared with placebo. Patients receiving statin therapy also had major reductions in LDL-C levels (mean 50%) and hs-CRP concentrations (mean 37%). In a subgroup analysis of the JUPITER trial, investigators evaluated outcomes in patients with moderate CKD, defined as estimated glomerular filtration rate (eGFR) <60 mL/min/1.73 m² ($n = 3,276$).

Cardiovascular events were significantly more common in patients with moderate CKD than in those with eGFR ≥60 mL/min/1.73 m², underscoring the role of CKD as a risk factor for CV morbidity. For patients with CKD, statin therapy significantly reduced the risk of CV events 45% and reduced all-cause mortality 44% compared with placebo. Findings from JUPITER therefore support use of statin therapy to reduce the risk of major CV events in patients with CKD and elevated markers of inflammation, one of the earliest signs of underlying atherosclerotic disease.

The Study of Heart and Renal Protection (SHARP) examines the effect of lowering plasma cholesterol using the combination of simvastatin and ezetimibe on the primary prevention of heart disease and stroke. SHARP was the first trial of lipid-lowering therapy to enroll only patients with primary CKD. It enrolled patients across a broad spectrum of CKD severity, including those who were not treated with maintenance dialysis.[57] Overall, SHARP included 9438 patients with CKD either on dialysis (n = 3023) or with a creatinine level of ≥1.7 mg/dL for men or ≥1.5 mg/dL for women (n = 6247). Importantly, patients had no history of MI or coronary revascularization at the time of enrollment. Initially, patients were randomly assigned to one of three groups: ezetimibe/simvastatin (10 mg/20 mg), simvastatin 20 mg or placebo. After 1 year of treatment, patients in the simvastatin monotherapy group were rerandomized to receive either ezetimibe/simvastatin or placebo. This reassignment was preplanned in the study protocol to occur if adverse events were no greater with ezetimibe/ simvastatin than with simvastatin alone after 1 year. The final analysis compared patients randomized to ezetimibe/simvastatin versus placebo. The primary end point was the occurrence of a major atherosclerotic event, defined as death due to coronary heart disease (CHD), nonfatal MI, nonhemorrhagic stroke or the need for arterial revascularization procedures. During a median follow-up of 4.9 years of patients not undergoing dialysis, treatment with ezetimibe/simvastatin reduced the risk of major atherosclerotic events by 17% compared with placebo (11.3 vs. 13.4%; P = 0.0021). Among the individual components of the composite end point, treatment with ezetimibe/simvastatin significantly reduced the risk of nonhemorrhagic stroke 25% (2.8 vs. 3.8%; P = 0.01) and reduced the need for arterial revascularization procedures 21% (6.1 vs. 7.6%; P = 0.0036). Ezetimibe/simvastatin also showed a nonsignificant trend toward a reduced risk of nonfatal MI or death from CHD compared with placebo. This study does not separate the beneficial effects of ezetimibe or simvastatin alone. However, if there is concern about the use of high-dose statins in advanced CKD or end-stage renal disease (ESRD), because of heightened risk of muscle- or liver-related adverse events, the SHARP trial does provide reassurance that a low, fixed-dose statin in combination with ezetimibe might be an effective and safe alternative. Moreover, statins may have other beneficial effects such as reducing inflammation, which is highly prevalent in patients with CKD and an independent predictor of CV events and death. An Assessment of Survival and Cardiovascular Events study examines the effect of rosuvastatin on the incidence of heart attacks, strokes and CV deaths in HD patients both with and without diabetes, irrespective of baseline lipid levels.

Two new studies, Prospective Evaluation of Proteinuria and Renal Function in Diabetic Patients with Progressive Renal Disease PLANET I (n = 325) and PLANET II (n = 220), enrolled patients with urinary protein/creatinine ratios of 500–5000 mg/g and a fasting LDL-C level of 90 mg/dL or higher.[58] The patients were stable on and had used angiotensin-converting enzyme inhibitors or angiotensin II receptor blockers for at least 3 months before enrollment. The patients were randomized to atorvastatin at 80 mg/day, rosuvastatin at 10 mg/day and rousvastatin at 40 mg/day. In PLANET I, atorvastatin was associated with a significant reduction on proteinuria by approximately 20%, but there was no effect on the rate of decline of GFR, whereas rosuvastatin worsened GFR by 8 mL/min/year but had no effect on proteinuria. A similar result was noted in the PLANET II study.[31] The incidence of common renal adverse reactions observed was higher with the use of rousvastatin compared with other statins.[148,149] Some studies have reported increased incidence of adverse effects (e.g., liver damage and rhabdomyolysis) with the use of statins in CKD. However, this concern was not substantiated by the 4D study[12] and most other large studies.[7,10,11] Notably, the risk for myopathy in patients with CKD seems to be increased when statins are used in combination with fibrates.[59,60]

Fibrates

Fibric acid derivatives are effective in reducing plasma TG concentrations and modestly increasing HDL-C concentrations in the general population.[61,62] The use of gemfibrozil was associated with a 20% reduction in CV events in those with creatinine clearances of 30–75 mL/min.[9] There are limited data on the effects of fibrates on clinical outcomes in patients with CKD or HD patients. Evidence is strong in support of an increased risk for myopathy that is associated with this class of drug in patients with advanced GFR impairment.[63,64]

Nicotinic Acid Derivatives

Nicotinic acid derivatives are the most suitable drugs that are available to produce a favorable impact on uremic dyslipidemia. They are effective in raising plasma HDL-C level and are the only drugs available to lower plasma Lp(a) significantly.[65] They reduce TG levels by 20–50%,[66] lower VLDL cholesterol and free fatty acids and shift the small, dense LDL fraction to larger, more buoyant particles.[67] They also lower plasma LDL-C levels. Common adverse effects are cutaneous flushing, pruritus, rashes, nausea and gastrointestinal adverse effects. These adverse effects are less often observed with the extended-release formulations. The compliance of patients can be increased by the coadministration of aspirin and gradual dosage escalation that decreases the adverse effects.[68] In the general population, nicotinic acid has been shown to improve cardiac and cerebrovascular outcomes.[69-72] However, recent data from the Heart Protection Study-Thrive study have negated these findings. Studies that used nicotinic acid in patients with CKD were mostly small with short durations of follow-up but showed the expected changes in lipid and lipoprotein profiles.[68] No studies have examined the impact of nicotinic acid on CVD outcomes in patients with CKD or HD patients.

Antioxidants

Dialysis patients in general are in a state of high oxidative stress. A beneficial effect of vitamin E on the oxidative susceptibility of LDL-C in dialysis patients has been shown.[73-75] Treatment with tocopherol also resulted in partial normalization of malondialdehyde modifications of LDL-C in dialysis patients.[76] Vitamin E may also exert an additive or synergistic effect with statins. In a study on dialysis patients, treatment with atorvastatin was found to be effective in lowering plasma total cholesterol, TGs, LDL-C, apoB and oxidized low-density lipoprotein (ox-LDL) levels by 30–40%, and the addition of tocopherol to atorvastatin further reduced in vitro LDL oxidation.[74] The Secondary Prevention with Antioxidants of Cardiovascular Disease in End-stage Renal Disease (SPACE) trial suggested that vitamin E supplementation lowers the incidence of major CV events in HD patients. However, total mortality[77] was not affected. The impact of antioxidants on the clinical outcomes of patients with CKD and dialysis patients is not conclusive and this needs further study.[78]

Sevelamer

This metal-free phosphate binder has also been shown to reduce plasma total and LDL-C concentrations by 18–22% and 30–37%, respectively, by acting as a bile acid sequestrant.[79] Whether this reduction in cholesterol contributes to the decreased progression of coronary calcification[80] is unclear.

Impact of Dialysis Membrane on Dyslipidemia

One interesting observation is the impact of type of dialysis membrane used in these patients Compared with high-flux modified cellulosic membrane, HD using high-flux polysulfone membranes was associated with a decrease in plasma total TGs by 10%, cholesterol in remnant particles by 21% and ox-LDL by 15%.[81] The mechanism of these reductions might be related to potential differences in dialysis membrane biocompatibility that affects inflammatory responses and/or differences in the removal of plasma lipase inhibitory molecules.

Use of vitamin E-coated membrane dialyzer results in a significant reduction in ox-LDL or malondialdehyde-rich LDL and an attenuation of the increase in aortic calcification index after 24 months.[75] Lipid apheresis is very effective in lowering plasma LDL-C, and, depending on the technique, can also lower plasma Lp(a), TGs and fibrinogen.[82] At present, the effects of these extracorporeal therapies on clinical outcomes are unclear.

Experimental Therapies

A number of novel therapeutic options are in various stages of development for modulating lipids and lipoproteins. They include lipase gene transfer,[83] apoA-I (Milano) infusion[84] and short interfering RNA for apoB.[85] However, at present, they are not ready for clinical use and must be considered experimental in uremic dyslipidemia.

CONCLUSION

Chronic kidney disease and nephrotic syndrome are associated with alteration in lipid parameters .The optimal targets for plasma lipids in patients with CKD and on HD are unknown. The commonly used clinical assays to measure TGs and total, LDL- and HDL-C may not capture the clinically relevant lipid abnormalities of uremia, such as elevated Lp(a), IDL cholesterol, modified LDL-C and alterations in HDL-C subfractions. Data from clinical trials support the beneficial effects of statins in early stages of CKD. However, there is a lack of data on the use of statins in stages 4 and 5 of CKD. Data in patients who are treated by PD as well as in nondiabetic HD patients are too sparse to draw any conclusion on these subpopulations. Statins are not very effective in correcting the elevated plasma concentrations of TGs and Lp(a) as well as decreased plasma concentrations of HDL-C, which are the major lipid abnormalities seen in uremia. The 4D study did not provide definitive evidence for statins to improve CV outcomes in HD patients with diabetes. Nicotinic acid derivatives and, to a lesser extent, fibrates may be more suitable to treat uremic dyslipidemia; however, this does not translate into better CV protection.

Physicians dealing with kidney disease should detect and treat dyslipidemia at early stages of CKD. Most of the experts believe that targeting lipoproteins may be important to decrease CVD in this high-risk population with adverse CV event risk. Adequately powered studies are required to elucidate the protective role of statin and other agents on the CV outcome in the population with CKD.

REFERENCES

1. Iseki K, Yamazato M, Tozawa M, et al. Hypocholesterolemia is a significant predictor of death in a cohort of chronic hemodialysis patients. Kidney Int. 2002;61:1887-93.
2. Degoulet P, Legrain M, Reach I, et al. Mortality risk factors in patients treated by chronic hemodialysis. Report of the Diaphane collaborative study. Nephron. 1982;31:103-10.
3. Kronenberg F, Neyer U, Lhotta K, et al. The low molecular weight apo(a) phenotype is an independent predictor for coronary artery disease in hemodialysis patients: a prospective follow-up. J Am Soc Nephrol. 1999;10:1027-36.
4. Ferramosca E, Burke S, Chasan-Taber S, et al. Potential antiatherogenic and anti-inflammatory properties of sevelamer in maintenance hemodialysis patients. Am Heart J. 2005;149:820-5.
5. Holdaas H, Wanner C, Abletshauser C, et al. The effect of fluvastatin on cardiac outcomes in patients with moderate to severe renal insufficiency: a pooled analysis of double-blind, randomized trials. Int J Cardiol. 2006;117:64-74.
6. Sever PS, Dahlof B, Poulter NR, et al. Prevention of coronary and stroke events with atorvastatin in hypertensive patients who have average or lower-than-average cholesterol concentrations, in the Anglo-Scandinavian Cardiac Outcomes Trial–Lipid Lowering Arm (ASCOT-LLA): a multicentre randomised controlled trial. Lancet. 2003;361:1149-58.
7. MRC/BHF Heart Protection Study of cholesterol lowering with simvastatin in 20 536 high-risk individuals: a randomised placebo-controlled trial. Lancet. 2002;360:7-22.
8. Lemos PA, Serruys PW, de Feyter P, et al. Long-term fluvastatin reduces the hazardous effect of renal impairment on four-year atherosclerotic outcomes (a LIPS substudy). Am J Cardiol. 2005;95:445-51.
9. Tonelli M, Collins D, Robins S, et al. Gemfibrozil for secondary prevention of cardiovascular events in mild to moderate chronic renal insufficiency. Kidney Int. 2004;66:1123-30.
10. Tonelli M, Isles C, Curhan GC, et al. Effect of pravastatin on cardiovascular events in people with chronic kidney disease. Circulation. 2004; 110:1557-63.
11. Tonelli M, Moye L, Sacks FM, et al. Pravastatin for secondary prevention of cardiovascular events in persons with mild chronic renal insufficiency. Ann Intern Med. 2003;138:98-104.
12. Wanner C, Krane V, Marz W, et al. Atorvastatin in patients with type 2 diabetes mellitus undergoing hemodialysis. N Engl J Med. 2005;353:238-48.
13. Kronenberg F, Kuen E, Ritz E, et al. Lipoprotein(a) serum concentrations and apolipoprotein(a) phenotypes in mild and moderate renal failure. J Am Soc Nephrol. 200;11:105-15.
14. Kronenberg F, Kuen E, Ritz E, et al. Apolipoprotein A-IV serum concentrations are elevated in patients with mild and moderate renal failure. J Am Soc Nephrol. 2002;13:461-9.
15. Krentz AJ. Lipoprotein abnormalities and their consequences for patients with type 2 diabetes. Diabetes Obes Metab. 2003;5 Suppl 1:S19-27.
16. Kronenberg F. Dyslipidemia and nephrotic syndrome: recent advances. J Ren Nutr. 2005;15:195-203.
17. Iseki K, Fukiyama K. Predictors of stroke in patients receiving chronic hemodialysis. Kidney Int. 1996;50:1672-5.
18. Liu Y, Coresh J, Eustace JA, et al. Association between cholesterol level and mortality in dialysis patients: role of inflammation and malnutrition. JAMA. 2004;291:451-9.
19. Longenecker JC, Klag MJ, Marcovina SM, et al. High lipoprotein(a) levels and small apolipoprotein(a) size prospec-tively predict cardiovascular events in dialysis patients. J Am Soc Nephrol. 2005;16:1794-802.
20. Koda Y, Nishi S, Suzuki M, et al. Lipoprotein(a) is a predictor for cardiovascular mortality of hemodialysis patients. Kidney Int Suppl. 1999;71:S251-3.
21. Zimmermann J, Herrlinger S, Pruy A, Metzger T, Wanner C: Inflammation enhances cardiovascular risk and mortal-ity in hemodialysis patients. Kidney Int 55: 648–658, 1999.
22. Ohashi H, Oda H, Ohno M, et al. Lipoprotein(a) as a risk factor for coronary artery disease in hemodialysis patients. Kidney Int Suppl. 1999;71:S242-4.

23. Shoji T, Emoto M, Shinohara K, et al. Diabetes mellitus, aortic stiffness, and cardiovascular mortality in end-stage renal disease. J Am Soc Nephrol. 2001;12:2117-24.

24. Hocher B, Ziebig R, Altermann C, et al. Different impact of biomarkers as mortality predictors among diabetic and nondiabetic patients undergoing hemodialysis. J Am Soc Nephrol. 2003;14:2329-37.

25. Schwaiger JP, Lamina C, Neyer U, et al. Carotid plaques and their predictive value for cardiovascular disease and all-cause mortality in hemodialysis patients considering renal transplantation: a decade follow-up. Am J Kidney Dis. 2006;47:888-97.

26. Cressman MD, Heyka RJ, Paganini EP, O'Neil J, Skibinski CI, Hoff HF: Lipoprotein(a) is an independent risk factor for cardiovascular disease in hemodialysis patients. Circu-lation. 1992;86: 475-482.

27. Stack AG, Bloembergen WE. Prevalence and clinical correlates of coronary artery disease among new dialysis patients in the United States: a cross-sectional study. J Am Soc Nephrol. 2001;12:1516-23.

28. Steinmetz A, Barbaras R, Ghalim N, et al. Human apolipoprotein A-IV binds to apolipoprotein A-I/A-II receptor sites and promotes cholesterol efflux from adipose cells. J Biol Chem. 1990;265:7859-63.

29. Cheung AK, Sarnak MJ, Yan G, et al. Atherosclerotic cardiovascular disease risks in chronic hemodialysis patients. Kidney Int. 2000;58:353-62.

30. Guz G, Nurhan Ozdemir F, Sezer S, et al. Effect of apolipoprotein E polymorphism on serum lipid, lipoproteins, and atherosclerosis in hemodialysis patients. Am J Kidney Dis. 2000;36:826-36.

31. Hocher B, Ziebig R, Altermann C, et al. Different impact of biomarkers as mortality predictors among diabetic and nondiabetic patients undergoing hemodialysis. J Am Soc Nephrol. 2003;14:2329-37.

32. Cressman MD, Heyka RJ, Paganini EP, O'Neil J, Skibinski CI, Hoff HF: Lipoprotein(a) is an independent risk factor for cardiovascular disease in hemodialysis patients. Circu-lation. 1992;86:475-482.

33. Dvorin E, Gorder NL, Benson DM, et al. Apolipoprotein A-IV. A determinant for binding and uptake of high density lipoproteins by rat hepatocytes. J Biol Chem. 1986;261:15714-8.

34. Nestel PJ, Fidge NH, Tan MH: Increased lipoprotein-remnant formation in chronic renal failure. N Engl J Med. 1982;307: 329-333.

35. Steinmetz A, Barbaras R, Ghalim N, et al. Human apolipoprotein A-IV binds to apolipoprotein A-I/A-II receptor sites and promotes cholesterol efflux from adipose cells. J Biol Chem. 1990;265:7859-63.

36. Stein O, Stein Y, Lefevre M, et al. The role of apolipoprotein A-IV in reverse cholesterol transport studied with cultured cells and liposomes derived from an ether analog of phosphatidylcholine. Biochim Biophys Acta. 1986;878:7-13.

37. Dvorin E, Gorder NL, Benson DM, et al. Apolipoprotein A-IV. A determinant for binding and uptake of high density lipoproteins by rat hepatocytes. J Biol Chem. 1986;261:15714-8.

38. Nestel PJ, Fidge NH, Tan MH: Increased lipoprotein-remnant formation in chronic renal failure. N Engl J Med. 1982;307: 329–333.

39. Seishima M, Muto Y: An increased apo A-IV serum concentration of patients with chronic renal failure on hemodialysis. Clin Chim Acta 167: 303–311, 1987

40. Dieplinger H, Lobentanz EM, Konig P, Graf H, Sandholzer C, Matthys E, Rosseneu M, Utermann G: Plasma apolipoprotein A-IV metabolism in patients with chronic renal disease. Eur J Clin Invest 22: 166–174, 1992.

41. Kronenberg F, Konig P, Neyer U, Auinger M, Pribasnig A, Lang U, Reitinger J, Pinter G, Utermann G, Dieplinger H: Multicenter study of lipoprotein(a) and apolipoprotein(a) phenotypes in patients with end-stage renal disease treated by hemodialysis or continuous ambulatory peritoneal dialysis. J Am Soc Nephrol 6: 110–120, 1995

42. Oi K, Hirano T, Sakai S, et al. Role of hepatic lipase in intermediate-density lipoprotein and small, dense low-density lipoprotein formation in hemodialysis patients. Kidney Int Suppl. 1999;71:S227-8.

43. Ikewaki K, Schaefer JR, Frischmann ME, Okubo K, Hosoya T, Mochizuki S, Dieplinger B, Trenk-walder E, Schweer H, Kronenberg F, Koenig P, Dieplinger H: Delayed in vivo catabolism of interme-diate-density lipoprotein and low-density lipoprotein in hemodialysis patients as potential cause of premature atherosclerosis. Arterioscler Thromb Vasc Biol 25: 2615–2622, 2005

44. Craig WY, Neveux LM, Palomaki GE, Cleveland MM, Haddow JE: Lipoprotein(a) as a risk factor for ischemic heart disease: Metaanalysis of prospective studies. Clin Chem 44: 2301–2306, 1998

45. Dieplinger H, Kronenberg F: Genetics and metabolism of lipoprotein(a) and their clinical implica-tions (Part 1). Wien Klin Wochenschr 111: 5–20, 1999

46. Kronenberg F, Konig P, Lhotta K, Ofner D, Sandholzer C, Margreiter R, Dosch E, Utermann G, Die-plinger H: Apoli- poprotein(a) phenotype-associated decrease in lipopro- tein(a) plasma concen-trations after renal transplantation. Arterioscler Thromb 14: 1399–1404, 1994

47. Kronenberg F, Lhotta K, Konig P, Margreiter R, Dieplinger H, Utermann G: Apolipoprotein(a) iso-form-specific changes of lipoprotein(a) after kidney transplantation. Eur J Hum Genet 11: 693–699, 2003

48. erschdorfer L, Konig P, Neyer U, Bosmuller C, Lhotta K, Auinger M, Hohenegger M, Riegler P, Mar-greiter R, Uter- mann G, Dieplinger H, Kronenberg F: Lipoprotein(a) plasma concentrations after renal transplantation: A pro- spective evaluation after 4 years of follow-up. Atheroscle- rosis 144: 381–391, 1999

49. Kronenberg F, Lingenhel A, Lhotta K, Rantner B, Kronenberg MF, Konig P, Thiery J, Koch M, von Eckardstein A, Dieplinger H: The apolipoprotein(a) size polymorphism is associated with nephrotic syndrome. Kidney Int 65: 606 – 612, 2004

50. Wilson PW, D'Agostino RB, Levy D, Belanger AM, Silber- shatz H, Kannel WB: Prediction of coro-nary heart disease using risk factor categories. Circulation 97: 1837–1847, 1998

51. Attman PO, Alaupovic P. Lipid and apolipoprotein profiles of uremic dyslipoproteinemia: relation to renal function and dialysis. Nephron. 1991;57:401-10.

52. Lowrie EG, Lew NL. Commonly measured laboratory variables in hemodialysis patients: relation-ships among them and to death risk. Semin Nephrol. 1992;12:276-83.

53. Lowrie EG, Lew NL. Death risk in hemodialysis patients: the predictive value of commonly measured variables and an evaluation of death rate differences between facilities. Am J Kidney Dis. 1990;15:458-82.

54. K/DOQI clinical practice guidelines for management of dyslipidemias in patients with kidney dis-ease. Am J Kidney Dis 41: S1–S91, 2003

55. Seliger SL, Weiss NS, Gillen DL, Kestenbaum B, Ball A, Sherrard DJ, Stehman-Breen CO: HMG-CoA reductase in- hibitors are associated with reduced mortality in ESRD patients. Kidney Int 61: 297–304, 2002

56. Ridker PM, MacFadyen J, Cressman M, Glynn RJ. Efficacy of rosuvastatin among men and women with moderate chronic kidney disease and elevated high-sensitivity C-reactive protein: a second-ary analysis from the JUPITER (Justification for the Use of Statins in Prevention–an Intervention Trial Evaluating Rosuvastatin) trial. J Am Coll Cardiol 2010;55:1266–73

57. Baigent C, Landry M. Study of Heart and Renal Protection (SHARP). Kidney Int 2003;84 Suppl:S207-10.

58. Prospective Evaluation of Proteinuria and Renal Function in Diabetic Patients With Progressive Renal Disease Trial. Available at: http://clinicaltrials.gov/ct2/show/NCT00296400?term-planet&rank-1. Accessed April 11, 2010.

59. Ballantyne CM, Corsini A, Davidson MH, Holdaas H, Jacobson TA, Leitersdorf E, Marz W, Reckless JP, Stein EA: Risk for myopathy with statin therapy in high-risk pa- tients. Arch Intern Med 163: 553–564, 2003

60. Shek A, Ferrill MJ: Statin-fibrate combination therapy. Ann Pharmacother 35: 908–917, 2001

61. Wanner C, Bartens W, Walz G, Nauck M, Schollmeyer P: Protein loss and genetic polymorphism of apolipopro- tein(a) modulate serum lipoprotein(a) in CAPD patients. Nephrol Dial Transplant 10: 75–81, 1995

62. Grundy SM, Vega GL. Fibric acids: effects on lipids and lipoprotein metabolism. Am J Med. 1987;83:9-20.
63. Knopp RH. Drug treatment of lipid disorders. N Engl J Med. 1999;341:498-511.
64. Schonfeld G: The effects of fibrates on lipoprotein and hemostatic coronary risk factors. Atherosclerosis. 1994;111:161-74.
65. Carlson LA, Hamsten A, Asplund A. Pronounced lowering of serum levels of lipoprotein Lp(a) in hyperlipidaemic subjects treated with nicotinic acid. J Intern Med. 1989;226:271-6.
66. McKenney J. New perspectives on the use of niacin in the treatment of lipid disorders. Arch Intern Med. 2004;164:697-705.
67. Superko HR, Krauss RM. Differential effects of nicotinic acid in subjects with different LDL subclass patterns. Atherosclerosis. 1992;95:69-76.
68. Kronenberg F. Epidemiology, pathophysiology and therapeutic implications of lipoprotein(a) in kidney disease. Expert Rev Cardiovasc Ther. 2004; 2:729-43.
69. Taylor AJ, Sullenberger LE, Lee HJ, et al. Arterial biology for the investigation of the treatment effects of reducing cholesterol (ARBITER) 2: a double-blind, placebo-controlled study of extended-release niacin on atherosclerosis progression in secondary prevention patients treated with statins. Circulation. 2004;110:3512.
70. Canner PL, Berge KG, Wenger NK, et al. Fifteen year mortality in Coronary Drug Project patients: long-term benefit with niacin. J Am Coll Cardiol. 1986;8:1245-55.
71. Carlson LA, Rosenhamer G. Reduction of mortality in the Stockholm Ischaemic Heart Disease Secondary Prevention Study by combined treatment with clofibrate and nicotinic acid. Acta Med Scand. 1988;223:405-18.
72. Brown BG, Zhao XQ, Chait A, et al. Simvastatin and niacin, antioxidant vitamins, or the combination for the prevention of coronary disease. N Engl J Med. 2001;345:1583-92.
73. Islam KN, O'Byrne D, Devaraj S, et al. Alpha-tocopherol supplementation decreases the oxidative susceptibility of LDL in renal failure patients on dialysis therapy. Atherosclerosis. 2000;150:217224.
74. Diepeveen SH, Verhoeven GW, Van Der Palen J, et al. Effects of atorvastatin and vitamin E on lipoproteins and oxidative stress in dialysis patients: a randomised-controlled trial. J Intern Med. 2005;257:438-45.
75. Mune M, Yukawa S, Kishino M, et al. Effect of vitamin E on lipid metabolism and atherosclerosis in ESRD patients. Kidney Int Suppl. 1999;71:S126-9.
76. Yukawa S, Hibino A, Maeda T, et al. Effect of alpha-tocopherol on in vitro and in vivo metabolism of low-density lipoproteins in haemodialysis patients. Nephrol Dial Transplant. 1995;10 Suppl 3:1-3.
77. Boaz M, Smetana S, Weinstein T, et al. Secondary prevention with antioxidants of cardiovascular disease in endstage renal disease (SPACE): randomised placebo-controlled trial. Lancet. 2000;356:1213-8.
78. Mann JF, Lonn EM, Yi Q, et al. Effects of vitamin E on cardiovascular outcomes in people with mild-to-moderate renal insufficiency: results of the HOPE study. Kidney Int. 2004;65:1375-80.
79. Chertow GM, Burke SK, Raggi P. Sevelamer attenuates the progression of coronary and aortic calcification in hemodialysis patients. Kidney Int. 2002;62:245-52.
80. Block GA, Spiegel DM, Ehrlich J, et al. Effects of sevelamer and calcium on coronary artery calcification in patients new to hemodialysis. Kidney Int. 2005;68:1815-24.
81. Wanner C, Bahner U, Mattern R, et al. Effect of dialysis flux and membrane material on dyslipidaemia and inflammation in haemodialysis patients. Nephrol Dial Transplant. 2004;19:2570-5.
82. Bosch T, Gahr S, Belschner U, et al. Direct adsorption of low-density lipoprotein by DALI-LDL-apheresis: results of a prospective long-term multicenter follow-up covering 12,291 sessions. Ther Apher Dial. 2006;10:210-18.

83. Rip J, Nierman MC, Sierts JA, et al. Gene therapy for lipoprotein lipase deficiency: working toward clinical application. Hum Gene Ther. 2005;16:1276-86.

84. Fazio S, Linton MF. Apolipoprotein AI as therapy for atherosclerosis: does the future of preventive cardiology include weekly injections of the HDL protein? Mol Interv. 2003;3:436-40.

85. Soutschek J, Akinc A, Bramlage B, et al. Therapeutic silencing of an endogenous gene by systemic administration of modified siRNAs. Nature. 2004;432:173-8.

Evolving Targets and Therapeutic Agents for Dyslipidemia

Tapan Ghose and Satya Nand Pathak

INTRODUCTION

Three most recent clinical trials, the TNT (Treat to New Target trial)[1], PROVE IT-TIMI-22 (Pravastatin or Atorvastatin Evaluation and Infection Therapy-Thrombolysis in Myocardial Infarction 22) trial[2] and the JUPITER (Justification for the Use of Statin in Prevention and Intervention Trial Evaluating Rosuvastatin) trial[3] have provided a valuable new information on the relationship between low-density lipoprotein (LDL) cholesterol level and cardiovascular (CV) event rate with demonstration that reduction in LDL-C to mean level of 77 mg/dL, 62 mg/dL and 55 mg/dL respectively was associated with greater reduction in the CV events. These studies show that a continued linear relationship exists between LDL-C and CV events. Lack of demonstrated of a definite threshold or plateau between LDL-C and CV risk generates a hypothesis that even further reduction in LDL-C beyond 55 mg/dL could provide additional benefit in CV events reduction. Cardiovascular experts have now begun to consider lower level of LDL-C values an ideal. For human beings value between 30 and 50 mg/dL represents the physiological ideal.[4-6] We also know that our brain could develop at very low level of LDL cholesterol. Human umbilical cord blood level of LDL is 35 mg/dL approximately total cholesterol in male neonates 62 mg/dL and female neonates 67 mg/dL. The problem with these ideal values is that significant number of high-risk patients fail to achieve their recommended target levels and most CV events are actually not prevented, leaving a huge residual risk for subsequent clinical events in these patients. Further, the IMPROVE IT (The Improved Reduction of Outcomes: a multicenter, randomized, double-blind, active-control trial, testing the addition of ezetimibe to simvastatin therapy on CV outcomes relative to simvastatin monotherapy in patients with acute coronary syndrome) trial also demonstrated an interesting finding. Total death, myocardial infarction and stroke could be further reduced by addition of a non-statin agent (ezetimibe) on the top of maximally tolerated dose of a well-studied statin (simvastatin). Thus, there is further scope of improvement in the pharmacotherapy of lipid disorders.

In this chapter, we shall focus mainly upon emerging approaches to modify six main targets of dyslipidemia namely: (1) LDL, (2) lipoprotein (a), (3) triglyceride-rich lipoproteins, (4) high-density lipoproteins (HDL), (5) nuclear receptors and (6) phospholipases.

PROPROTEIN CONVERTASE SUBTILISIN/KEXIN TYPE 9 (PCSK9) INHIBITOR

Proprotein convertase subtilisin/kexin type 9 is a protein that is expressed in the liver and regulates hepatic LDL receptor dissociation. Once PCSK9 is secreted in the plasma it directly binds to LDL-R and enhances its degradation. The increased degradation of LDL-R leads to reduced LDL-C removal and thus higher circulating LDL-C in the plasma.[7,8] The PCSK9 inhibitor acts by inhibiting the PCSK9 and thus preventing degradation of LDL-R that leads to increased LDL-C removal from plasma.

The lead came from the mutation studies. Two types of PCSK9 mutation have been identified: (1) gain of function mutation (rare form) that leads to autosomal dominant form of severe hypercholesterolemia that increases the risk of coronary heart disease (CHD), (2) loss of function mutation (common form) that leads to reduced plasma level of LDL-C that confers protection from CV disease.

Approved PCSK9 inhibitor for clinical usage is alirocumab and evolocumab. Both are given by injection.

ODYSSEY trial (Evaluation of Cardiovascular Outcomes After an Acute Coronary Syndrome During Treatment With Alirocumab) shows that alirocumab, when added to statin therapy at the maximum tolerated dose, significantly reduced LDL cholesterol levels and there was an evidence of a reduction in the rate of CV events with alirocumab.

CHOLESTERYL ESTER TRANSFER PROTEIN (CETP) INHIBITORS

Cholesteryl ester transfer protein facilitates the transfer of esterified cholesterol from HDL to VLDL (very low-density lipoprotein) and LDL particles, in exchange for triglyceride. Lower CETP activity has been associated with higher HDL-C levels.[9,10] Common CETP inhibitors are torcetrapib, dalcetrapib, anacetrapib and evacetrapib. Development of torcetrapib was halted prematurely due to increased CV morbidity and mortality. This effect of torcetrapib is due to upregulation of cortisol and aldosterone synthesis that leads to elevation of blood pressure.[11] Dalcetrapib is a CETP inhibitor with no effects on neurohormones and minimal effect on blood pressure and LDL-C. However, despite increasing HDL-C it had no effect on vascular endothelial function, or CV events. Anacetrapib and evacetrapib are two CETP inhibitors that have pronounced LDL-lowering as well as HDL-raising effects.[12,13]

SQUALENE SYNTHASE INHIBITOR

Squalene synthase converts farnesyl pyrophosphate to squalene, which is an important step in cholesterol biosynthesis. Inhibition of squalene synthase lowers plasma cholesterol levels. Lapaquistat acetate is a squalene synthase inhibitor that decreases LDL-C by 20% and C-reactive protein levels by 25%. However, development of lapaquistat was halted due to reported cases of severe liver enzyme elevation.[14]

INHIBITOR OF APOLIPOPROTEIN B100 EXPRESSION

Apolipoprotein (ApoB)-containing lipoproteins are LDL, VLDL, and VLDL remnants. Since these lipoproteins are atherogenic strategies to prevent expression of ApoB are useful in the treatment of dyslipidemia. Mipomersen is an antisense oligonucleotide that targets mRNA encoding ApoB100. It reduces circulating levels of all lipoprotein species containing ApoB100 in humans. Mipomersen is currently approved for the treatment of homozygous familial hypercholesterolemia. Advantage of mipomersen is that it does not significantly affect intestinal ApoB48 expression, so intestinal fat absorption is unaffected and intestinal steatosis does not occur.[15]

MICROSOMAL TRIGLYCERIDE TRANSFER PROTEIN (MTP) INHIBITOR

Microsomal triglyceride transfer protein transfers neutral lipids to nascent ApoB and thus affects the rate of VLDL and chylomicron synthesis. Loss-of-function mutation of MTP causes abetalipoproteinemia, which is characterized by defective fat absorption and the absence of circulating ApoB-containing lipoproteins. Lomitapide is an inhibitor of MTP that lowers LDL-C levels by 50% in patients with homozygous familial hypercholesterolemia (FH). It is thus approved for the treatment of homozygous FH. Although lomitapide is effective in lowering LDL-C, its use rarely extends beyond FH because of a high incidence of gastrointestinal symptoms related to malabsorption of fat and hepatic steatosis related to inhibition of hepatic lipid export.[16]

DIACYLGLYCEROL ACYLTRANSFERASE (DGAT) INHIBITORS

Diacylglycerol acyltransferase (DGAT) is an enzyme present in small intestine, liver and adipose tissue. Diacylglycerol acyltransferase isozyme 1 is involved in a final step of triglyceride synthesis from diacylglycerol. Inhibition of this enzyme leads to reduction in serum triglyceride level. DGAT inhibitor in the phase III clinical development is LCQ-908, AZD7687 and PF-04620110.[17]

THYROMIMETICS OR TIROMES

Thyroid hormone receptor b1 isoforms (TR b1) predominant in liver and its activation increased biliary cholesterol excretion and intracellular cholesterol depletion, leading to increased expression of the LDL receptor in hepatocytes. TR b1 agonists such as eprotirome on a background of statin treatment lowered LDL-C up to 32%.[18] However, a recent eprotirome phase III trial was terminated because of liver injury associated with this drug.

APOLIPOPROTEIN E MIMETIC PEPTIDES

Apolipoprotein E acts as a ligand for receptor-mediated clearance of chylomicron and VLDL remnants that promote atherosclerosis. Apolipoprotein E also helps in the biogenesis of HDL. Apolipoprotein E mimetic peptides thus exert anti-inflammatory and antiatherosclerotic effect.[19] One ApoE mimetic peptide, AEM-28, has been approved by the US Food and Drug Administration for clinical use.

APOLIPOPROTEIN A-I (APOA1) SYNTHESIS INDUCER

Hepatic production of ApoA-I results in generation of nascent, lipid-depleted HDL particles, which enter the systemic circulation and carry out reverse cholesterol transport. RVX-208, induces hepatic ApoA-I synthesis, thus increases circulating level of HDL-C.[20] One of the drawbacks of RVX-208 is that it Increases in hepatic transaminase levels.

HDL-MIMETIC PEPTIDE

CER-001, an HDL-mimetic peptide made up of ApoA-I and phospholipids, has been associated with reduction in vascular inflammation and regression of atherosclerosis.[21]

NUCLEAR RECEPTORS

Three nuclear receptors including liver X receptors (LXRs), peroxisome proliferator-activated receptors (PPARs) and farnesoid X receptors play an important role in lipid metabolism.

LIVER X RECEPTOR AGONISTS

Liver X receptors serve as cholesterol sensors, when they are activated they increase biliary cholesterol excretion, reduce intestinal cholesterol absorption, and promote reverse cholesterol transport. Thus, LXR agonists attenuate atherosclerosis. However, a potentially limiting factor in the treatment of LXR agonists is that they also stimulate hepatic lipogenesis. Clinically studied LXR agonist is LXR-623.[22]

PEROXISOME PROLIFERATOR-ACTIVATED RECEPTORS AGONISTS

There are three principal PPARs (alpha, gamma and delta) that regulate fatty acid and lipoprotein metabolism. Peroxisome proliferator-activated receptor alpha (PPAR-α) promotes fatty acid oxidation in liver and muscle, lowers circulating triglycerides and ApoC-III and raises HDL-C. Peroxisome proliferator-activated receptor gamma (PPAR-γ) promotes fatty acid uptake by adipocytes and lowers circulating fatty acids. Peroxisome proliferator-activated receptor delta (PPAR-δ) promotes fatty acid oxidation in muscle and adipose tissue. Saroglitazar (Lipaglyn) is the world's first approved dual PPAR-α and γ agonist. It is approved for the treatment of diabetic

Table 20.1: Evolving targets and therapeutic agents

Evolving targets	Evolving therapies
PCSK9 inhibitor	Alirocumab and evolocumab
CETP inhibitor	Torcetrapib, dalcetrapib, anacetrapib and evacetrapib
Squalene synthase inhibitor	Lapaquistat acetate
Inhibitor of apolipoprotein B100 expression	Mipomersen
MTP inhibitor	Lomitapide
DGAT inhibitor	LCQ-908, AZD7687, PF-04620110
Thyromimetics or tircmes	Eprotirome
Apolipoprotein E mimetic peptides	AEM-28
Apolipoprotein A-I (ApoA1) synthesis inducer	RVX-208
HDL-mimetic peptide	CER-001
Liver X receptor agonists (LXRs)	LXR-623
PPAR-α and γ agonist	Saroglitazar (Lipaglyn)
PPAR-α agonist	Fibrate (Gemfibrozil)
PPAR-γ agonist	Thiazolidinedione
Phospholipase inhibitors	Varespladib and darapladib
Lipoprotein (a) lowering agents	Niacin, PCSK9 antibodies and antisense oligonucleotides mipomersen

dyslipidemia not controlled with statin.[23] It has linear pharmacokinetics, with Tmax of <1 hour and has half liter of 5.6 h. Saroglitazar is primarily eliminated through hepatobiliary route. The recommended dose is 4 mg once daily. Phase III studies [PRESS (prospective, randomized, efficacy and safety of saroglitazar) V & PRESS VI]. Saroglitazar reduced triglycerides upto 47% from baseline in these two trials. Saroglitazar also significantly reduced non-HDL-C and ApoB. Saroglitazar significantly improves insulin sensitivity. The effect of saroglitazar on glycosylated hemoglobin in diabetic dyslipidemia patients was found to be comparable with pioglitazone in PRESS V study. The most commonly reported adverse events are gastritis, dyspepsia, pyrexia and asthenia. It is not associated with weight gain or edema.[24,25]

Fibrate and thiazolidinedione drugs are ligands of PPAR-α and PPAR-γ respectively. Early studies showed that gemfibrozil, a fibrate, reduced CV morbidity and mortality. However, subsequent studies evaluating the addition of fibrates to statins have not demonstrated clinical benefit.[26] Although meta-analysis indicates that fibrates may confer clinical benefit in patients with triglyceride levels at least 200 mg/dL, even with statin co-treatment.

PHOSPHOLIPASE INHIBITORS

Secretory phospholipase A2 (sPLA2) activation leads to generation of smaller, more athero-genic LDL particles within the arterial wall. However, a phase III study evaluating the sPLA2 inhibitor varespladib in patients with acute coronary syndrome demonstrated increased risk of recurrent myocardial infarction.[27] Lipoprotein-associated phospholipase A2 (Lp-PLA2) is also associated with elevation of LDL particle. In early phase studies, the Lp-PLA2 inhibitor, darapladib, shows favorable effects on lipid and inflammatory biomarkers and a reduction in the volume of necrotic core within atherosclerotic plaques.[28] However, a large outcome trial failed to demonstrate a benefit of darapladib on CV death, myocardial infarction or stroke.[29]

LIPOPROTEIN (A) LOWERING AGENTS

High level of lipoprotein (a) (Lp(a)) is an independent risk factor for the development of CV disease.[30] Serum levels of Lp(a) are influenced by genetic factors,[31] but not by diet or lifestyle factors. There are three well-studied drugs that lower Lp(a). These are niacin, PCSK9 antibodies and antisense oligonucleotides mipomersen.

HDL INFUSION THERAPY

Infusion of lipid-depleted forms of HDL has favorable effects on atherosclerotic plaque, endothelial function and markers of reverse cholesterol transport. It has been observed that intravenous infusions of complexes containing the ApoA-I variant, ApoA-I Milano and phospholipid (ETC-216) resulted in regression of coronary atherosclerosis measured by serial intravascular ultrasound in patients with recent acute coronary syndrome.[32]

CONCLUSION

With rapid advancement in biochemistry and molecular biology of lipid disorders, several new targets have been identified. Manipulation of these ligands with various agonists or antagonists has produced clinically significant beneficial effect in dyslipidemia. All these therapeutic agents are at various stages of development. Few of these molecules have been approved for usage in addition to statin or when statins are not tolerated. However, mortality reduction with these agents is yet to be shown. Further research in these fields is required because these agents have the potential of life-time exposure of the individual to them.

REFERENCES

1. LaRosa JC, Grundy SM, Waters DD, et al. ,Treating to New Targets(TNT) Investigators. Intensive lipid lowering with atorvastatin in patients with stable coronary artery disease. N Engl J Med. 2005;352(14):1425-35.
2. Cannon CP, Braunwald E, Mc Cabe CH et al, for the Pravastatin or Atorvastatin Evaluation and Infection Therapy-Thrombolysis in Myocardial Infarction 22 Investigators. Intensive versus moderate lipid lowering with statin after acute coronary syndrome. N Engl J Med. 2004;350:1495-1504.
3. Ridker PM, Danielson E, Fonseca FA, et al.; JUPITAR Study Group. Rosuvastatin to prevent vascular events in men and women with elevated C-reactive protein. N Engl J Med. 2008;359(21):2195-207.
4. Brown MS, Goldstein JL. A receptor mediated pathway for cholesterol homeostasis. Science. 1986;232:34-47.
5. Hochholzer W, Giugliano RP. Lipid lowering goals: back to nature? Ther Adv Cardiovasc Dis. 2010;4(3):185-91.
6. Cordain L, Eaton SB, Mann N, et al. The paradoxical nature of hunter-gatherer diets: meat based, yet nonatherogenic. Eur J Clin Nutr. 2002;56,Suppl 1:S 42-S 52.

7. Akram ON, Bernier A, Petrides F, et al. Beyond LDL cholesterol, a new role for PCSK9. Arterioscler Thromb Vasc Biol. 2010;30:1279-81.

8. Do RQ, Vogel RA, Schwartz GG. PCSK9 Inhibitors: potential in cardiovascular therapeutics. Curr Cardiol Rep. 2013;3:345.

9. Thompson A, Di AE, Sarwar N, et al. Association of cholesteryl ester transfer protein genotypes with CETP mass and activity, lipid levels, and coronary risk. JAMA. 2008;299:2777-88.

10. Ritsch A, Scharnagl H, Eller P, et al. Cholesteryl ester transfer protein and mortality in patients undergoing coronary angiography: the Ludwigshafen Risk and Cardiovascular Health study. Circulation. 2010;121:366-74.

11. Forrest MJ, Bloomfield D, Briscoe RJ, et al. Torcetrapib-induced blood pressure elevation is independent of CETP inhibition and is accompanied by increased circulating levels of aldosterone. Br J Pharmacol. 2008;154:1465-73.

12. Nicholls SJ, Brewer HB, Kastelein JJ, . Effects of the CETP inhibitor evacetrapib administered as monotherapy or in combination with statins on HDL and LDL cholesterol: a randomized controlled trial. JAMA. 2011a;306:2099-2109.

13. Gotto AM Jr, Cannon CP, Li XS, et al. Evaluation of lipids, drug concentration, and safety parameters following cessation of treatment with the cholesteryl ester transfer protein inhibitor anacetrapib in patients with or at high risk for coronary heart disease. Am J Cardiol. 2014;113:76-83.

14. Stein EA, Bays H, O'Brien D, et al. Lapaquistat acetate: development of a squalene synthase inhibitor for the treatment of hypercholesterolemia. Circulation. 2011;123:1974-85.

15. Crooke RM, Graham MJ, Lemonidis KM, et al. An apolipoprotein B antisense oligonucleotide lowers LDL cholesterol in hyperlipidemic mice without causing hepatic steatosis. J Lipid Res. 2005;46:872-84.

16. Cuchel M, Meagher EA, du Toit TH, et al. Efficacy and safety of a microsomal triglyceride transfer protein inhibitor in patients with homozygous familial hypercholesterolaemia: a single-arm, open-label, phase 3 study. Lancet. 2013;381:40-46.

17. Denison H, Nilsson C, Lofgren L, et al. Diacylglycerol acyltransferase 1 inhibition with AZD7687 alters lipid handling and hormone secretion in the gut with intolerable side effects: a randomized clinical trial. Diabetes Obes Metab. 2014;4:334-43.

18. Ladenson PW, Kristensen JD, Ridgway EC, et al. Use of the thyroid hormone analogue eprotirome in statin-treated dyslipidemia. N Engl J Med. 2010;362:906-16.

19. Zhao W, Du F, Zhang M, et al. A new recombinant human apolipoprotein E mimetic peptide with high-density lipoprotein binding and function enhancing activity. Exp Biol Med (Maywood). 2011;236:1468-76.

20. Bailey D, Jahagirdar R, Gordon A, et al. RVX-208: a small molecule that increases apolipoprotein A-I and high-density lipoprotein cholesterol in vitro and in vivo. J Am Coll Cardiol. 2010;55:2580-89.

21. Tardy C, Goffinet M, Boubekeur N, et al. CER-001, a HDL-mimetic, stimulates the reverse lipid transport and atherosclerosis regression in high cholesterol diet-fed LDL-receptor deficient mice. Atherosclerosis. 2014;1:110-18.

22. Katz A, Udata C, Ott E, . Safety, pharmacokinetics, and pharmacodynamics of single doses of LXR-623, a novel liver X-receptor agonist, in healthy participants. J Clin Pharmacol. 2009;49:6439.

23. Shetty SR, Kumar S, Mathur RP, et al. Observational study to evaluate the safety and efficacy of saroglitazar in Indian diabetic dyslipidemia patients. Indian Heart J. 2014;6723-26.

24. Pai V, Paneerselvam A, Mukhopadhyay S, et al. A multicenter, prospective, randomized, double-blind study to evaluate the safety and efficacy of saroglitazar 2 and 4 mg compared to pioglitazone 45 mg in diabetic dyslipidemia (PRESS V). J Diabetes Sci Technol. 2014;8(1):132-41.

25. Jani RH, Pai V, Jha P, et al. A multicenter, prospective, randomized, double-blind study to evaluate the safety and efficacy of saroglitazar 2 and 4 mg compared with placebo in type 2 diabetes mellitus patients having hypertriglyceridemia not controlled with atorvastatin therapy (PRESS VI). Diabetes Technol Ther. 2014;16(2):63-71.

26. ACCORD Study Group, Ginsberg HN, Elam MB, et al. Effects of combination Lipid therapy in type 2 diabetes mellitus. N Engl J Med. 2010;17:1563-74.

27. Nicholls SJ, Kastelein JJ, Schwartz GG, et al. Varespladib and cardiovascular events in patients with an acute coronary syndrome: the VISTA-16 randomized clinical trial. JAMA. 2014;311:2252-62.

28. Serruys PW, Garcia-Garcia HM, Buszman P, et al. Effects of the direct lipoprotein-associated phospholipase A(2) inhibitor darapladib on human coronary atherosclerotic plaque. Circulation. 2008;118:1172-82.

29. STABILITY Investigators. Darapladib for preventing ischemic events in stable coronary heart disease. N Engl J Med. 2014;370:1702-11.

30. Erqou S, Kaptoge S, Perry PL, et al. Lipoprotein(a) concentration and the risk of coronary heart disease, stroke, and nonvascular mortality. JAMA. 2009;302:412-23.

31. Boerwinkle E, Leffert CC, Lin J, et al. Apolipoprotein(a) gene accounts for greater than 90% of the variation in plasma lipoprotein(a) concentrations. J Clin Invest. 1992;90:52-60.

32. Nissen SE, Tsunoda T, Tuzcu EM, et al. Effect of recombinant ApoA-I Milano on coronary atherosclerosis in patients with acute coronary syndromes: a randomized controlled trial. JAMA. 2003;290:2292-2300.

Fibrates in Dyslipidemia

Jeet Ram, Sunil Kumar Verma and Sundeep Mishra

- Introduction
- Effect of fibrates on lipoproteins metabolism
- Mechanism of action
- Clinical use
- Effect of fibrates on cardiovascular risk
- Metabolic syndrome and effect of fibrates
- Who are the candidates for fibrates?
- Selection among different fibrates
- Conclusion

INTRODUCTION

Hypercholesterolemia is a well-established major risk factor for cardiovascular diseases (CVDs). In addition, high triglycerides (TGs) and low high-density lipoprotein cholesterol (HDL-C) levels alone or in combination have also been found to be associated with significant CV risk.[1-3] Current guidelines recommend modification of high TGs and low HDL as secondary therapeutic target to provide additional vascular protection.[4] Fibrates were introduced in clinical practice about 35 years ago in Europe, based on favorable effect on the lipids. However, their clinical efficacy remains controversial. Food and Drug Administration (FDA) first approved fenofibrate (TRICOR) for severe hypertriglyceridemia in 1993 and in 1999 it was also approved for reducing low density lipoprotein cholesterol (LDL-C), TGs, total cholesterol (TC) and apolipoprotein levels in patients with primary hypercholesterolemia or mixed dyslipidemia.[5]

The main indications for the use of fibrates are the treatment of hypertriglyceridemia when diet and life style changes are not sufficient. Another potential indication is for the prevention of CVD in patients with elevated plasma TG and low HDL-C levels, although the data supporting their use are weaker than those for statins.

EFFECT OF FIBRATES ON LIPOPROTEINS METABOLISM

Fibric acid derivatives are the class of drugs that have been shown to inhibit the production of very low-density lipoproteins (VLDLs) and increase its clearance as well, primarily by increasing the activity of lipoprotein lipase (LPL). This increase in LPL activity occurs as a result of inhibition of hepatic LPL inhibitors apolipoprotein C-III (apoC-III) and to some extent by enhancing apolipoprotein lipase gene expression. Because apoC-III delays the catabolism of TG-rich lipoproteins (TRLs), its inhibition provides a further mechanism by which peroxisome proliferator-activated receptor alpha (PPAR-α) activators such as fibrates lower the concentration of plasma TG.[6] The main effect of these drugs is reduction in plasma TGs and some increase in HDL. The precise mechanisms of increase in HDL-C are not known; however, fibrates increase the expression of apoA-I and apoA-II genes.[7,8] Generally, the increase in plasma apoA-II is greater than that of apoA-I.[9,10] This results in an increase in the concentration of HDL particles containing both apoA-I and apoA-II, but a decrease in those containing apoA-I without apoA-II.[10,11] Other potential mechanisms by which fibrates increase the level of HDL-C include an enhancement of cell cholesterol efflux secondary to an induction of cell ABCA1 expression.[12] Their effects on LDL are less marked and variable. These drugs also are known to modify intracellular metabolism of lipids through increase in transport of fatty acids (FAs) into mitochondria and then improved catabolism inside the mitochondria and peroxisomes.[13,14]

The combination of small dense LDL (sdLDL), decreased HDL-C and increased TG has been called the "atherogenic lipoprotein phenotype". Small LDLs are significantly associated with increased CV risk and they are associated with raised TG and decreased HDL-C levels. It has been shown that plasma lipoprotein profile with a predominance of sLDL particles is associated with approximately a threefold increased risk of coronary artery disease (CAD). Treatment with fibrates has beneficial effects on LDL size and subclasses in patients with type 2 diabetes mellitus (DM) or metabolic syndrome, that is, those who have high CV risk. Treatment with fibrate therapy can lead to changes in the number of plasma LDL and HDL particles that may occur independently of any change in the cholesterol content of these lipoproteins.

MECHANISM OF ACTION

These drugs act via the ligation and activation of ligand-activated transcription factor PPAR-α and to some extent also exert PPAR-β/δ and PPAR-γ activity. Peroxisome proliferator-activated receptors regulate gene expression by forming heterodimers with activated retinoid-X-receptor and binding to specific peroxisome proliferator response elements in the promoter region of the target gene.[15,16] Expression of the different subtypes varies in different tissues, with PPAR-α being highly expressed in liver, heart, kidney, muscle, brown adipose tissue and vascular cells.[17,18] Peroxisome proliferator-activated receptor alpha is activated by endogenous molecules, such as FAs and also by synthetic compounds such as fibrates.[19] As far as the mode of action is concerned, all fibrates have a similar mode of action, although reports of variations in their clinical effects indicate that there must be some differences in the mechanism of action between the individual members of the class.

Peroxisome proliferators-activated receptors are a group of specific transcription factors that play a role in transcription of genes involved in the peroxisomal β-oxidation. Peroxisome proliferator-activated receptors represent the family of 3 nuclear receptor isoforms, namely PPAR-α,-γ, and-δ/β, which are encoded by different genes. These receptors play a key role as regulation of glucose and lipid metabolism. These receptors are also involved in the cell proliferation, differentiation and inflammatory responses. Fibrates action is linked to the induction of transcription of genes involved in the peroxisomal β-oxidation mediated by PPARs. Peroxisome proliferator-activated receptors and fibrates primary involvement in lipid metabolism and subsequently in inflammation and atherosclerosis are the main concerns regarding their role in atherosclerotic CVD. The mechanism of action of fibrates can be divided into five groups: (1) induction of lipoprotein lipolysis, (2) induction of hepatic FA uptake and reduction in hepatic TG production, (3) increased removal of LDL particles, (4) reduction in neutral lipids and (5) increase in HDL production and stimulation of reverse cholesterol transport.

The action of fibrates on TGs combines both effect on LPL activity and apoC-III expression (a strong inhibitor of LPL). Changes in LPL activity can lead to increased lipolysis of plasma TRLs as well as increased accessibility of TRLs for the action of LPL, with a reduction in TRL apoC-III content. Both these mechanisms of LPL expression induction and inhibition of apoC-III gene transcription are mediated by PPAR-α. Reduced apoC-III synthesis results in enhanced LPL-mediated catabolism of VLDL particles. Therefore, reduction in VLDL particles, with induced TRLs catabolism, represents the most likely hypolipidemic mechanism of fibrates. In addition, fibrates can reduce postprandial lipemia in patients with primary hyper-cholesterolemia and also in patients with type 2 DM.

Another potential mechanism of action of fibrates is the increased FA uptake by the stimu-lation of FA transporter protein and conversion to acyl-CoA by induction of acyl-CoA synthe-tase activity. Fibrate-induced enhancement of β-oxidation and decrease in FA synthesis may lower FAs availability for TG synthesis.

Fibrates cause synthesis of LDL molecules that have higher affinity for the LDL recep-tors. These LDL molecules are catabolized more rapidly. Also, the cholesterol ester content of the LDL increases in all LDL subclasses, thereby forming larger, less-dense LDL particles. A decrease in neutral lipid (cholesteryl ester and TG) exchange between VLDL and HDL may result from decreased plasma levels of TRL. Fibrate-induced lowering of TRLs levels reduces net cholesterol ester transfer from HDL to TRLs; this leads to an increase in cholesterol ester and a decrease in TG content of HDL, also mediated by unchanged lecithin: cholesterol acyl transferase activity. The LPL-mediated lipolysis of TRLs and increased apoA-I and apoA-II synthesis may also contribute to the rise in HDL levels following fibrate treatment by promoting the formation of HDL precursors. The liver production of apoA-I and apoA-II increases with fibrate treatments. These two are the major constituents of the HDL. This leads to the increase in plasma HDL concentrations as well as a more efficient reverse cholesterol transport.

CLINICAL USE

Fibrates and the agonists of PPAR-α have been found to decrease TGs level and raise HDL levels.[20] In addition to their lipid-modifying effects, they also exhibit anti-inflammatory prop-erties, which may also confer some vascular protection.[21] The effect of fibrates depends upon the baseline levels of TGs and HDL-C. Patients with high baseline TGs and low HDL have the highest benefit. This was shown in one of the trials using gemfibrozil in which the decrease in the plasma TG level and increase in the concentration of HDL-C were found to be most pronounced in patients with higher fasting plasma TG levels.[22] Similarly the other trial using fenofibrate showed greatest increase in HDL-C in patients with low baseline HDL-C levels.[23]

As far as the lipid-modifying effects of different fibrates on TGs are concerned, there have been many studies, and most showing only minor differences in TG levels, with reductions of 30–50% being reported for most agents.[27-31] In contrast, the HDL-C raising effect of fibrates varies widely between different studies, ranging from as little as 2% to as much as 25%. Some reports have suggested that the HDL-C raising effect of fenofibrate is superior to the others members of the class.[32] However, this was not apparent in the Fenofibrate Intervention and Event Lowering in Diabetes (FIELD) study in which fenofibrate increased HDL-C by only about 2%[4] and did not raise the level of apoA-I at all.[18] However, the cardioprotective properties of fibrates may be largely independent of their effects on plasma lipid levels, especially in people with features of the metabolic syndrome.

From a clinical point of view, six randomized control trials of major fibrates (gemfibrozil, fenofibrate, bezafibrate) have looked at the clinical benefit in different scenarios. The earliest and the most successful of these trials is the Helsinki Heart Study (HHS), which was done with gemfibrozil; most of the benefits were seen among patients who had atherogenic dyslipidemia without any significant effects in other subgroups.[24] Similar observations were made in the Bezafibrate Infarction Prevention (BIP) trial for bezafibrate,[25] for fenofibrate in the Action to Control Cardiovascular Risk in Diabetes-Lipid (ACCORD-Lipid) trial[26] and for gemfibrozil in the Veterans Affairs High-Density Lipoprotein Intervention Trial (VA-HIT).[27] The following are the results of some of the trials carried out in human.

The World Health Organization (WHO) Clofibrate Study

The WHO Clofibrate Study (started in 1962 with average follow-up of 13.2 years) included 10,627 men with hypercholesterolemia but without any information on TG and HDL-C levels. It tested the hypothesis that whether the effectiveness of clofibrate in reducing hypercholesterolemia and hypertriglyceridemia would reduce the incidence of ischemic heart disease and mortality. Coronary heart disease (CHD) events in this trial were reduced from 7.4% in the placebo group to 5.9% in the clofibrate group, a relative risk reduction of 20% ($P = 0.05$). There was no reduction in mortality from ischemic heart disease with clofibrate treatment. However, there was also a small but significant excess of noncoronary deaths in the clofibrate group. This excess of noncoronary deaths led to arguments against the continued use of this drug. The increased all-cause mortality rate during clofibrate treatment did not continue after treatment was stopped. However, the subsequent trials did not show significant excess of noncoronary deaths with gemfibrozil (HHS and VA-HIT), bezafibrate (BIP) or fenofibrate (FIELD).[28] Clofibrate is still available in some centers, although its use has declined since the introduction of newer molecules.

The Helsinki Heart Study

The HHS was a double-blind placebo-controlled trial that included 4081 men aged 40–55 years free of clinically manifest CHD at enrolment to the study with a non-HDL-C values >200 mg/dL. This randomized double-blind control trial tested the efficacy of simultaneously elevating HDL-C and lowering levels of non-HDL-C with gemfibrozil in reducing the risk of CAD. Over the 5 years of the study, gemfibrozil increased the concentration of HDL-C by a mean of 11% and decreased serum TC, LDL-C and TGs by 10%, 11% and 35% respectively. The cumulative rate of total cardiac end points [nonfatal myocardial infarction (MI), fatal MI, sudden cardiac death or unwitnessed death] at 5 years was 27.3 per 1000 in the gemfibrozil group and 41.4 per 1000 in the placebo group, which translates into a 34.0% reduction in the incidence of total coronary events ($P < 0.02$). The difference between the gemfibrozil and placebo groups became evident in the second year and continued throughout the study. There was no significant difference between the groups in the total death rate nor did the treatment influence the cancer rate. A subgroup analysis of HHS addressed the effect of body mass index (BMI) (BMI >26 kg/m^2 vs. BMI <26 kg/m^2) on the response to gemfibrozil.[29,30] The benefits of treatment with gemfibrozil were much greater in the subjects with BMI >26 kg/m^2. In the group of subjects with a BMI >26 kg/m^2, the net difference in cardiac end points between the gemfibrozil and placebo groups was 21 events (25 of 1119 vs. 46 of 1081 respectively). This represented a risk reduction in the overweight subjects of 47.5%. In marked contrast, in the group of people whose BMI was <26 kg/m^2, the difference in cardiac end points between the gemfibrozil and placebo groups was 7 events (31 of 927 subjects vs. 38 of 954 subjects), representing a risk reduction of only 16% in this leaner subgroup. There were some additional analyses from the outcomes of the HHS that have evaluated the ability of baseline lipid levels to predict CHD events in the placebo group and also the benefits of treatment with gemfibrozil. Surprisingly the concentration of LDL-C was found to be a poor predictor of risk in this population. The levels of HDL-C and serum TG, however, were strong predictors. A concentration of HDL-C <1.08 mmol/L (<42 mg/dL) was associated with a relative risk 1.73 times greater than that in subjects whose HDL-C level was >1.08 mmol/L (>42 mg/dL). Likewise, subjects whose serum TG was >2.3 mmol/L (>204 mg/dL) had a relative risk 1.81 times greater than that in subjects with a serum TG level <2.3 mmol/L (<204 mg/dL). The excess risk associated with lower HDL-C and higher serum TG was essentially abolished by treatment with gemfibrozil.

The Veterans Affairs High-Density Lipoprotein Intervention Trial

The VA-HIT was a multicenter randomized double-blind placebo-controlled trial that included 2531 men with known clinical CHD and aged <74 years.[31] It assessed the effects of gemfibrozil at a dose of 1200 mg/day versus dietary therapy on the incidence of CV events. To be eligible for inclusion, subjects had to have a low level of both HDL-C (≤1.03 mmol/L, ≤40 mg/dL) and LDL-C (<3.6 mmol/L, <140 mg/dL) and a plasma TG ≤3.4 mmol/L (≤300 mg/dL). The active treatment was gemfibrozil 1200 mg per day and the mean follow-up was 5.1 years. One year after randomization, the concentration of HDL-C was increased by 6% ($P < 0.001$) and the plasma TG was decreased by 31% ($P < 0.001$). These changes were sustained for the duration of the study. Gemfibrozil therapy resulted in minimal alterations in TC and LDL-C levels. The primary end point (nonfatal MI or death attributable to CHD) was reduced by 22% in the gemfibrozil group that was statistically significant ($P < 0.006$), with a benefit of therapy becoming apparent during the third year of follow-up.[31] There were 220 (17.4%) deaths from all causes in the placebo group compared with 198 (15.7%) in the gemfibrozil group, although this difference did not reach statistical significance. There were 51 cancer deaths in the placebo group and 45 in the gemfibrozil group, a difference that was not statistically different. There was no significant difference between the two groups in the rate of death from any specific cause.

There was an interesting observation from the subsequent paper from the VA-HIT study. It discussed the relationship between the different lipoproteins blood levels and CV events.[32] The baseline plasma concentrations of HDL-C, TG, apoB, apoA-I and HDL3-C (although not LDL-C or HDL2-C) were all significant predictors of CHD events during the trial period. The magnitude of benefit from gemfibrozil therapy was predicted by the baseline plasma TG levels.

The Bezafibrate Infarction Prevention Study

The BIP study was a double-blind, placebo-controlled trial that included 3090 subjects with clinically manifest CHD (2825 men, 265 women) aged <74 years.[33] It was designed and initiated in 1990 to test the hypothesis that whether bezafibrate, which raises HDL-C and reduces TGs, would reduce CAD mortality and nonfatal MI in patients with established CADs. The study population was having TC of 180–250 mg/dL, HDL-C <45 mg/dL, TG <300 mg/dL and

LDL-C <180 mg/dL. The active treatment was bezafibrate 400 mg per day and the mean follow-up was 6.2 years. There was no significant effect of bezafibrate on the combined incidence of nonfatal MI or death from CHD (the primary end point of the study). Compared with placebo, bezafibrate increased HDL-C of 14% and decreased TGs of 25%. About 7.3% ($P = 0.24$) was the reduction in the cumulative probability of the primary end point after the end of the study. However, a subsequent post-hoc subgroup analysis postulated the possibility of a substantially greater risk reduction with bezafibrate in the small subgroup of the patients with the elevated entry concentration of plasma TGs (>2.25 mmol/L or >200 mg/dL). In this subgroup, the event rate was 19.7% in the placebo group and 12.0% in the bezafibrate group, indicating a relative reduction of 39% ($P < 0.02$).[33] A further post hoc, subgroup analysis of the BIP study found that in 1470 patients with the metabolic syndrome, bezafibrate was associated with reduced risks of any MI (hazard ratio 0.71, $P < 0.02$) and nonfatal MI (hazard ratio 0.67 ($P < 0.009$).[34] These finding added to the observations from both the HHS and the VA-HIT studies that a higher baseline TG level, such as in patients with the metabolic syndrome, identifies a group of people who derive a substantial additional CV benefit. So this trial established that bezafibrate is safe and effective in elevated HDL-C and reducing TGs. This trial also pointed out that bezafibrate may have prominent role in the management of dyslipidemia and CAD when targeted to the subgroup of the patients with high TGs.

The Fenofibrate Intervention and Event Lowering in Diabetes Study

The FIELD study was a randomized, double-blind, placebo controlled parallel-group trial among 9795 middle-aged to elderly people with type 2 DM.[35] The rationale for the FIELD was to determine whether early intervention with fenofibrate could prevent CV events in middle aged to elderly patients with type 2 DM. After a placebo run-in phase followed by a fenofibrate run-in phase, patients with a TC of 3.0–6.5 mmol/L (116 to 252 mg/dL) plus either total/HDL-C ratio >4.0 or plasma TG >1.0 to 5.0 mmol/L (87 to 435 mg/dL) were randomized to micronized fenofibrate 200 mg/d or matching placebo. All other treatments, including statins after randomization, were at the discretion of the physician. The primary outcome was CHD events (CHD death or nonfatal MI); for prespecified subgroup analyses the outcome was total CVD events (the composite of CVD death, MI, stroke and coronary and carotid revascularization). Follow-up was a median of 5.0 years. Treatment with fenofibrate reduced the plasma TG by 29% and LDL-C by 12%; these effects were apparent for the duration of the trial. Fenofibrate increased the level of HDL-C by 5% at 4 months, but this was reduced to an increase over placebo of about 2% at the conclusion of the study. The explanation for such attenuation in the effect of fenofibrate on HDL-C is not known.

The primary composite end point of CHD death or non fatal MI was 5.9% in the placebo group and 5.2% in the fenofibrate group, a relative reduction of 11%, ($P ≤ 0.16$). This reflected a significant 24% reduction in nonfatal MI ($P < 0.010$) and a nonsignificant 19% increase in CHD mortality ($P ≤ 0.22$). Total CVD events were reduced by 11% from 13.9% to 12.5% ($P < 0.035$); this included a significant 21% reduction in coronary revascularization ($P < 0.003$) and a nonsignificant 10% reduction in stroke ($P ≤ 0.36$). Total mortality was 6.6% in the placebo group and 7.3% in the fenofibrate group ($P ≤ 0.18$). Among patients with no prior CVD, total CVD events were reduced by 19% ($P < 0.004$) but this was not the case in patients with prior CVD in whom there was a nonsignificant 2% increase in events ($P ≤ 0.85$). The secondary composite end point of total CV events was significantly lower in fenofibrate group compared with placebo group (12.5% vs. 13.9% respectively, $P = 0.035$). Cardiovascular mortality

(2.9% vs. 2.6% respectively, $P = 0.41$), total mortality (7.3% vs. 6.9% respectively, $P = 0.18$) and stroke (3.2% vs. 3.6% respectively, $P = 0.36$) were not significantly different between the fenofibrate and placebo groups. Patients allocated to the fenofibrate group had less progression of albuminuria ($P < 0.002$) and a significantly lower rate of laser treatment for retinopathy (5.2% vs. 3.6%, $P < 0.001$); the mechanism underlying these renal and retinal effects is not known. The rate of statin drop-in in the fenofibrate group averaged 8%, whereas it averaged 17% in the placebo group. Fenofibrate was associated with a slightly increased risk of pancreatitis (0.5% vs. 0.8%) and pulmonary embolism (0.7% vs. 1.1%), but no other significant adverse effects were observed. Treatment with fenofibrate in the FIELD study increased the plasma homocysteine level by 35% from a median of 11.2 μmol/L in the placebo group to 15.1 μmol/L in the treated group. On the basis of the results from epidemiological studies, an increase in homocysteine of this magnitude could theoretically translate into a 10–20% increase in CV events.[36] It is noteworthy that the fenofibrate induced increase in HDL-C in the FIELD study (<2% at study end) and the reduction in CV events (11%) were both much less than predicted from the results of trials using other fibrates that have a smaller effect on levels of homocysteine. Recent studies demonstrating that homocysteine inhibits the synthesis of apo-I in the liver suggest that the less than expected CV benefits of treatment with fenofibrate in the FIELD study may well have been the consequence of a sustained increase in the plasma concentration of homocysteine inhibiting the synthesis of apoA-I and thus opposing the expected increase in the concentration of HDL-C. In line with the earlier trials, there was a trend toward greater event reduction with fenofibrate in FIELD participants who had lower baseline levels of HDL-C.[37]

The Action to Control Cardiovascular Risk in Diabetes

The ACCORD-Lipid substudy was designed to determine whether combination therapy with a statin plus fenofibrate would reduce the risk of CV events as compared with statin monotherapy: it had been observed that at any given LDL-C level, patients with diabetes have excess CV risk, and it seemed possible that the addition of a fibrate that lowers the TG and raises the HDL-C would improve lipid composition and could transform the outcomes in this population in terms of additional reduction in CV mortality. A total of 5518 men and women with type 2 DM were enrolled in the ACCORD Lipid trial. All participants received simvastatin (20–40 mg/day) and were also randomly assigned to masked fenofibrate (160 or 54 mg/day, depending on renal function) or placebo. The primary outcome was the first post randomization occurrence of a nonfatal MI, nonfatal stroke or CV death. After a mean follow-up of 4.7 years, fenofibrate plus simvastatin had not significantly decreased the rate of the primary outcome of fatal CV events, nonfatal MI or nonfatal stroke as compared with simvastatin alone.[38] However, a prespecified subgroup analysis showed a 31% reduction in the rate of the primary outcome among the 17% of patients with baseline TG levels above 204 mg/dL and HDL-C levels below 34 mg/dL. This finding is consistent with subgroup analyses from previous fibrate-monotherapy trials and suggests that elevated TG and low HDL-C levels may be required for these agents to be clinically effective.

EFFECT OF FIBRATES ON CV RISK

Fibrates particularly target atherogenic dyslipidemia, thus reducing residual CVD risk. Fibrates have been found to decrease TC by 8%, LDL-C by 8% and TG by 15–50%, and to raise HDL-C by 9%. These improvements in lipid profile were associated with significant reduction in CVD morbidity and mortality (i.e., relative risk decrease of 27 to 65% in nonfatal MI and CVD death) especially in those patients with increased TG and/or reduced HDL-C at baseline. Fibrate-related significant reductions in nonfatal and/or fatal CVD events were observed in the HHS, the VA-HIT, the Lower Extremity Arterial Disease Event Reduction (LEADER) study and FIELD study. Furthermore, the Bezafibrate Coronary Atherosclerosis Intervention Trial (BECAIT), the Lipid Coronary Angiography Trial (LOCAT) and the Diabetes Atherosclerosis Intervention Study (DAIS) reported that fibrate treatment prevented coronary atherosclerosis prevention. In the BIP study, bezafibrate significantly decreased the risk of fatal or nonfatal MI or sudden death only in those patients with TG>200 mg/dL and HDL <35 mg/dL. However, meta-analyses showed reductions in coronary events following fibrate treatment, but no effect on nonvascular or CVD death.

Like statins, fibrates also have several "pleiotropic" effects that provide cardioprotection by mechanism other than lipid-lowering properties. In this regard, fibrates have been reported to reduce inflammatory markers including C-reactive protein, tumor necrosis factor alpha and interleukin-2. Fibrate treatment also results in improvement in flow-mediated dilation and insulin sensitivity. Fibrates also have antioxidant properties that prevent endothelial dysfunction.

However, ACC/AHA 2013 Blood Cholesterol Guidelines have identified four major statin benefit groups for whom the atherosclerotic CVD (ASCVD) risk reduction clearly outweighs the risk of adverse events: (1) individuals with clinical ASCVD, (2) primary elevations of LDL-C ≥190 mg/dL, (3) diabetes aged 40–75 years with LDL-C 70–189 mg/dL and without clinical ASCVD or (4) without clinical ASCVD or diabetes with LDL-C 70–189 mg/dL and estimated 10-year ASCVD risk ≥7.5%. "High-intensity," "moderate intensity" and "lower intensity" statin therapy definitions are used by the expert panel to define the intensity of statin therapy on the basis of average expected LDL-C response to a specific statin and dose. Classifying specific statins and doses by the percent reduction in LDL-C level is based on the evidence that the relative reduction in ASCVD risk from statin therapy is related to the degree by which LDL-C is lowered. However, expert panel did not find evidence to support titrating cholesterol-lowering drug therapy to achieve optimal LDL-C or non-HDL-C levels for the primary or secondary prevention of ASCVD. These guidelines emphasize the adherence to lifestyle and to statin therapy before the addition of a nonstatin drug (fibrate, niacin cholesterol-absorption inhibitors and omega-3 fatty acids) in patients who have insufficient response to statin therapy or who have statin intolerance. The panel could find no data supporting the routine use of nonstatin drug combined with statin therapy to reduce further ASCVD events. The expert panel recommends that the clinicians treating high-risk patients who have a less-than-anticipated response to statin, who are unable to tolerate a less-than-recommended intensity of statin or who are completely statin intolerant may consider the addition of a nonstatin cholesterol-lowering therapy. High-risk individuals include those with ASCVD, those with LDL-C≥190 mg/dL and those with diabetes. In these guidelines, the only fibrate recommended in fenofibrate that can be considered concomitantly with a low- or moderate-intensity statin only if the benefit from ASCVD risk reduction or TG lowering when TGs are >500 mg/dL are judged to outweigh the potential risk of adverse effect.

METABOLIC SYNDROME AND EFFECT OF FIBRATES

An elevated baseline level of plasma TG identifies patients in whom treatment with a fibrate produces a reduction in CHD events that is substantially greater than in the study population as a whole. This was apparent with gemfibrozil in the HHS and VA-HIT studies and with bezafibrate in the BIP study. This contrasts with the results in statin trials in which there is no evidence that the baseline levels of TG predict the magnitude of treatment benefit. Despite the fact that an elevated baseline plasma TG level identifies subjects in whom fibrates achieve a marked reduction in CHD events, the magnitude of the fibrate-mediated reduction in TG does not predict the CHD reduction.[39] This suggests that an elevated level of plasma TG is a marker for a condition in which fibrates are especially effective in reducing CHD risk. It also indicates that the elevated TG is not a direct causative factor of CHD. The relationship between fibrate-induced HDL-C increase and CHD events is complex. In prospective population studies, a 1% increase in HDL-C equates with an approximate 1% lower risk of CHD.[40] An identical relationship has been observed in at least two intervention studies in which most of the subjects appeared to lack features of the metabolic syndrome. Consistent with the epidemiology, in the Lipids Research Clinics Coronary Primary Prevention Trial with cholestyramine[41,42] the changes in concentration of HDL-C contributed significantly to the CHD risk reduction, with each 1% increase in HDL-C accounting for a 1% decrease in CHD events. The same relationship between CHD risk reduction and HDL-C was reported in the Scandinavian Simvastatin Survival Study (4S).[43] In contrast, when subjects with features of the metabolic syndrome (specifically overweight, high TG, and low HDL-C) are treated with a fibrate, the decrease in CHD risk is much greater than predicted by the observed changes in plasma lipid concentrations, suggesting that there may be additional mechanisms by which fibrates protect in such people. Indeed, in the HHS and VA-HIT studies, the decrease in plasma TG levels did not predict benefit and in the VA-HIT study, the increase in concentration of HDL-C in the gemfibrozil group accounted for only about one quarter of the risk reduction observed in this group. The precise nature of these additional protective mechanisms is not known. It has been suggested (but not proven) that fibrates stimulate reverse cholesterol transport to an extent that is greater than can be explained by increases in the concentration of HDL-C.[20] It has also been suggested (but again not proven) that fibrates protect by inhibiting inflammation. If the high CV risk in people with the metabolic syndrome were to be linked in some way to inflammation in the liver or visceral fat, it is possible that an inhibition of inflammation in these sites may be one of the mechanisms by which fibrates reduce CV risk in people with the metabolic syndrome. When these observations are considered together, it is apparent that, despite the large body of research into fibrates over the past 20 years or more, there are still substantial areas of ignorance. It is not known, for example, why some fibrates increase creatinine and homocysteine levels more than others. Nor is it known whether such increases are clinically important and, if they are, by what mechanism. At an even more fundamental level, the mechanism by which fibrates reduce CV risk in people with the metabolic syndrome is not known. And in practical terms, is it not known whether treatment with fibrates reduces the residual CV risk that persists despite effective statin treatment in many people with the metabolic syndrome.

WHO ARE THE CANDIDATES FOR FIBRATES?

Given that statins have been shown to reduce CV risk in all groups in whom they have been studied (including people with the metabolic syndrome), it is apparent that fibrates have a therapeutic role only if they have additional benefits in people already on statins. Because statins reduce risk in everyone, although the benefits of fibrates are largely confined to people with features of the metabolic syndrome, it is likely that the mechanisms by which stains and fibrates protect are distinct. If this is the case, it is possible that fibrates will reduce the residual risk in patients with diabetes or the metabolic syndrome who are already well treated with statins. The balance of (circumstantial) evidence favors treatment with the combination of a fibrate and a statin in high-risk overweight people who also have an elevated plasma TG and low level of HDL-C.

SELECTION AMONG DIFFERENT FIBRATES

The HHS and VA-HIT studies have shown that gemfibrozil is extremely effective in reducing CV risk in people with features of the metabolic syndrome such as overweight, hypertriglyceridemia and low HDL-C. It has been proposed that gemfibrozil may exert additional antiatherogenic effects by decreasing sLDL. However, concerns about muscle problems associated with the addition of gemfibrozil to a statin tend to limit the use of this combination. Evidence supporting the use of bezafibrate is less robust, although the subgroup analysis of those with the metabolic syndrome in the BIP study provided results remarkably similar to those with gemfibrozil in the HHS and VA-HIT studies. The observation that muscle problems appear to be less of an issue when fenofibrate is combined with a statin has led to suggestions that fenofibrate is the agent of choice if a fibrate is to be added to a statin. However, the evidence in support of the cardioprotective benefits of fenofibrate is less robust than has been reported for gemfibrozil. The practicing physicians will have to make their decisions about whether to use the combination of fibrates and statins on the basis of circumstantial evidence. The choice of which fibrate then becomes an assessment of the relative efficacies of the different agents in the clinical trials against which must be balanced factors such as the muscle problems associated with gemfibrozil and the greater increase in homocysteine and creatinine associated with the use of fenofibrate. The ideal will be to develop a PPAR-α agonist that has the cardioprotective properties of gemfibrozil, the safety of co-administration with statins of fenofibrate and no other potentially adverse effects such as an elevation of homocysteine and creatinine.

Reduction in microvascular complications of diabetes (in terms of diabetic retinopathy, progression of microalbuminuria and the risk of limb amputations) has also been studied with different fibrates, and fenofibrate was the most in-depth studied molecule.[44,45] Bezafibrate demonstrated significant reduction in severity of intermittent claudication for up to 3 years in LEADER study.[46]

Bezafibrate is pan-(α, β and γ) PPAR balanced activator. This unique action differentiates bezafibrate from other fibrates. This is related to the bezafibrate effect on glucose metabolism and insulin resistance. Serum adiponectin levels have been shown to be increased significantly with bezafibrate therapy.[47] Bezafibrates lead to long-term stabilization of insulin sensitivity and pancreatic β-cell function and reduced blood glucose levels and hemoglobin A1c.[48,49] Many studies have shown that bezafibrate reduced the incidence of type 2 DM by 30–40% compared to placebo or other fibrates during a long-term follow-up period.[50,51]

Fenofibrate-associated creatinine increase (i.e., a rise in serum creatinine of at least 20% from baseline to 4th month of therapy) may occur in certain diabetic patients such as those who are older, have a history of CVD and are treated with an ACE-I at baseline or a thiazolidinedione at 4 months, as reported in a post-hoc analysis of the ACCORD trial. However, this effect is reversible after fibrate discontinuation.

CONCLUSION

While summarizing the available data till now, it can be said fibrate molecules certainly have important place in the management of dyslipidemia and ASCVD. Also, there promising mechanism toward insulin sensitization will make them more demanding in metabolic syndrome in near future. Cardiovascular disease along with diabetes is one of the most important considerations of the fibrate treatment as this class of drug appears to act on the final common pathway. Fibrates are able to improve several lipid and lipoprotein parameters such as decreasing TG, TC and LDL-C levels, increasing HDL-C concentrations and reducing sLDL particles. Currently, there is lack of data that if these beneficial effects are associated with a reduction in CV events.

REFERENCES

1. Bansal S, Burring JE, Rifai N, et al. Fasting compared with non fasting triglycerides and risk of cardiovascular events in women. JAMA. 2007;298(3):309-16.
2. Barter P, Gotto AM, La Rossa AC, et al. HDL cholesterol and very low levels of LDL cholesterol and cardiovascular events. N Engl J Med. 2007;357(13):1301-10.
3. de Goma EM, Leeper NJ, Heidenreich PA. Clinical significance of high density lipoprotein cholesterol in patients with low LDL cholesterol. J Am Coll Cardiol. 2008;51(1):49-55.
4. Stone NJ, Robinson J, Lichtenstein AH, et al. 2013 ACC/AHA guideline on the treatment of blood cholesterol to reduce atherosclerotic cardiovascular risk in adults: a report of the American College of Cardiology/American Heart Association Task Force on Practice Guidelines. Circulation (online).
5. Goldfine AB, Kaul S, Hiatt WR. Fibrates in the treatment of dyslipidemia—time for reassessment. N Engl J Med. 2011 Aug 11;365(6):481-4.
6. Staels B, Vu-Dac N, Kosykh VA, et al. Fibrates downregulate apolipoprotein C-III expression independent of induction of peroxisomal acyl coenzyme A oxidase. A potential mechanism for the hypolipidemic action of fibrates. J Clin Invest. 1995;95:705-12.
7. Malmendier CL, Delcroix C. Effects of fenofibrate on high and low density lipoprotein metabolism in heterozygous familial hypercholesterolemia. Atherosclerosis. 1985;55:161-9.
8. Mellies MJ, Stein EA, Khoury P, et al. Effects of fenofibrate on lipids, lipoproteins, and apolipoproteins in 33 subjects with primary hypercholesterolemia. Atherosclerosis. 1987;63:57-64.
9. Knopp RH, Walden CE, Warnick GR, et al. Effect of fenofibrate treatment on plasma lipoprotein lipids, high-density lipoprotein cholesterol subfractions, and apolipoproteins B, AI, AII, and E. Am J Med. 1987;83:75-84.
10. Hiukka A, Leinonen E, Jauhiainen M, Sundvall J, Ehnholm C, Keech AC, Taskinen MR. Long-term effects of fenofibrate on VLDL and HDL subspecies in participants with type 2 diabetes mellitus. Diabetologia. October 2007;50(10):2067-75. First online: 26 July 2007.
11. Bard JM, Parra HJ, Camare R, et al. A multicenter comparison of the effects of simvastatin and fenofibrate therapy in severe primary hypercholesterolemia, with particular emphasis on lipoproteins defined by their apolipoprotein composition. Metabolism. 1992;41:498-503.
12. Chinetti G, Lestavel S, Bocher V, et al. PPAR-alpha and PPAR-gamma activators induce cholesterol removal from human macrophage foam cells through stimulation of the ABCA1 pathway. Nat Med. 2001;7:53-8.
13. Knopp RH. Drug treatment of lipid disorders. N Engl J Med. 1999;341:498-511.
14. Tenenbaum A, Fisman EZ, Motro M, et al. Optimal management of combined dyslipidemia: what have we behind statins monotherapy? Adv Cardiol. 2008;45:127-53.

15. Schoonjans K, Staels B, Auwerx J. The peroxisome proliferator activated receptors (PPARS) and their effects on lipid metabolism and adipocyte differentiation. Biochim Biophys Acta. 1996;1302:93-109.

16. Staels B, Dallongeville J, Auwerx J, et al. Mechanism of action of fibrates on lipid and lipoprotein metabolism. Circulation. 1998;98:2088-93.

17. Auboeuf D, Rieusset J, Fajas L, et al. Tissue distribution and quantification of the expression of mRNAs of peroxisome proliferator-activated receptors and liver X receptor-alpha in humans: no alteration in adipose tissue of obese and NIDDM patients. Diabetes. 1997;46:1319-27.

18. Marx N, Duez H, Fruchart JC, et al. Peroxisome proliferator-activated receptors and atherogenesis: regulators of gene expression in vascular cells. Circ Res. 2004;94:1168-78.

19. Latruffe N, Vamecq J. Peroxisome proliferators and peroxisome proliferator activated receptors (PPARs) as regulators of lipid metabolism. Biochimie. 1997;79:81-94.

20. Abourbih S, Filion KB, Joseph L, et al. Effects of Fibrates on lipid profile and cardiovascular outcome: a systematic review. Am J Med. 2009;122(10):e 961-8.

21. Staels B, Koenig W. Habib A, et al. Activation of human aortic smooth muscle cell is inhibited by PPAR-alpha but not by PPAR-gamma agonists. Nature. 1998;393(6687):790-3.

22. Miller M, Bachorik PS, McCrindle BW, et al. Effect of gemfibrozil in men with primary isolated low high-density lipoprotein cholesterol: a randomized, double-blind, placebo-controlled, crossover study. Am J Med. 1993;94:7-12.

23. Despres JP, Lemieux I, Salomon H, et al. Effects of micronized fenofibrate versus atorvastatin in the treatment of dyslipidaemic patients with low plasma HDL-cholesterol levels: a 12-week randomized trial. J Intern Med. 2002;251:490-99.

24. Landray MJ, Townend JN, Martin S, et al. Lipid lowering drugs and homocysteine. Lancet. 1999;353:1974-5.

25. Westphal S, Dierkes J, Luley C. Effects of fenofibrate and gemfibrozil on plasma homocysteine. Lancet. 2001;358:39-40.

26. Jones PH, Davidson MH. Reporting rate of rhabdomyolysis with fenofibrate +statin versus gemfibrozil + any statin. Am J Cardiol. 2005;95:120-22.

27. Bissonnette R, Treacy E, Rozen R, et al. Fenofibrate raises plasma homocysteine levels in the fasted and fed states. Atherosclerosis. 2001;155:455-62.

28. A co-operative trial in the primary prevention of ischaemic heart disease using clofibrate. Report from the Committee of Principal Investigators. Br Heart J. 1978;40:1069-1118.

29. Frick MH, Elo O, Haapa K, et al. Helsinki Heart Study: primary-prevention trial with gemfibrozil in middle-aged men with dyslipidemia. Safety of treatment, changes in risk factors, and incidence of coronary heart disease. N Engl J Med. 1987;317:1237-45.

30. Tenkanen L, Manttari M, Manninen V. Some coronary risk factors related to the insulin resistance syndrome and treatment with gemfibrozil. Experience from the Helsinki Heart Study. Circulation. 1995;92:1779-85.

31. Rubins HB, Robins SJ, Collins D, et al. Gemfibrozil for the secondary prevention of coronary heart disease in men with low levels of high-density lipoprotein cholesterol. Veterans Affairs High-Density Lipoprotein Cholesterol Intervention Trial Study Group. N Engl J Med. 1999;341:410-18.

32. Robins SJ, Collins D, Wittes JT, et al. Relation of gemfibrozil treatment and lipid levels with major coronary events: VA-HIT: a randomized controlled trial. JAMA. 2001;285:1585-91.

33. Goldenberg I, Boyko V, Tennenbaum A, Tanne D, Behar S, Guetta V. Long-term benefit of high-density lipoprotein cholesterol-raising therapy with bezafibrate: 16-year mortality follow-up of the bezafibrate infarction prevention trial. Arch Intern Med. 2009;169:508-14.

34. Tenenbaum A, Motro M, Fisman EZ, et al. Bezafibrate for the secondary prevention of myocardial infarction in patients with metabolic syndrome. Arch Intern Med. 2005;165:1154-60.

35. Keech A, Simes RJ, Barter P, et al. Effects of long-term fenofibrate therapy on cardiovascular events in 9795 people with type 2 diabetes mellitus (the FIELD study): randomised controlled trial. Lancet. 2005;366:1849-61.

36. Stampfer MJ, Malinow MR, Willett WC, et al. A prospective study of plasma homocyst(e) ine and risk of myocardial infarction in US physicians. JAMA. 1992;268:877-81.
37. Liao D, Tan H, Hui R, et al. Hyperhomocysteinemia decreases circulating high-density lipoprotein by inhibiting apolipoprotein A-I Protein synthesis and enhancing HDL cholesterol clearance. Circ Res. 2006;99:598-606.
38. Ginsberg HN, Elam MB, Lovato LC, et al. Effects of combination lipid therapy in type 2 diabetes mellitus. N Engl J Med. 2010;362:1563-74. [Erratum, N Engl J Med 2010;362: 1748.]
39. Manninen V, Tenkanen L, Koskinen P, et al. Joint effects of serum triglyceride and LDL cholesterol and HDL cholesterol concentrations on coronary heart disease risk in the Helsinki Heart Study. Implications for treatment. Circulation. 1992;85:37-45.
40. Gordon DJ, Probstfield JL, Garrison RJ, et al. High-density lipoprotein cholesterol and cardiovascular disease. Four prospective Am studies. Circulation. 1989;79:8-15.
41. The Lipid Research Clinics Coronary Primary Prevention Trial results. I. Reduction in incidence of coronary heart disease. JAMA. 1984;251:351-64.
42. The Lipid Research Clinics Coronary Primary Prevention Trial results. II. The relationship of reduction in incidence of coronary heart disease to cholesterol lowering. JAMA. 1984;251:365-74.
43. Pedersen TR, Olsson AG, Faergeman O, et al. Lipoprotein changes and reduction in the incidence of major coronary heart disease events in the Scandinavian Simvastatin Survival Study (4S). Circulation. 1998;97:1453-60.
44. ACCORD Study Group. Effect of combination lipid therapy in type 2 diabetes mellitus. N Eng J Med. 2010;362:1563-74.
45. Scott R, O'Brien R, Fulcher G, et al. FIELD Study investigators: Effects of fenofibrate treatment on cardiovascular disease risk in 9795 individuals with type 2 diabetes and various components of metabolic syndrome; the Fenofibrate Intervention and Event Lowering in Diabetes (FIELD) study. Diabetes Care. 2009;32:493-8.
46. Meade T, Zuhrie R, Cook C, et al. Bezafibrate in men with lower extremity arterial disease: randomised controlled trial. BMJ. 2002;325(7373):1139.
47. Hiuge A, Tenenbaum A, Maeda N, et al. Effects of peroxisome proliferator-activated receptor ligands, bezafibrate and fenofibrate on adiponectin level. Arterioscler Thromb Vasc Biol. 2007;27:635-44.
48. Tenenbaum H, Behar S, Boyko V, et al. Long-term effect of bezafibrate on pancreatic beta cell function and insulin resistance in patients with diabetes. Atherosclerosis. 2007;194:265-71.
49. Teramoto T, Shirai K, Daida H, et al. Effects of bezafibrate on lipid and glucose metabolism in dyslipidemic patients with diabetes: the J-BENEFIT study. Cardiovasc Diabetol. 2012; 11:29.
50. Tenenbaum A, Motro M, Fisman EZ, et al. Effect of bezafibrate on incidence of type 2 diabetes mellitus in obese patients. Eur Heart J. 2005;26:2032-8.
51. Flory JH, Ellenberg S, Szapary PO, et al. Antidiabetic action of bezafibrate in a large observational database. Diabetes Care. 2009; 32:547-51.

Index

Page numbers followed by *f* refer to figure, and *t* refer to table